The HSC Handbook of Pediatrics

EIGHTH EDITION

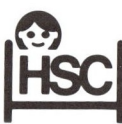

The Hospital for Sick Children
Toronto, Canada

Editor
Alison G. Shefler, M.D., FRCPC
Formerly, Chief Resident, Department of Pediatrics
The Hospital for Sick Children, Toronto, Canada
Currently, Senior Registrar, Intensive Care Unit
The Children's Hospital
Camperdown, Sydney, Australia

Associate Editor
Patricia C. Parkin, M.D., FRCPC
Assistant Professor, Department of Pediatrics
University of Toronto Faculty of Medicine
Staff Physician, Division of General Pediatrics
The Hospital for Sick Children, Toronto, Canada

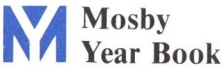

St. Louis Baltimore Boston Chicago London
Philadelphia Sydney Toronto

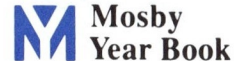

Mary Mansor

r: Leslie Fenton
da J. Daly

by Mosby–Year Book, Inc.
f Mosby–Year Book, Inc.

rt of this publication may be reproduced,
n, or transmitted, in any form or by any
nical, photocopying, recording, or otherwise,
mission from the publisher.

d States of America
k, Inc.
tline Industrial Drive, St. Louis MO 63146

n to photocopy or reproduce solely for internal or personal use
itted for libraries or other users registered with the Copyright
nce Center, provided that the base fee of $4.00 per chapter plus
.10 per page is paid directly to the Copyright Clearance Center, 21
Congress Street, Salem, MA 01970. This consent does not extend to
other kinds of copying, such as copying for general distribution, for
advertising or promotional purposes, for creating new collected works,
or for resale.

Library of Congress Cataloging-in-Publication Data

The HSC handbook of pediatrics / editor, Alison G. Shefler; associate
  editor, Patricia C. Parkin. — 8th ws.
    p. cm
  Rev. ed. of: Residents handbook of pediatrics / William H.
Abelson, R. Garth Smith. 7th ed. 1987.
  Includes bibliographical references and index.
  ISBN 1-55664-325-X
  1. Pediatrics—Handbooks, manuals, etc. I. Shefler, Alison G.
II. Parkin, Patricia C. III. Abelson, William H. Residents
handbook of pediatrics. IV. Hospital for Sick Children. V. Title:
Handbooks of pediatrics.
  [DNLM: 1. Pediatrics—handbooks. WS 39 H873]
RJ48.H78   1991
618.92—dc20
DNLM/DLC
for Library of Congress   91-28663
                                                                   CIP

92 93 94 95 96   CL/MA/MA   9 8 7 6 5 4 3 2

Contributors

Peter F. Armstrong, M.D., FRCSC, F.A.C.S.
Assistant Professor, Department of Surgery, University of Toronto; Faculty of Medicine; Staff Surgeon, Division of Orthopedic Surgery and Associate Director, Pediatric Trauma Unit, The Hospital for Sick Children, Toronto, Canada.
Orthopedics

P. Ann Bayliss, B.A.Sc., M.D., FRCPC
Formerly, Associate Chief Resident; currently, Fellow, Developmental Pediatrics, The Hospital for Sick Children, Toronto, Canada.
Growth and Development

Jennifer Blake, M.D., FRCSC
Formerly, Assistant Professor, Department of Obstetrics and Gynecology, University of Toronto Faculty of Medicine; Head, Division of Gynecology, The Hospital for Sick Children, Toronto, Canada; currently, Chair Undergraduate M.D. Program, McMaster University Health Sciences Centre, Hamilton, Canada.
Genitourinary Disease

Scott M. Bryson, M.Sc., Phm.
Formerly, Co-ordinator Therapeutic Drug Monitoring, Department of Pharmacy, The Hospital for Sick Children, Toronto, Canada; currently, Assistant Director, Department of Pharmacy, British Columbia Children's Hospital, Vancouver, British Columbia, Canada.
Formulary

Joe T.R. Clarke, M.D., Ph.D., FRCPC
Associate Professor, Department of Pediatrics, University of Toronto Faculty of Medicine; Head, Division of Clinical Genetics, The Hospital for Sick Children, Toronto, Canada.
Metabolic Disease

Natalie Dayneka, B.Sc., Phm.
Therapeutic Drug Monitoring Pharmacist, Department of Pharmacy, The Hospital for Sick Children, Toronto, Canada.
Formulary

Bruno diGravio, M.D., FRCPC
Formerly, Fellow, Division of Neonatology, The Hospital for Sick Children, Toronto, Canada; Currently, Consulting Pediatrician, Kitchener, Ontario, Canada.
Neonatology

Lee Dupuis, M.Sc., Phm.
Assistant Professor, University of Toronto Faculty of Pharmacy; Coordinator, Drug Information Service and Education, Department of Pharmacy, The Hospital for Sick Children, Toronto, Canada.
Formulary

James Elder, M.B., B.S.
Formerly, Fellow, Pediatric Ophthalmology, The Hospital for Sick Children, Toronto, Canada; currently, Pediatric Ophthalmologist, Royal Children's Hospital, Melbourne, Victoria, Australia.
Ophthalmology

Graham Ellis, Ph.D., F.C.A.C.B., M.R.C.Path., D.A.B.C.C.
Associate Professor, Department of Clinical Biochemistry, University of Toronto Faculty of Medicine; Assistant Biochemist, Department of Biochemistry, The Hospital for Sick Children, Toronto, Canada.
Laboratory Reference Values

Robert W. Ezenauer, M.D., M.P.H.
Formerly, Fellow, Pediatric Ophthalmology, The Hospital for Sick Children, Toronto, Canada; currently, Staff Ophthalmologist, USA Army Fitzsimmons Army Medical Center, Aurora, Colorado.
Ophthalmology

Annette Feigenbaum, M.B., Ch.B., FRCPC
Fellow, Division of Genetic and Metabolic Disease, The Hospital for Sick Children, Toronto, Canada.
Genetics

Contributors

Brian M. Feldman, M.D., FRCPC
Formerly, Associate Chief Resident, Department of Pediatrics; currently, Fellow, Division of Rheumatology, The Hospital for Sick Children, Toronto, Canada.
Endocrinology

Vito Forte, M.D., FRCSC
Assistant Professor, Department of Otolaryngology, University of Toronto Faculty of Medicine; Staff Surgeon, Division of Otolaryngology, The Hospital for Sick Children, Toronto, Canada.
Otolaryngology

Katryn Furuya, M.D., FRCPC
Senior Fellow, Division of Gastroenterology, The Hospital for Sick Children, Toronto, Canada.
Hepatology

Michael Harbord, M.B., B.S., F.R.A.C.P.
Formerly, Fellow, Division of Neurology, The Hospital for Sick Children, Toronto, Canada; currently, Pediatric Neurologist, Flinders Medical Centre, Lecturer in Pediatrics, Flinders University, Bedford Park, South Australia.
Neurology

Stephen P. Hardy, B.Sc., M.D., FRCPC
Formerly, Associate Chief Resident, The Hospital for Sick Children, Toronto, Canada; Currently, Pediatrician, Kitchener, Ontario, Canada.
Growth and Development

Elizabeth Harvey, M.D., FRCPC
Assistant Professor, Department of Pediatrics, University of Toronto Faculty of Medicine; Staff Physician, Division of Nephrology, The Hospital for Sick Children, Toronto, Canada.
Fluids and Electrolytes

Kurt Heiss, M.D.
Chief Resident, Department of Surgery, The Hospital for Sick Children, Toronto, Canada.
Surgery

Martin C.K. Hosking, M.D., FRCPC
Fellow, Division of Cardiology, The Hospital for Sick Children, Toronto, Canada.
Cardiology

David Hummel, M.B., Ch.B., FRCPC
Staff Physician, Department of Pediatrics, Markham-Stouffville Hospital, Markham, Ontario, Canada; Associate Staff Physician, Division of Immunology, The Hospital for Sick Children, Toronto, Canada.
Allergy and Immunology

Douglas Johnston, D.D.S., M.Sc., Dip. Paed.
Assistant Professor, University of Toronto Faculty of Dentistry; Head, Division of Pediatric Dentistry, The Hospital for Sick Children, Toronto, Canada.
Dentistry

Miriam Kaufman, R.N., M.D., FRCPC
Assistant Professor, Department of Pediatrics, University of Toronto Faculty of Medicine; Staff Physician, Division of Adolescent Medicine, The Hospital for Sick Children, Toronto, Canada.
Adolescent Medicine

James Kellner, M.D., FRCPC
Formerly, Assistant Professor, Department of Pediatrics, University of Toronto Faculty of Medicine, Staff Physician, Division of Emergency Medicine, The Hospital for Sick Children, Toronto, Canada; currently, Assistant Director, Emergency Department, Alberta Children's Hospital, Edmonton, Alberta, Canada.
Emergencies

Anthony Khoury, M.B., B.Ch., FRCSC
Assistant Professor, Department of Surgery, University of Toronto Faculty of Medicine; Staff Surgeon, Division of Urology, The Hospital for Sick Children, Toronto, Canada.
Genitourinary Disease

Bernice R. Krafchik, M.B., Ch.B., FRCPC
Associate Professor, Department of Pediatrics, University of Toronto Faculty of Medicine; Staff Physician, Division of Dermatology, The Hospital for Sick Children, Toronto, Canada.
Dermatology

Stephen P. Kraft, M.D., FRCSC
Assistant Professor, Department of Ophthalmology, University of Toronto Faculty of Medicine; Staff Ophthalmologist, Division of Ophthalmology, The Hospital for Sick Children, Toronto, Canada.
Ophthalmology

Ivan Krajbich, M.D., (Hon.) B.Sc., FRCSC
Assistant Professor, Department of Surgery, University of Toronto Faculty of Medicine; Staff Surgeon, Division of Orthopedic Surgery, The Hospital for Sick Children, Toronto, Canada.
Orthopedics

Alex Levin, M.D., B.S.
Formerly, Fellow, Pediatric Ophthalmology, The Hospital for Sick Children, Toronto, Canada; currently, Pediatric Ophthalmologist, Wills Eye Hospital, Philadelphia, Pennsylvania.
Ophthalmology

Suzanne Lewis, M.D., B.Sc.
Fellow, Department of Clinical Genetics, Chedoke-McMaster University & Hospital, Hamilton, Ontario, Canada.
Metabolic Disease

Andrew Lynk, M.Sc., M.D., FRCPC
Formerly, Fellow, Division of Infectious Diseases, The Hospital for Sick Children, Toronto, Canada; currently, Pediatrician, Sydney, Nova Scotia, Canada.
Infectious Disease

David R. Mack, M.D., FRCPC
Formerly, Fellow, Division of Gastroenterology, The Hospital for Sick Children, Toronto, Canada; currently, Assistant Professor, Department of Pediatrics and Staff Physician, Combined Section of Pediatric Gastroenterology and Nutrition, University of Nebraska School of Medicine and Creighton University School of Medicine, Omaha, Nebraska.
Gastroenterology

Michael A. McGuigan, M.D., C.M.
Assistant Professor, Department of Pediatrics, University of Toronto Faculty of Medicine; Medical Director, Poison Information Centre, The Hospital for Sick Children, Toronto, Canada.
Poisoning, Adolescent Medicine

Marcellina Mian, M.D., C.M., FRCPC
Assistant Professor, Departments of Pediatrics and Behavioral Sciences, University of Toronto Faculty of Medicine; Director, Suspected Child Abuse and Neglect Program, Hospital for Sick Children, Toronto, Canada.
Child Abuse

Christine Newman, M.D., FRCPC
Assistant Professor, Department of Pediatrics, University of Toronto Faculty of Medicine; Staff Physician, Division of Neonatology, The Hospital for Sick Children, Toronto, Canada.
Neonatology

Anne Niec, M.D., FRCPC
Formerly, Chief Resident, Department of Pediatrics, The Hospital for Sick Children, Toronto, Canada; currently, Fellow, Ambulatory Pediatrics, Children's Hospital, Boston, Massachusetts.
Adolescent Medicine

Martin Petric, Ph.D.
Assistant Professor, Department of Microbiology, University of Toronto Faculty of Medicine; Staff Virologist, The Hospital for Sick Children, Toronto, Canada.
Laboratory Reference Values

Annette O. Poon, M.B., B.Ch., FRCPC
Assistant Professor, Department of Pediatrics, University of Toronto Faculty of Medicine; Medical Director, Hematology Diagnostic Laboratories and Blood Bank, The Hospital for Sick Children, Toronto, Canada.
Laboratory Reference Values

Rashid Rajah, M.B., Ch.B.
Formerly, Fellow, Division of Gastroenterology, The Hospital for Sick Children, Toronto, Canada; currently, Pediatrician, Brandon, Manitoba, Canada.
Nutrition

Mercer Rang, M.B., B.S., FRCSC
Professor, Department of Surgery, University of Toronto Faculty of Medicine; Staff Surgeon, Division of Orthopedic Surgery, The Hospital for Sick Children, Toronto, Canada.
Orthopedics

Joe Reisman, B.A., M.D., FRCPC
Assistant Professor, Department of Pediatrics, University of Toronto Faculty of Medicine; Staff Physician, Division of Chest Diseases, The Hospital for Sick Children, Toronto, Canada.
Respiratory Disease

Rayfel Schneider, M.B., B.Ch., FRCPC
Assistant Professor, Department of Pediatrics, University of Toronto Faculty of Medicine; Director, Undergraduate Medical Education and Staff Physician, Divisions of General Pediatrics and Rheumatology, The Hospital for Sick Children, Toronto, Canada.
Rheumatology

Dennis Scolnik, M.B., Ch.B.
Formerly, Fellow, Division of Nephrology; currently, Fellow, Division of Clinical Pharmacology and Toxicology; The Hospital for Sick Children, Toronto, Canada.
Nephrology

Donna Secker, B.Sc., R.P.Dt.
Dietitian-Nutritionist, Department of Food Services, The Hospital for Sick Children, Toronto, Canada.
Nutrition

Alison G. Shefler, M.D., FRCPC
Formerly, Chief Resident, Department of Pediatrics, The Hospital for Sick Children, Toronto, Canada; currently, Senior Registrar, Intensive Care Unit, The Children's Hospital, Camperdown, Sydney, Australia.
Neonatology, Procedures

Robert H. Taylor, M.B., B.Ch., F.F.A.R.C.S.
Formerly, Fellow, Department of Critical Care, The Hospital for Sick Children, Toronto, Canada; currently, Anesthetist, The Hospital for Sick Children, Belfast, Northern Ireland.
Procedures

Peter Wilson, M.B., B.S., F.R.A.C.P.
Formerly, Fellow, Division of Hematology and Oncology, The Hospital for Sick Children, Toronto, Canada.
Haematology and Oncology

Ronald M. Zuker, M.D., FRCSC, F.A.C.S.
Associate Professor, Department of Surgery, University of Toronto Faculty of Medicine; Head, Division of Plastic Surgery, The Hospital for Sick Children, Toronto, Canada.
Plastic Surgery

Notice

Every effort has been made to ensure that the drug dosage schedules are accurate and in accord with standards accepted at the time of printing. However, we think it important to mention that the doses we use do not necessarily conform to the manufacturer's recommendations. Nonetheless, the reader is cautioned to check the product information sheet included in the package of each drug and to verify indications, contraindications, and recommended dosages.

Foreword

Each pediatric resident and pediatrician is confronted with a wide array of medical conditions from acute life-threatening disorders to common problems encountered in the everyday practice of pediatrics. Over the years, *The HSC Handbook of Pediatrics* has provided a reliable source of information which is practical, easy to find and most important, available when the information is most needed. *The Handbook* is not intended to be a comprehensive textbook of pediatrics but, rather, a useful guide to initiate the diagnostic or management process.

The eighth edition of *The HSC Handbook of Pediatrics* provides a concise, management-oriented approach to the investigation and treatment of many pediatric conditions. *The Handbook* has been adapted to provide essential pediatric information for medical students, residents and practicing physicians. The book consists of 27 condensed systems-oriented chapters as well as sections on emergency procedures, laboratory reference values, and a drug formulary. In addition, *The Handbook* includes useful tables, graphs, and nomograms which will assist in the evaluation of the pediatric patient.

The HSC Handbook of Pediatrics was written and edited by senior residents and subspecialty fellows with extensive input and guidance from the faculty and staff of The Hospital for Sick Children. I should like to especially acknowledge the efforts of associate editor, Dr. Patricia Parkin, and the tremendous contribution of the editor, Dr. Alison Shefler, who deserves the major credit for creating the eighth edition of *The Handbook*. Congratulations for a job well done!

Robert H. A. Haslam, M.D., FRCPC
Professor and Chairman
Department of Pediatrics

Preface

With echoes of "keep it thin" resounding through the halls of the Hospital for Sick Children, the task of editing the eighth edition of *The HSC Handbook of Pediatrics* was enthusiastically undertaken. The final product represents the collective effort of a great number of pediatric trainees, subspecialty fellows, and faculty. The handbook was originally designed to provide a practical reference and guide to the management of pediatric patients. Although the philosophy of the book remains unchanged, much of the exhaustive detail on pathogenesis has been eliminated in order to streamline and facilitate information retrieval. Each chapter has been extensively revised and expanded to parallel new developments in diagnostic and therapeutic approaches to pediatric clinical problems.

The section on Emergencies and chapters on Neonatology, Hematology and Oncology, and Infectious Diseases have been extensively revised and updated, reflecting the changing face of the pediatric population. The material in Nutrition, Metabolic Disease, and Genetics has been shifted from purely reference information to a problem-based approach to interpretation and management of these complex patients. New features include a chapter devoted to Hepatology, and the remodeling of the Genitourinary Disease chapter to include both gynecology and urologic disease. Pharmacologic therapeutics remains a significant aspect of patient management; all relevant information on drug dosing and monitoring is contained in the comprehensive Formulary section. This, along with the Laboratory Reference Values, has been thoroughly updated in keeping with the growing body of material available. The sections on Poisoning, Endocrinology, and Neurology continue to take full advantage of the problem-oriented approach to pediatric diagnostics and therapeutics.

The wide range of topics spans primary, secondary, and tertiary care, and has broadened the scope and practicability of the eighth edition of *The HSC Handbook of Pediatrics*. It should continue to serve as a reference and guide to pediatric trainees, practicing physicians, nurses, and paramedical personnel in the wide diversity of settings in which pediatric care is provided.

Acknowledgments

When a publication originates from a large tertiary care institution, there is an ever-increasing number of contributors whose expertise and support have been lent to its production. The editorial staff would especially like to thank the following individuals: Dr. Robert Gow (Cardiology), Dr. Anne Curtis (Dermatology), Dr. Dennis Daneman, Dr. Robert Ehrlich, Dr. Jack Holland, Dr. Sang-Wey Kooh (Endocrinology), Dr. Anna Jarvis, Dr. John Edmonds (Emergencies), Dr. Eve Roberts (Hepatology), Dr. Nancy Olivieri, Dr. John Doyle (Hematology-Oncology), Dr. E. Lee Ford-Jones, Dr. Ronald Gold (Infectious Disease), Dr. Max Perlman, Dr. Haresh Kirpalani (Neonatology), Dr. Daune Macgregor, Dr. Jeff Kobayashi (Neurology), Dr. Peter Cox (Procedures), Dr. B. Anne Eberhard (Rheumatology), Dr. Gerard Canny (Respiratory Disease), Dr. Prashant Joshi (Formulary).

The thorough revision and update of the Formulary and associated sections by Lee Dupuis is gratefully acknowledged. No book reaches the publisher until it has been keyed in, corrected, and modified innumerable times, a job superbly executed by Mrs. Eva Mcgrath and her staff in the word processing department. All additional artwork was provided by Dr. Ricki Heller. Special thanks to the superior nursing staff on the Hematology-Oncology ward for providing a communications base and large measure of good humor during the bulk of the editing stages. Finally, the infectious enthusiasm and continued support of Dr. Alan Goldbloom, especially in his role as an overseas correspondent, was the "glue" that held the book together in its final proofing and production stages.

Alison G. Shefler, M.D., FRCPC
Patricia C. Parkin, M.D., FRCPC

Contents

I SYSTEMS, 1

1. Adolescent Medicine, 2
2. Allergy and Immunology, 14
3. Cardiology, 28
4. Dentistry, 56
5. Dermatology, 60
6. Endocrinology, 72
7. Fluids and Electrolytes, 87
8. Gastroenterology, 102
9. Genetics, 123
10. Genitourinary Disease, 127
11. Growth and Development, 152
12. Hematology and Oncology, 180
13. Hepatology, 208
14. Infectious Diseases, 228
15. Metabolic Disease, 288
16. Neonatology, 300
17. Nephrology, 348
18. Neurology, 374
19. Nutrition, 391
20. Ophthalmology, 411
21. Orthopedics, 424
22. Otolaryngology, 446
23. Plastic Surgery, 457
24. Poisoning, 464
25. Respiratory Disease, 484
26. Rheumatology, 509
27. Surgery, 520

- II **EMERGENCIES,** 529
- III **PROCEDURES,** 561
- IV **LABORATORY REFERENCE VALUES,** 581
- V **FORMULARY,** 639

ONE

SYSTEMS

ONE

Adolescent Medicine

- History
  1. H = *home,* including relations with parents, family responsibilities, family stresses, independence
  2. E = *education,* including present performance in school and career goals
  3. A = *activities,* including special interests, relationships with friends, job
  4. D = *drugs* including smoking, alcohol
  5. S = *sexuality*
- Physical examination
  1. Growth parameters
  2. Vision and hearing, using standard screening methods
  3. Sexual maturity rating (Tanner stage) (see pp 174-176)
  4. Blood pressure
  5. Assessment of thyroid
  6. Assessment of scoliosis (see p 440)
  7. Examination of external genitalia in all adolescents
  8. Pelvic examination in sexually active females or in those with menstrual problems
  9. Skinfold thickness
  10. Breast examination: Be sure to explain the importance of self-examination in a female or gynecomastia if present in a male
  11. Testicular examination in males: Teach self examination

- Laboratory investigations
    1. CBC, Fe studies as indicated (not uncommon)
    2. Rubella immune status
    3. Sexually active females: Pap smear, serologic test for syphilis, microscopic examination of discharge, and cultures for gonorrhea, *Chlamydia,* and *Trichomonas* should be done yearly and PRN
    4. Sexually active males: VDRL and cultures when indicated
    5. In "street kids," consider screening for hepatitis and HIV
- Check immunization status. TB test if indicated, Td booster every 10 yr

TABLE 1-1 Clinical Features of Patients with Anorexia Nervosa and Bulimia

Anorexia	Bulimia
Psychological	
High achievers with average or above average intelligence	Good peer relations
Perfectionistic	High energy
Low self-esteem	Talkative
Distorted perceptions, particularly body image	
Behavioral	
Relentless pursuit of thinness	Self-induced vomiting
Preoccupation with food, calories, and exercise	Laxative abuse
Decreased sexual interest	Diuretic abuse
Denial of weight problem	Substance abuse more common
	Secretive overeating
	More likely to be sexually active
	Distressed by symptoms
General physical features	
Hypothermia and cold intolerance	Eroded enamel on posterior aspect of upper incisors, parotid enlargement
Dry skin	
Lanugo	
Easy bruising	
Gastrointestinal	
Slowed gastric emptying	Acute gastric dilation, rarely rupture
Constipation	Esophagitis, Mallory-Weiss tears

TABLE 1-1 Clinical Features of Patients with Anorexia Nervosa and Bulimia (Cont'd)

Anorexia	Bulimia
Cardiovascular	
Bradycardia, dysrhythmias Hypotension	Possible ipecac poisoning (cardiac toxicity: check CPK)
Hematologic	
Vitamin B_{12} deficiency Pancytopenia	
Metabolic	
Features of dehydration ↓ GFR ↑ Renal stones ↑ Carotene	Hypokalemia Hypochloremia Hyponatremia, metabolic alkalosis (may be secondary to vomiting, diuretics, or laxatives)
Endocrine	
Amenorrhea Growth retardation (if prolonged starvation during growth spurt) "Senile" vaginitis Partial diabetes insipidus Sick euthyroid syndrome (TSH normal; N- ↓ T4, ↓ T3, ↑ rT3) GH level N- ↑ (somatomedin C level ↓) Estradiol-testosterone levels ↓ Basal FSH and LH levels ↓	Menstrual irregularities

TABLE 1-2 Commonly Abused Substances*

Substance	Characteristics	Effects

Alcohol	Absorption
	  Stomach
	  Small intestine
	Metabolism
	  95% liver
	  5% excreted in kidney
		Relaxation, euphoria
		Blood alcohol levels (BAL):
		0.075-0.15%
		(75-150 mg/dl)
		  Sedation
		  Hypnotic
		  Impaired judgment
		  Slurred speech
		  Ataxia
		0.25-0.4%
		(250-400 mg/dl)
		  Apathy
		  Stupor
		  Coma
		  Hypothermia
		  Respiratory distress
		0.45-0.5%
		(450-500 mg/dl)
		  Death in 50%

Amphetamines	Absorption
	  Oral
	  Inhalation
	  IV
	Metabolism
	  Liver
	Excreted in urine
		CNS:
		  ↑ Physical and mental alertness, euphoria, gregariousness, hallucinations, intracranial hemorrhages, Gilles de la Tourette syndrome, seizures
		CVS:
		  ↑ BP, ↑ HR, palpitations, arrhythmias
		GI:
		  Nausea/vomiting

*See p 345 for a discussion of neonatal drug withdrawal.

Withdrawal	Fetal Effects	Treatment Principles

Acute alcoholic hallucinoses
Wernicke's encephalopathy (thiamine deficiency)
Delirium tremens
  Confusion
  Hallucinations
  Sweating
  Ataxia
  Seizures
	Fetal alcohol syndrome (FAS)
	  Mental retardation
	  Microcephaly
	  Dysmorphic facies
	  Childhood hyperactivity
	  Short stature
	  Cardiac abnormality
		Overdose:
		  Airway protection
		  IV fluids, glucose
		Associated diagnostic possibilities: head injury, hypoglycemia
		Coexisting illness: GI ulcers, hepatitis, STD
		Psychological features: dependency, suicide risk, concomitant drug use

Apathy Depression Lethargy Anxiety Sleep disturbance Myalgias Abdominal pain Voracious appetite	Unknown	Stabilization of vital signs (VS) Supportive care for agitation, psychosis Seizure control

Continued.

TABLE 1-2 Commonly Abused Substances (Cont'd)

Substance	Characteristics	Effects
Amphetamines—cont'd		Metabolic: Hyperthermia, cardiomyopathy, pulmonary edema, endocarditis GI: Anorexia Pulmonary: Granulomas, fibrosis Musculoskeletal: Rhabdomyolysis Chronic: Anxiety dysphoria, confusion, depression, nausea, vomiting, headache, sweating, apprehension, confusion, fatigue

Cocaine
Erythroxylon coca
"Cadillac"
"Speedball" (heroin and cocaine)
Liquid lady (alcohol and cocaine)
"Crack" (free-base cocaine, adulterants removed)
	Absorption
	  Nasal
	  Oral
	  Pulmonary
	Metabolized in liver and plasma
	Excreted in urine (↑ with acidic pH), bile
		"Fight or flight" response
		Vasoconstriction
		Local anesthetic
		CNS: Euphoria, restlessness, excitement, emotional instability, tremors, seizures
		Respiratory: ↑ RR → respiratory depression
		CVS: Tachycardia, VF, hypertension

Withdrawal	Fetal Effects	Treatment Principles
Agitation, depression	Prematurity	Stabilization of VS
Anorexia → hyperphagia	IUGR	May need activated charcoal, lavage
Insomnia → hypersomnolence	↓ Interactive behavior	Rx of arrhythmias
Anhedonia	Poor response to external stimuli	Seizure control
Lack of energy	Neonatal cerebral infarction	Temperature control
Anxiety		Suicide precautions

Continued.

TABLE 1-2 Commonly Abused Substances (Cont'd)

Substance	Characteristics	Effects

Cocaine
Erythroxylon
coca—cont'd
		GI:
		  Nausea/vomiting
		Metabolic:
		  Hyperthermia
		Eyes:
		  Mydriasis

Heroin	Synthesized from morphine
	Absorption
	  Inhalation
	  Oral
	  IV
	  SC
	Converted to MAM (6-monacetylmorphine) in liver, brain, kidney, blood, lungs
	Excreted in urine
		CNS:
		  Coma, seizures, ↑ ICP, acute delirium, chronic organic brain damage
		Musculoskeletal:
		  Rhabdomyolysis, myoglobinuria
		Pulmonary:
		  Pulmonary edema, respiratory depression, pulmonary arteritis, pulmonary hypertension
		CVS:
		  Tachy- and bradycardia, paroxysmal atrial tachycardia, VF, QT prolongation
		Renal:
		  Nephrotic syndrome, amyloidosis
		Eyes:
		  Miosis

LSD
(Lysergic acid diethylamide)
"Acid"
"Sunshine"
"White Lightning"
	Absorption
	  Oral (mainly)
	  Nasal
	  IV
	Metabolism
	  Liver
		Visual illusions
		Perceptual distortion and synesthesia
		Mydriasis
		Hyperthermia
		Depersonalization and derealization
		Acute anxiety attacks
		Seizures

Adolescent Medicine

Withdrawal	Fetal Effects	Treatment Principles
Anxiety Yawning Perspiration Lacrimation Insomnia Hypertension Fever Weight loss Vomiting and diarrhea	IUGR Neonatal withdrawal (Note: secreted in breast milk) ↑ SIDS	Stabilization of VS Gut decontamination Antidote: naloxone Supportive care
Withdrawal symptoms		Stabilization of VS Supportive care, seizure control Reassurance Reduction of sensory stimuli

Continued.

TABLE 1–2 Commonly Abused Substances (Cont'd)

Substance	Characteristics	Effects
Marijuana (Cannabis sativa) "Grass" "Pot" Cannabis Hashish (dried resin of plant flower tops) Bhang (dried leaves and stems)	Psychoactive component: tetrahydrocannabinol (THC) Absorption inhalation > oral Metabolized in liver Excreted in feces, urine	Acute: Bronchodilation, tachycardia, pupillary constriction, ↓ intraocular pressure, euphoria, relaxation, sleepiness, lethargy, dry mouth, ↑ appetite Chronic: Large A/W irritation, gynecomastia, ↓ sperm count Amotivation syndrome: Apathy, passivity, loss of productivity, ↓ energy, tiredness, ↓ frustration tolerance
Toluene	Present in paints, lacquers, thinners, coatings Clear, colorless, flammable liquid Absorption Inhalation (mainly) Oral Skin Lipid soluble Elimination 80% metabolized in liver Small amounts in urine, bile 18% by lungs	Exposure to: *100 ppm:* impaired psychomotor and perceptual performance *500–800 ppm:* progressively ↑ headache, drowsiness, nausea, fatigue, weakness, confusion *> 800 ppm:* severe fatigue, convulsions, ataxia, staggered gait *> 10,000 ppm:* anesthesia within 1 min Renal: Renal tubular acidosis CVS: Sudden death, ↓ AV conduction Chronic encephalopathy, recurrent headaches, permanent cerebellar ataxia

Withdrawal	Fetal Effects	Treatment Principles
Restlessness Sleeplessness ↓ Appetite Nausea Irritability Sweating Dreaming	FAS-like clinical presentation Tremulousness IUGR Facial dysmorphism ↑ Fetal mortality	Stabilization of VS Watch for ARDS, acute renal failure Activated charcoal, gastric lavage Monitor level of consciousness Psychological features: dependency, suicide risk, concomitant drug use
		Stabilization of VS Supportive care

TWO

Allergy and Immunology

Allergy

INVESTIGATIONS

Skin Testing
- Skin testing should be carried out with allergens implicated by the allergy history. The results must be interpreted in the context of the history
- The preferred method of skin testing is the prick method. Intradermal tests are used less often, but are indicated when the history is highly suggestive and the prick test is negative
- A positive wheal and erythema reaction occurs within 15 min and enables detection of specific IgE antibodies to the applied antigen
- Skin testing is most useful for the identification of specific allergens in allergic rhinitis, asthma, insect sting allergy, immediate food reactions and specific drug allergy; it is less useful for the identification of specific allergens in chronic urticaria angioedema and delayed food reactions
- Most antihistamines should be withheld 72 hr prior to skin testing. Astemizole should be withheld for 4 weeks. A positive histamine control ensures that testing is reliable.

In Vitro Testing-Radioallergosorbent Test (RAST)
- Most useful for detection of specific IgE antibodies in patients with life-threatening reactions (anaphylaxis), extensive dermatitis, or severe dermatographism where skin is excessively reactive
  - No need to discontinue antihistamines prior to testing
  - The tests are expensive and not more reliable than skin testing

Challenge Testing
- Useful for immunologic and nonimmunologic sensitivities to drugs, food, and other biologic products, such as vaccines and insulin
- Because of the risk of anaphylaxis, tests should be undertaken in a controlled setting

Suspicion of Allergic Disorder
- Eosinophilia of >5% or $>0.25 \times 10^9$/L (>250/mm^3)
- Smear of nasal secretions or bronchial mucus for eosinophils
- Elevated total serum immunoglobulin E level

MANAGEMENT

Allergen Avoidance
- Complete avoidance advised where possible (e.g., cat allergy)
- For house dust mite allergy, dust control in the child's bedroom is important (regular vacuuming, dusting with a damp cloth, removal of feather pillows and duvets, encasing mattress and pillows in plastic covers, maintaining humidity at 40%, removal of carpeting or using an ascaricide on the carpets, frequent cleaning of filters on heating or air-conditioning systems)
- For outdoor allergens, air-conditioning with a closed circuit will help reduce exposure

Immunotherapy
- Consider in patients poorly controlled on optimal environmental manipulation and pharmacotherapy
- Most important indication: insect venom anaphylaxis
- Not indicated for eczema or food allergy

Other Measures
- Medic Alert bracelet
- Epipen/Anakit and written instruction regarding their use for anaphylaxis

Pharmacologic Management

TABLE 2-1 Pharmacologic Management of Allergic Disorders

Condition	Medication	Comments
Allergic rhinitis	*Antihistamines* 　Chlorpheniramine 　Terfenadine 　Astemazole 　Loratidine	Newer antihistamines are nonsedating; may be given once daily
	Sympathomimetics 　Oral 　　Pseudoephedrine	
	Topical 　　oxymetazoline HCl 　　Xylometazoline HCl	Limit use to 3–5 days only; risk of rebound vasodilation
	Topical steroids 　Beclomethasone 　Flunisolide 　Budesonide	Effective in allergic and nonallergic rhinitis
	Cromolyn sodium	
	Anticholinergics 　Ipratropium bromide	Especially for rhinorrhoea of vasomotor rhinitis
Atopic dermatitis, urticaria	Hydroxyzine Diphenhydramine HCl Ketotifen fumarate Astemazole	
Anaphylaxis	Epinephrine Diphenhydramine HCl	
Allergic conjunctivitis	*Cromolyn Sodium* *Antihistamines*	As for allergic rhinitis

FOOD ALLERGY

- Must distinguish between intolerance, pharmacologic effects, metabolic, and true allergy (uncommon, incidence 5%)
- Most common foods causing food allergy: egg, milk, wheat, peanut, soybean, seafood, nuts
- Clinical manifestations include gastrointestinal symptoms; urticaria, atopic dermatitis, and angioedema; less commonly other symptoms like allergic rhinitis, asthma, anaphylaxis
- Symptoms diminish with time, especially milk and egg; peanut and shellfish allergy is lifelong
- No scientific evidence of immunologic food sensitivity with the following: attention-deficit disorder with hyperactivity, tension-fatigue syndrome, most headaches
- Symptoms occurring soon after ingestion (within 2 hr) more likely a true allergy
- Physical examination—usually noncontributory
- Food challenge
- Skin tests for IgE mediated reactions

Therapy

- Strict elimination of the specific food is the only proven therapy
- Generalized elimination diets should be restricted

ALLERGIC RHINITIS

- Perennial or seasonal sneezing, rhinorrhea, nasal congestion, and often sore throats
- Consider in the differential diagnosis of recurrent colds or pharyngitis
- Therapy: avoidance, pharmacotherapy, immunotherapy (see above)

ADVERSE DRUG REACTIONS

- Predictable reactions: usually dose dependent, related to known pharmacologic actions of drugs and occur in otherwise healthy patients
  1. Overdose or toxicity: may be expected in any patient, provided a threshold level has been exceeded
  2. Side effects: therapeutically undesirable but often unavoidable effects of drugs at pharmacologic doses
  3. Secondary effects: indirect but not inevitable effects of pharmacologic actions of drugs, e.g., pseudomembranous colitis after antibiotic use
  4. Drug interactions: two or more drugs given together augment or diminish the expected response or result in unintended reaction
- Unpredictable reactions: often dose independent, related to individual's immunologic response or genetic susceptibility
  1. Intolerance: lowered threshhold to normal pharmacologic action of drugs in susceptible persons
  2. Idiosyncratic reactions: qualitative abnormal response in genetically susceptible persons
  3. Allergic reactions: mediated by definite or presumed immunologic reactions
  4. Pseudoallergic reactions: minor allergic reactions but no immunologic mechanism exists, e.g., radiocontrast material, aspirin sensitivity
- Immediate allergic reactions occur within 1 hr and consist of pruritis, urticaria, flushing, and other manifestations of anaphylaxis
- Accelerated reactions occur within 1-72 hr of drug administration and consist primarily of pruritus and urticaria, but laryngeal edema may be seen
- Delayed reactions start 3 days after initiation of therapy and usually involve the skin with urticarial, exanthematous, or fixed drug eruptions, erytherma multiforme or serum-sickness-like reactions; one or more organ systems may be involved

Investigations
- Few diagnostic tests available; therefore, history is extremely important
- Note nature and duration of the reaction, time of onset of the symptoms relative to the initiation of therapy, to previous use of the particular medications, and to the patient's symptoms prior to commencement of the medication. Note all prescription and non-prescription medicines taken around the time of the reaction.

Treatment
- Discontinue suspected medication
- Provide symptomatic relief (epinephrine, antihistamines, corticosteroids)
- Avoid further use of offending drug unless a life-threatening condition exists. Desensitization should then be undertaken in a controlled clinical setting.

Specific Drug Allergy
- Penicillin (see Fig. 2-1)
- Cephalosporins: usual incidence of cross-reactivity with penicillins is 10-15%; should generally be avoided in proven penicillin sensitivity
- Sulfonamide: up to 5% of patients have side effects; most common are skin rashes
  1. Urticaria: occurs 1-2 days after initiation of treatment. History of previous sulfonamide use. Rash resolves 1-2 days after discontinuation of medication. Antihistamines useful. IgE mechanism thought to be involved. Reaction may be to other components of the medication. No in vivo or in vitro diagnostic tests available.
  2. Idiosyncratic reaction: less common; occurs later in course of therapy (10-12 days). Starts with high fever and rashes, e.g., erythema multiforme, Stevens-Johnson syndrome, toxic epidermal necrolysis; occasional systemic involvement, including hepatitis, nephritis, myocarditis, pneumonitis, transient hypothyroidism. May occur with first exposure. Lymphocytotoxicity tests may be done in affected individual and in carriers.

Allergy and Immunology

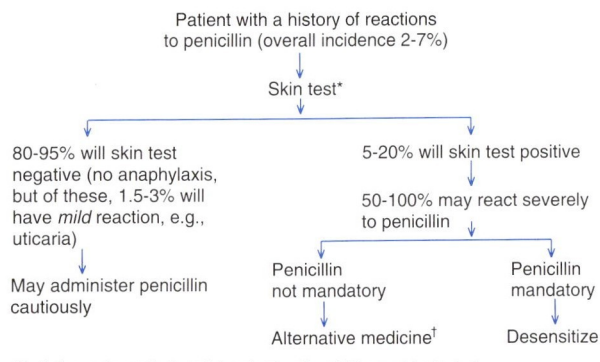

```
Patient with a history of reactions
to penicillin (overall incidence 2-7%)
            ↓
         Skin test*
         ↓        ↓
```

80-95% will skin test negative (no anaphylaxis, but of these, 1.5-3% will have *mild* reaction, e.g., uticaria)
↓
May administer penicillin cautiously

5-20% will skin test positive
↓
50-100% may react severely to penicillin
↓   ↓
Penicillin not mandatory   Penicillin mandatory
↓   ↓
Alternative medicine†   Desensitize

*Both the major and minor determinants of penicillin must be tested
†Sensitivity to penicillin is a contraindication to use of any semisynthetic analogues of penicillin

Figure 2-1 **Management of suspected penicillin sensitivity.**

Immunology

IMMUNODEFICIENCY DISORDERS (IDDs)

Clinical

- Recurrent pyogenic infections in different sites, or more than one severe pyogenic infection, e.g., meningitis, osteomyelitis
- Prolonged infection with poor response to antibiotics
- Unusually severe infections
- Infection with unusual organisms, e.g., *Pneumocystis carinii, Aspergillus*
- Illness following live virus vaccination, e.g., MMR
- Failure to thrive
- Chronic diarrhea, often with malabsorption
- Absence of lymph nodes and tonsils
- Persistent candidiasis
- Positive family history of early infant deaths, increased susceptibility to infection, collagen vascular disease

Differential Diagnosis

- Allergy, e.g., asthma, allergic rhinitis
- Foreign body associated with infection, e.g., foreign body aspiration, central venous line infections
- Cystic fibrosis
- Integument defects, e.g., immotile cilia syndrome
- Infection with resistant organisms
- Continuous reinfection, e.g., contaminated water supply

Investigation

- Initial screening
  1. Hematologic: hemoglobin, platelet count and morphology, total white blood count and differential
  2. Quantative immunoglobulin levels: IgG, IgA, IgM
  3. Functional antibody assays: tetanus, polio, measles, mumps, rubella, diphtheria antibody levels (for IgG function); Schick test for diphtheria neutralizing antibodies; isohemagglutinins (for IgM function-useful after 1 yr of age
  4. Delayed hypersensitivity skin tests, e.g., *Candida,* PPD, dermatophyton (measures specific T-cell and macrophage response to antigens)
  5. CXR for thymic shadow (<1 yr of age)
  6. Include HIV testing in high-risk groups
- Further investigations should be done if there is an abnormality detected on screening, or convincing clinical evidence of immunodeficiency disorder even if screening tests are negative.
- Causes of anergy include malnutrition, primary or secondary to immunodeficiency (including immunosuppressive therapy), viral infection (acute or postlive viral vaccination, e.g., measles, rubella) or granulomatous disease (Wegener's, Crohn's, sarcoidosis)
- More advanced testing include determination of IgG subclasses, specific antibody responses to administered antigens (B cells), lymphocyte subtype enumeration, proliferation response to mitogens (T cells), thymic biopsy (T cells), tests of complement pathways (C3, C4; CH50-classical, alternative), tests of neutrophil chemotaxis (Rebuck window), metabolic function (nitroblue tetrazolium)

Management

- General measures: family studies and genetic counselling. Prenatal diagnosis is available for some primary IDDs
- Antibiotics: prophylactic, e.g., trimethoprim-sulfamethoxazole in neutropenia, selective IgA or IgG subclass deficiencies, or postsplenectomy
- Avoid exposure to infectious diseases
- Immunizations
  1. Avoid live vaccines in T-cell and B-cell disorders and in some secondary IDDs (e.g., generalized malignant disease and immunosuppressive agents, including high-dose corticosteroids). Live vaccines can be given when there are neutrophil and complement disorders.
  2. Active immunization with pneumococcal vaccine, e.g., prior to splenectomy or in sickle cell disease
  3. Passive immunization with gamma globulin, especially after exposure to varicella (B cell, T cell, and some of the secondary IDDs)
  4. Caution with blood transfusions
     - Selective IgA deficiency: washed packed cells to avoid anaphylaxis
     - T-cell defects: irradiated blood products to prevent graft-versus-host reaction; use cytomegalovirus free blood because of risk of infection
- Specific therapy
  1. Gamma globulin replacement for B-cell defects
  2. Bone marrow transplantation for T-cell and combined defects

TABLE 2-2 Clinical Differentiation of the Major Immunodeficiency Syndrome Subgroups

Immune Deficiency	B-Cell (Antibody) Defects	T-Cell (Cellular) Defects	Neutrophil Disorders	Complement Deficiencies
Relative incidence*	50%	30% (10% cellular, 20% combined)	18%	2%
Infecting organisms	Common pyogenic organisms, e.g., pneumococcus, *H. influenzae*	Bacteria, fungi, viruses, protozoa	*Staphylococcus*, Gram-negative organisms, fungi	Bacteria (*Neisseria* with C6, C7 and C8 deficiency)
Common sites and types of infection	Sinopulmonary, middle ear infections most commonly; also skin, gastrointestinal tract involvement	Candidiasis of skin, mucous membranes and nails; pneumonitis; enteritis	Skin, lymph nodes, liver (abscess), lung, bone, periodontal, perirectal	Meningitis, disseminated gonococcal infection

| Specific features | DiGeorge syndrome: tetany, congenital heart disease, unusual facies
Ataxia–telangiectasia: ataxia, telangiectasia of skin and conjunctivae
Wiskott-Aldrich syndrome: thrombocytopenia (with petechiae and bleeding)
Cartilage-hair hypoplasia: short-limb dwarfism, fine, light-colored hair | Delayed umbilical cord detachment (>3 wk)
Chédiak-Higashi syndrome: partial oculocutaneous albinism | Associated autoimmune disorders |

*Excludes asymptomatic IgA deficiency. IgA deficiency occurs in 1:400 normal individuals.

TABLE 2-3 Classification of Immunodeficiency Disorders

Primary immunodeficiencies
  Predominant B-cell defects (50%)
    X-linked agammaglobulinemia (congenital hypogammaglobulinemia)
    Transient hypogammaglobulinemia of infancy
    Selective IgG subclass deficiencies
    Common variable immunodeficiency (acquired hypogammaglobulinemia)
    Selective IgA deficiency
    Immunodeficiency with increased IgM
  Combined T-cell and B-cell defects (20%)
    Severe combined immunodeficiency
    Severe combined immunodeficiency with adenosine deaminase (ADA) deficiency
    Purine nucleoside phosphorylase (PNP) deficiency
    Combined immunodeficiency with abnormal immunoglobulin synthesis (Nezelof syndrome)
    Ataxia-telangiectasia (IgA)
    Wiskott-Aldrich syndrome (IgA, IgE, IgM)
    Immunodeficiency with short-limb dwarfism
  Predominant T-cell defects (10%)
    DiGeorge syndrome—congenital thymic aplasia
    Chronic mucocutaneous candidiasis
  Phagocytic disorders (18%)
    Defective production
      Cyclic neutropenia
      Aplastic anemia
      Kostmann's syndrome
      Schwachman-Diamond syndrome

TABLE 2-3 Classification of Immunodeficiency Disorders (Cont'd)

  Disorders of cell movement
    Lazy leukocyte syndrome
    Hyperimmunoglobulin E syndrome
  Disorders of cell membrane
    LFA-1 glycoprotein deficiency
  Disorders of phagocytosis
    Actin dysfunction
  Defective microbiocidal activity
    Chronic granulomatous disease
    Chediak-Higashi syndrome (defective degranulation)
 Deficiency of complement components (2%)
    Early components (C1-C4)— associated with collagen vascular disease
    Late components (C5-C9)— associated with recurrent Neisseria infection

Secondary immunodeficiency
  Infections, e.g., HIV, EBV
  Protein-losing states, e.g., nephrotic syndrome, protein-loading enteropathy
  Malignant disease, e.g., leukemia, lymphoma
  Immunosuppressive agents, e.g., antineoplastic drugs, corticosteroids, radiation
  Hematologic disorders, e.g., sickle cell disease
  Metabolic disorders, e.g., diabetes mellitus, severe uremia, galactosemia
  Nutritional deficiencies, e.g., protein-calorie malnutrition
  Splenectomy
  Prematurity

THREE

Cardiology

Abbreviations

AET	atrial ectopic tachycardia
AI	aortic insufficiency
AS	aortic stenosis
ASD	atrial septal defect
AVM	arteriovenous malformation
AVNRT	atrioventricular nodal reentry tachycardia
CAVSD	complete atrioventricular septal defect
CHB	congenital heart block
CHD	congenital heart disease
CHF	congestive heart failure
CMP	cardiomyopathy
CMV	cytomegalovirus
CRF	chronic renal failure
EFE	endocardial fibroelastosis
HLHS	hypoplastic left heart syndrome
JET	junctional ectopic tachycardia
ICP	intracranial pressure
IDM	infant of a diabetic mother
IHSS	idiopathic hypertrophic subaortic stenosis
LAD	left axis deviation
MR	mitral regurgitation
MS	mitral stenosis
NSR	normal sinus rhythm
PA	pulmonary atresia
PAPVR	partial anomalous pulmonary venous return
PAT	paroxysmal atrial tachycardia
PDA	patent ductus arteriosus
PFC	persistent fetal circulation
PS	pulmonary stenosis
RAD	right axis deviation
RBBB	right bundle branch block
RDS	respiratory distress syndrome

SBE	subacute bacterial endocarditis
SSS	sick sinus syndrome
SVT	supraventricular tachycardia
TA	tricuspid atresia
TAPVR	total anomalous pulmonary venous return
D-TGA	transposition of great arteries
L-TGA	corrected transposition of great arteries
TMI	transient myocardial ischemia
ToF	tetralogy of Fallot
VPB	ventricular premature beats
VSD	ventricular septal defect
VT	ventricular tachycardia

Congestive Heart Failure

Clinical Features and Investigations

- Usually difficult to distinguish right from left-sided failure
- General features include tachycardia, tachypnea (often earliest signs), cardiomegaly, gallop rhythm (S_3), weak pulse, cardiomegaly, and diaphoresis. N.B. normal RR up to 40 in newborn; 30-40, <6 mo; 20-30, 6 mo-1 yr, 20 thereafter
- Additional signs of right-sided (or combined) failure include hepatomegaly, facial edema, sacral edema
- Left-sided failure, or pulmonary congestion, is manifested by exertional dyspnea (major example: feeding), orthopnea, wheezing, and crackles
- CXR: cardiomegaly ± venous congestion
- ECG: may be normal, but does not rule out presence of CHF
- See Table 16-10, p 334 for additional features in the neonatal period

Management

- General measures
  1. Sitting up to relieve respiratory distress, NPO
  2. Humidified oxygen, monitor O_2 saturation or arterial blood gases
- Digoxin
  1. Use of digoxin individualized, in consultation with cardiologist. Initial IV administration in severe CHF; less distressed infants may be treated orally. All patients should be switched to oral therapy as soon as feasible. See p 659 for digitalization dose. *Note: IV dosage is only 70-80% of amount used orally*
  2. Myocarditis or cardiomyopathy, e.g., rheumatic, viral, myocardial ischemia, iron overload in thalassemia:
     - Digitalization dose reduced to 50%, maintenance dose reduced to 33-50%
     - Monitor with ECG plus serum digoxin levels
  3. Reduce dose in renal failure and in presence of drugs that increase digoxin levels, e.g., quinidine, amiodarone, propafenone. Start with 50% of usual dose and monitor levels and ECG
  4. Contradicted in IHSS, cardiac tamponade, and complete heart block
- Diuretics
  1. Acutely: furosemide PO or IV (watch for ↓ K^+)
  2. Chronically: hydrochlorothiazide-spironolactone, metalazone
- Pulmonary edema
  1. O_2
  2. Furosemide 1.0 mg/kg IV—slowly over 5-10 min
  3. Morphine 0.2 mg/kg; maximum dose, 10 mg
  4. Digoxin IV, depending on underlying cause
- Vasodilators: captopril

Electrocardiography

- Refer to Table 3-1 for the proper placement of leads in electrocardiography.
- Analyze ECG systematically: rate, rhythm, axis, chamber enlargement, ST and T wave changes, and strain-infarction
- A Q wave may normally appear in leads II, III, AVF, V_5 and V_6
- From birth to 3 days, T wave is upright over the right precordium and may be negative over the left precordium. By 4 days, the T wave is negative in V_1. From this time until age 4-5 yr, an upright T wave in V_1 implies abnormal right ventricular hypertrophy.
- Rate (Fig. 3-1): estimated by dividing 300 by number of large squares (each 0.2 sec) between each QRS, assuming regular rhythm. Normal heart rates: 0-3 mo, ~100→180; 3 mo-2 yr, ~80→150; 2-10 yr, ~70-110; >10 yr, 55→90. Subtract 20 bpm for rates obtained when child is asleep. Most rates in children will go up to 200-220 with exercise or fever.
- Rhythm and conduction (see Fig. 3-1):
  1. Check for P before each QRS
  2. Check for QRS after each P
  3. Measure PR interval
  4. Measure QRS interval
  5. Measure QT (calculate QTc):

$$\text{corrected QT (QTc)} = \sqrt{\frac{\text{measured QT}}{\text{R-R interval}}}$$

Cardiology

6. QTc should not exceed
   - 0.45 in infant <6 mo
   - 0.44 in children
   - 0.425 in adolescents and adults
- Differential diagnosis of long QT syndrome
  1. Drugs, e.g., quinidine, amiodarone, sotolol
  2. Electrolyte disturbances, e.g., decreased K^+, Ca^{2+}, or Mg^{2+} (Fig. 3-2, Table 3-2)
  3. CNS damage
  4. Myocarditis
  5. Jervell-Lange-Nielsen syndrome (long QT plus congenital deafness)
  6. Romano-Ward syndrome (long QT, normal hearing, autosomal dominant)
  7. Severe heart failure
- Axis determination (check lead I and AVF) (Figs. 3-3 and 3-4)
- Chamber enlargement (Table 3-3)
- ST/T changes

Text continued on p. 41.

TABLE 3-1 Lead Placement for Electrocardiography

Lead	Positioning of Electrodes*
I	RA-LA
II	RA-LL
III	LA-LL
AVR	RA
AVL	LA
AVF	LL
V_1	4th RIC at RSB
V_2	4th LIC at LSB
V_3	Between V_2 and V_4
V_4	5th LIC at midclavicular line
V_5	5th LIC at anterior axillary line
V_6	5th LIC at midaxillary line
V_3R	V_3 on right chest
V_4	V_4 on right chest
V_7	Posterior axillary line

*RA = right arm; LA = left arm; LL = left leg; RIC = right intercostal space; LIC = left intercostal space; RSB = right sternal border; LSB = left sternal border.

Modified from Park MK. Pediatric cardiology for practitioners. Chicago: Year Book, 1984:36; and from Garson A Jr. The electrocardiogram in infants and children. Philadelphia: Lea & Febiger, 1983:32.

TABLE 3-2 Electrocardiogram-Related Electrolyte Disturbances

Hyperkalemia	Tall, narrow, "tented" T waves Widening QRS complexes Wide, flattened P waves Ectopic rhythms and intraventricular block
Hypokalemia	↑ QTc interval with broad flat T wave ST segment depression T wave flattened or inverted U wave Ectopic beats, supraventricular-ventricular
Hypercalcemia	Short QTc interval Myocardial irritability ↑ PR interval, QRS duration, ±AV block
Hypocalcemia	↑ QTc interval
Hypomagnesemia	↑ QTc interval

Modified from Park MK. Pediatric cardiology for practitioners. Chicago: Year Book, 1984:250.

TABLE 3-3 Criteria for Chamber Enlargement (Hospital for Sick Children)

RVH
1. R in V_1 20 mm or more at all ages
2. S in V_6 0-7 days 14 mm, 8-30 days 10 mm, 1-3 mo 7 mm, 3 mo-16 yr 5 mm (or more)
3. R/S ratio in V_1 0-3 mo 6.5, 3-6 mo 4.0, 6 mo-3 yr 2.4, 3-5 yr 1.6, 6-15 yr 0.8 (or more)
4. T positive in V_1 if R/S more than 1.0

LVH
1. S in V_1 more than 20 mm at all ages
2. R in V_6 20 mm or more
3. Secondary T inversion in V_5 or V_6
4. Q 4 mm or more in V_5, V_6, or V_7

Right atrial
1. Peaked P wave 3 mm or more in any lead

Left atrial
1. Bifid P in any lead
2. P duration of more than 0.09 sec
3. Late inversion of P in V_1 of more than 1.5 mm

Combined ventricular
Direct evidence of RVH + LVH *or* RVH + (a) Q of 2 mm or more in V_5 or V_6 (b) inverted T in V_6 (after positive in right chest leads)

From Davignon A, et al. Normal ECG standards for infants and children. Pediatr Cardiol 1979; 1:123-131.

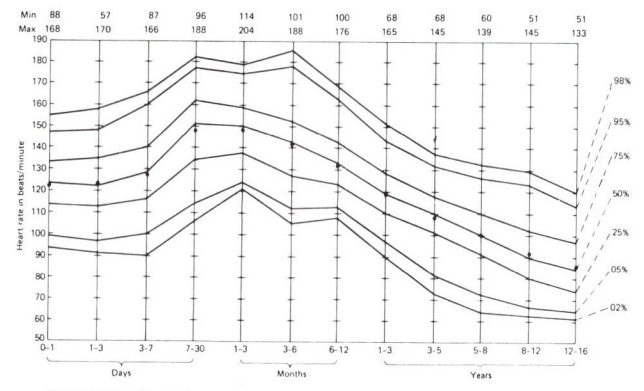

Cardiology

A Heart rate vs. age (● = mean)

B PR duration vs. age in lead II (● = mean)

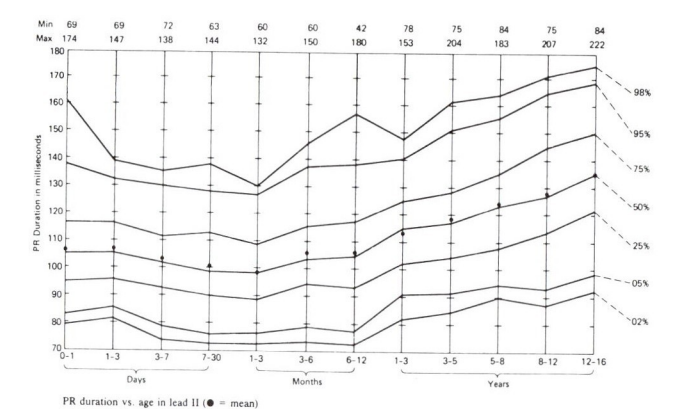

Figure 3-1 **Normal ECG standards in pediatrics.** (From Davignon A, et al. Normal ECG standards for infants and children. Pediatr Cardiol 1979; 1:123-131.)

Continued.

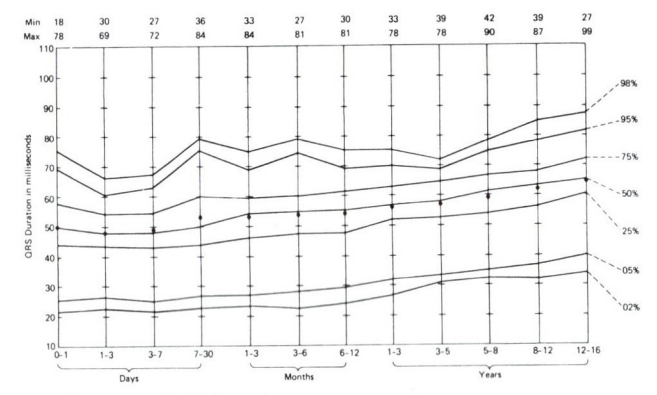

QRS duration vs. age in lead V5 (● = mean)

C

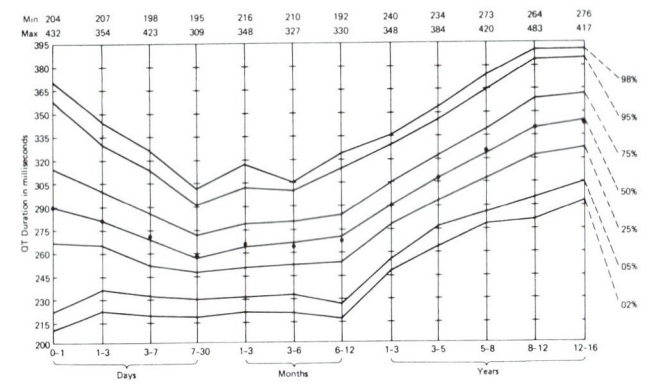

QT duration vs. age in lead V5 (● = mean)

D

Figure 3-1, continued.

Cardiology

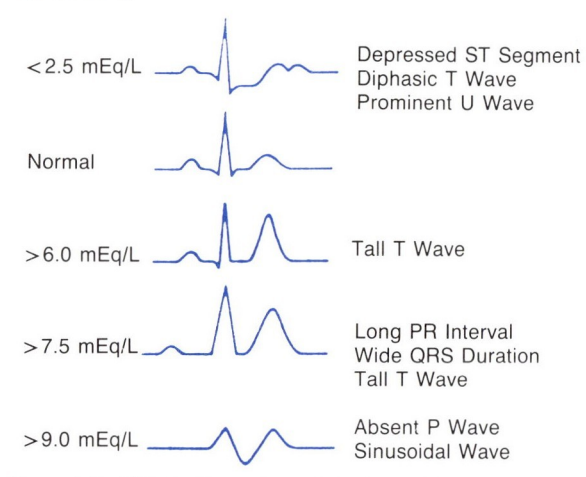

SERUM K

< 2.5 mEq/L		Depressed ST Segment Diphasic T Wave Prominent U Wave
Normal		
> 6.0 mEq/L		Tall T Wave
> 7.5 mEq/L		Long PR Interval Wide QRS Duration Tall T Wave
> 9.0 mEq/L		Absent P Wave Sinusoidal Wave

Figure 3-2 **ECG findings of hypokalemia and hyperkalemia.** (From Park MK, Guntheroth WG. How to read pediatric ECGs. 2nd ed. Copyright © 1987 by Year Book Medical Publishers, Inc, Chicago.)

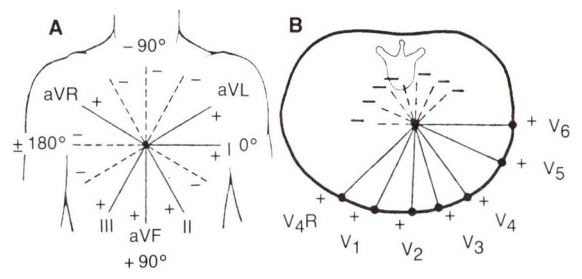

Figure 3-3 **Hexaxial *(A)* and horizontal *(B)* reference systems.** (From Park MK, Guntheroth WG. How to read pediatric ECGs. 2nd ed. Copyright © 1987 by Year Book Medical Publishers, Inc, Chicago.)

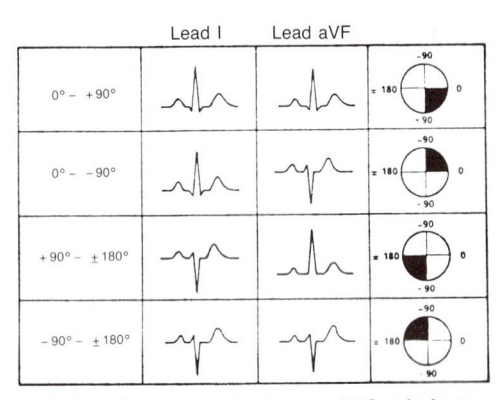

Lead I axis	Lead I	Lead aVF	Quadrant
0° – +90°			
0° – –90°			
+90° – ±180°			
–90° – ±180°			

Figure 3-4 **Locating quadrants of mean QRS axis from leads I and aVF.** (From Park MK, Guntheroth WG. How to read pediatric ECGs. 2nd ed. Copyright © 1987 by Year Book Medical Publishers, Inc, Chicago.)

Identification of Cardiac Dysrhythmias

1. Regular sinus rhythm

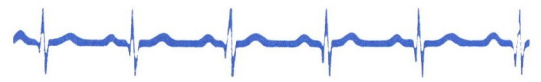

Figure 3-5 **Regular sinus rhythm.** (From Park MK, Guntheroth WG. How to read pediatric ECGs. 2nd ed. Copyright © 1987 by Year Book Medical Publishers, Inc, Chicago.)

2. Premature atrial contraction (PAC)

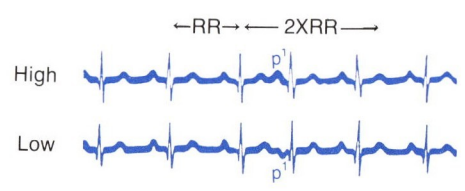

Figure 3-6 **Atrial premature beat.** (From Park MK, Guntheroth WG. How to read pediatric ECGs. 2nd ed. Copyright © 1987 by Year Book Medical Publishers, Inc, Chicago.)

- Premature beat with abnormal P wave (ectopic focus), usually normal QRS; not followed by a compensatory pause
- Premature beat with aberrancy: like a PAC but with QRS of wide complex morphology resembling RBBB
- Normal variation, postcardiac surgery, digitalis toxicity

3. Atrial ectopic tachycardia (Table 3-4)

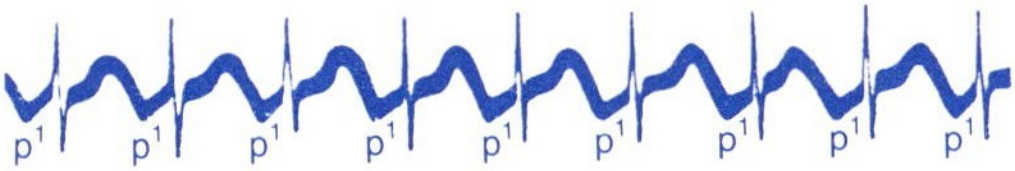

Figure 3-7 **Atrial tachycardia.** (From Park MK, Guntheroth WG. How to read pediatric ECGs. 2nd ed. Copyright © 1987 by Year Book Medical Publishers, Inc, Chicago.)

- Rapid bursts or sustained atrial tachycardia, with the P wave usually abnormal, showing warm-up and cool-down characteristics. May have periods of A-V block
- Management (see Table 3-4)
4. Supraventricular tachycardia (SVT or PAT)
- Rapid rate with normal QRS complex, with or without discernible P waves. *If broad QRS complex, think ventricular tachycardia.*
- Management (see p 47 and Table 3-4 on pp 48-49)
5. Atrial flutter

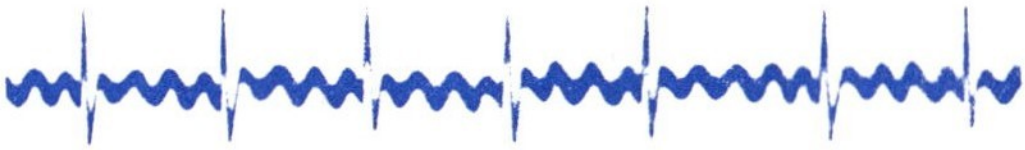

Figure 3-8 **Atrial flutter.** (From Park MK, Guntheroth WG. How to read pediatric ECGs. 2nd ed. Copyright © 1987 by Year Book Medical Publishers, Inc, Chicago.)

- Normal QRS with "flutter waves"
- Congenital heart disease with dilated atria, myocarditis, digitalis toxicity, post-Mustard, Senning and Fontan procedure
- Even with a well-controlled ventricular rate, must treat the atrial flutter. Medical therapy frequently not successful in acute situations so often need to rely on physical methods—i.e., DC cardioversion, esophageal overdrive pacing.

- Maintenance medical therapy; digitalization, sotalol, propafenone, amiodarone, procainamide, and quinidine can all be used.
6. Atrial fibrillation

Rapid Ventricular Response

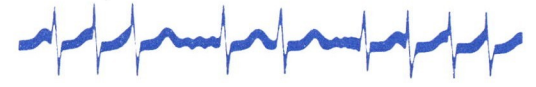

Slow Ventricular Response

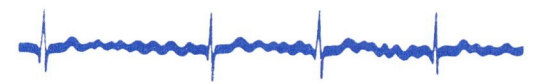

Figure 3-9 **Atrial fibrillation.** (From Park MK, Guntheroth WG. How to read pediatric ECGs. 2nd ed. Copyright © 1987 by Year Book Medical Publishers, Inc, Chicago.)

- Normal QRS with irregularly irregular R-R interval. No discernible P waves
- Causes same as for atrial flutter, plus thyrotoxicosis; treat as for flutter
7. First-degree heart block; PR interval > normal (see Fig. 3-1 for normal values)

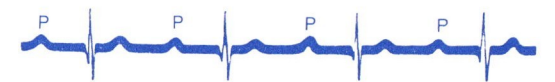

Figure 3-10 **First-degree AV block.** (From Park MK, Guntheroth WG. How to read pediatric ECGs. 2nd ed. Copyright © 1987 by Year Book Medical Publishers, Inc, Chicago.)

- Seen in healthy children and those with acute rheumatic fever, cardiomyopathies, congenital heart disease (ASD, Ebstein's, CAVSD), postcardiac surgery, digoxin toxicity; treat underlying cause

8. Second-degree heart block

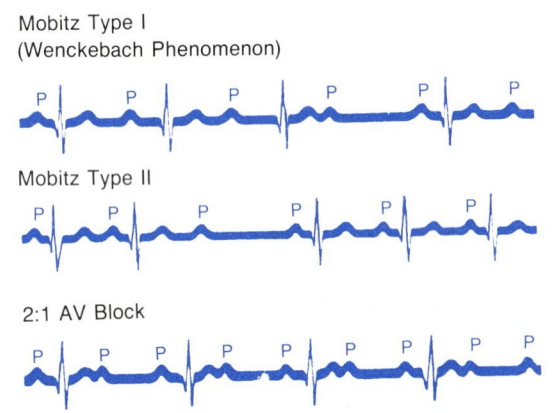

Mobitz Type I
(Wenckebach Phenomenon)

Mobitz Type II

2:1 AV Block

Figure 3-11 **Second-degree AV block.** (From Park MK, Guntheroth WG. How to read pediatric ECGs. 2nd ed. Copyright © 1987 by Year Book Medical Publishers, Inc, Chicago.)

- Mobitz I (Wenckebach): progressive lengthening of PR interval until atrial beat nonconducted (2:1, 3:1, 4:1)
- Mobitz II: dropped beats without PR lengthening (2:1, 3:1, 4:1)
- Seen in healthy children, myocarditis, cardiomyopathy, myocardial infarction, postcardiac surgery, congenital heart disease, digoxin toxicity; Generally, treat underlying cause; pacemaker occasionally required.

9. AV dissociation (third-degree heart block)

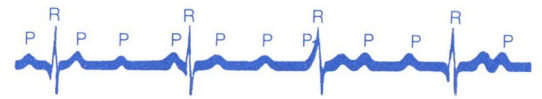

Figure 3-12 **Complete (third-degree) AV block.** (From Park MK, Guntheroth WG. How to read pediatric ECGs. 2nd ed. Copyright © 1987 by Year Book Medical Publishers, Inc, Chicago.)

- No relation between atrial and ventricular impulse, with atrial rate faster and presence of a slow junctional or ventricular rhythm
    1. Congenital: idiopathic, maternal systemic lupus erythematosus, L-TGA
    2. Acquired: cardiac surgery, myocarditis, post-MI
    3. Treatment: depends on rate, cause. Usually requires pacemaker; may require atropine or isoproterenol in interim
- AV dissociation with junctional ectopic tachycardia (JET): nonconduction of atrial impulse with a fast independent junctional rhythm, AV dissociation (see Table 3-4)

10. Ventricular premature beat (VPB)

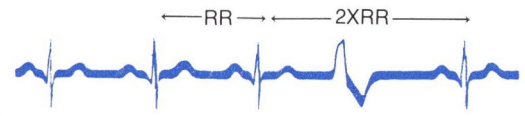

Figure 3-13 **Ventricular premature beat.** (From Park MK, Guntheroth WG. How to read pediatric ECGs. 2nd ed. Copyright © 1987 by Year Book Medical Publishers, Inc, Chicago.)

- Usually prolonged QRS complex and always different from NSR complex. T wave deflection opposite to QRS. Compensatory pause follows PVC.
- Causes and treatment—see ventricular tachycardia

11. Ventricular tachycardia

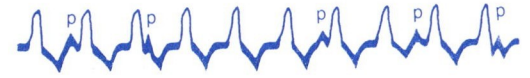

Figure 3-14 **Ventricular tachycardia (or SVT with aberrant ventricular conduction).** (From Park MK, Guntheroth WG. How to read pediatric ECGs. 2nd ed. Copyright © 1987 by Year Book Medical Publishers, Inc, Chicago.)

- Defined as greater than 3 VPB's/min at a rate greater than 120 beats/min. Presence of fusion beats prior to onset and capture beats during tachycardia usually diagnostic. QRS duration usually broad. If morphology different from NSR, must consider VT. *Ninety-five percent of broad complex tachycardias are VT.*
- Fusion beat arises from fusion of normal beat with VPB.
- Capture beat: with AV dissociation present in VT, the occasional P wave is conducted giving an occasional normal sinus beat interspersed in the tachycardia
- Causes and treatment (see Table 3-4)

12. Wolff-Parkinson-White syndrome
    - Short PR interval with initial slurring of the QRS upstroke (delta wave) due to pre-excitation. QRS slightly prolonged
    - Treatment (see p 47)

13. Bundle branch block (commonest cause: postsurgery)
    - Occurs if QRS is one of the following (see Fig. 3-1):
      a. >0.08 seconds if <2 yr
      b. >0.09 seconds if 2-8 yr
      c. >0.10 seconds if >8 yr
    - Right bundle branch
      a. Wide S wave in I, V_6
      b. RSR' (M shape) in V_1
      c. RAD
    - Left bundle branch
      a. LAD
      b. Loss of Q wave in I, V_5, V_6
      c. Slurred wide R wave in I, AVL, V_5, V_6
      d. Wide S wave in V_1, V_2

Treatment of Supraventricular Tachycardia

Acute Treatment
- Vagal maneuvres: Valsalva, carotid sinus massage, gag, *do not use ocular pressure*
- Facial immersion, ice water, or ice bag (in infants do this first)
- Esophageal pacing in infants if available
- Adenosine 0.05 mg/kg IV push. May be repeated in the following doses at 2-min intervals if no response: 0.1 mg/kg; 0.15 mg/kg; 0.2 mg/kg; 0.25 mg/kg. Maximum dose, 25 mg. Check BP at 1 and 2 min.
- Neostigmine 0.01-0.04 mg/kg IV bolus; have atropine ready (0.01 mg/kg) in case of cholinergic excess

  or
- Edrophonium 0.2 mg/kg IV bolus over 3 min; keep atropine ready
- Phenylephrine 0.01-0.10 mg/kg IV bolus (not first choice); Use in 0.01-mg/kg increments
- Synchronized cardioversion, 0.25-1.0 joules/kg; should be first choice when there is severe hemodynamic compromise

Chronic Treatment
- Wolff-Parkinson-White syndrome
  1. β-blockers
     - Propranolol 2-10 mg/kg/day in three or four divided doses
     - Metoprolol 2-5 mg/kg/day in two or three divided doses
  2. Verapamil 2-10 mg/kg/day in three or four divided doses *(> age 5)*
  3. Propafenone 300-600 mg/m^2/day in three or four doses
  4. Digoxin should not be used without consultation with cardiology
  5. Amiodarone 10 mg/kg × 10 days loading, 5 mg/kg/day as a single dose maintenance
- For other forms of SVT, any of the above drugs may be used, usually in combination with digoxin

TABLE 3-4 **Differentiation of Tachycardia in Children**

	Sinus	SVT	Atrial Flutter
Clinical Features	Fever Sepsis Hypovolemia Shock CHF Catecholamines	Usually normal heart 50% Parkinson-Wolff-White (Delta waves seen only after conversion to sinus rhythm) 25% AVNRT Ebstein's anomaly L-TGA, single ventricle	90% structural with dilated atria Post-Mustard, Senning Myocarditis Digoxin toxicity
Rate	Usually <200 beats/min	Infants: up to 300 beats/min Children: <240 beats/min	Atrial often >250-400 beats/min with 1:2, 1:3, 1:4 block
P wave	Normal	May not see visible P waves 60% retrograde P wave	Constant
QRS wave	Normal	Normal after initial 10-20 beats unless abberation present	Normal
Treatment	Treat underlying cause	See p 47	Digoxin Propafenone Amiodarone D/C cardioversion 1. Acute decompensation 2. Postoperative Fontan

Cardiology

AET	JET	Ventricular Tachycardia
Usually normal heart	Post-bypass surgery	>70% abnormal heart Myocarditis Long QT Post-surgery Digoxin toxicity Catecholamines Amphetamines
>200 beats/min	Atrial rate < ventricle rate Ventricle 200-300 beats/min	Usually <250 beats/min Infants: up to 200-500 beats/min
Initial P wave may be abnormal, but remains constant May have multiple P wave morphology	Retrograde P waves	A-V dissociation may be seen Usually no P wave or retrograde P wave
Normal	Normal, as in AV dissociation	Wide
Unaffected by vagal maneuvre, overdrive 33% spontaneous regression Digoxin has little effect Propranolol Amiodarone Procainamide Difficult to control	Unable to overdrive Cool down body temperature Ensure optimal volume status, normal pH Propafenone loading dose: 0.2 mg/kg/IV every 2 min, × 10 days then maintenance 300-600 mg/m^2/day IV	If unstable, cardioversion If stable: 1. Correct pH, electrolytes 2. Lidocaine 1 mg/kg IV 3. Procainamide 5 mg/kg IV Chronic therapy 1. Mexilitine 2. Propranolol

Endocarditis (Subacute bacterial endocarditis [SBE])

- Streptococcal commonest (α-hemolytic, non-hemolytic *S. viridans, S. faecalis*). *Staphylococcus aureus:* often normal heart, accounts for >50% of SBE in IV drug users. *S. epidermidis* in postoperative cardiac anomalies and prosthetic valves. Gram-negative, fungal infection rare, and found usually in immunosuppressed

Investigations
- Blood cultures taken from three separate sites for culture in 24-hr
- CBC, ESR, BUN, creatinine
- Increased immunoglobulins, rheumatoid factor, decreased complement in up to 40%
- Urine microscopy (hematuria in 30%)
- 2D-ECHO—vegetations: lesions ≥2 mm; may get false-negative results
- Negative cultures in up to 10-15%: previous antibiotics, unusual organism, anaerobes, right-sided endocarditis

Management
- Prior to culture results
  1. Penicillin 6-20 million U/day IV in six divided doses ± aminoglycoside

  or

  2. Cloxacillin 100 mg/kg/day IV in six divided doses

  and

  3. Streptomycin 20 mg/kg/day IM in one or two divided doses
- Organism isolation and antibiotic specificity to guide therapy—usually 4-6 wk in total.
- Follow-up: generally no change in 2D-ECHO findings during acute management
- Prevention (p 716)

Rheumatic Fever

TABLE 3-5 Revised Jones Criteria for Guidance in Diagnosis of Rheumatic Fever*

Major manifestations
1. Carditis
   Murmur
   Cardiomegaly
   Pericarditis
   Congestive heart failure
2. Polyarthritis
3. Chorea
4. Erythema marginatum
5. Subcutaneous nodules

Minor manifestations
1. Clinical evidence
   History of previous rheumatic fever
   Arthralgia
   Fever
2. Laboratory
   Increased ESR, C-reactive protein, WBC count, anemia
   Prolonged P-R and Q-T intervals on ECG

Supportive evidence
1. Recent scarlet fever
2. Throat culture positive for group A streptococci
3. Increased ASO or other streptococcal antibodies

*Two major manifestations or one major and two minor manifestations with supportive evidence of recent streptococcal infection indicate a high probability of rheumatic fever. However, failure to meet the Jones criteria does not exclude rheumatic fever.

Modified from Rudolph AM, ed. Pediatrics. 17th ed. Norwalk: Appleton-Century-Crofts; 1982:446.

Management

- Antibiotic therapy
  1. Benzathine penicillin G 1.2 million U IM given as a single dose (half the dose if <30 kg); *or* penicillin V 200,000-400,000 U PO tid-qid × 10 days; *or* erythromycin 20-40 mg/kg/day (÷ bid or tid) × 10 days
  2. For continued prophylaxis, benzathine penicillin G 1.2 million U IM monthly; *or* penicillin V 200,000 U PO bid; *or* sulfadiazine 1 g PO daily (half the dose if <30 kg)

- Uncomplicated disease
  1. ASA 70-100 mg/kg/day 6 wk
  2. Bed rest, then gradual ambulation after 2 wk
- With carditis
  1. Bed rest: duration dependent on severity of carditis
  2. Prednisone, 1-2 mg/kg/day, if cardiomegaly present
  3. ASA if no cardiomegaly

Corrective Cardiac Procedures Defined

- Blalock-Hanlon: surgical atrial septectomy
- Brock: infundibulectomy or closed pulmonary valvulotomy
- Fontan: connection of right atrium to left pulmonary artery either by atrial-appendage to pulmonary artery anastomosis or use of conduit-graft between them
- Mustard: intra-atrial baffle or patch (pericardium) for palliation of simple transposition
- Park: creation of atrial septostomy by use of knife-tipped catheter after passage through foramen ovale
- Rashkind: balloon atrial septostomy with cardiac catheter
- Rastelli
  1. Placement of valved conduit-graft between right ventricle and pulmonary artery
  2. Repair of CAVSD by resuspension of mitral valve and tricuspid valve on newly created atrial septum
- Senning: a type of repair of simple TGA by intra-atrial baffle, using flaps of native atrial septum and atrial wall
- Jatene: arterial switch for correction of TGA
- Norwood: two-stage palliation for hypoplastic left heart syndrome and other forms of complex CHD with systemic outflow obstruction
- Shunts
  1. Blalock-Taussig: subclavian artery to pulmonary artery
  2. Glenn: superior vena cava to R pulmonary artery (e.g., for tricuspid atresia)
  3. Potts: descending aorta to L pulmonary artery
  4. Waterston: ascending aorta to R pulmonary artery

Myocarditis

- Newborns and infants may present with lethargy, anorexia, vomiting, and signs of CHF
- ECG may show low voltages, ST-T changes, prolonged QT, and dysrhythmias
- CXR examination may show cardiomegaly
- Increased ESR ± increased AST

Management
- Anti-CHF measures (reduced dosage of digoxin; p 30)
- Role of biopsy, steroids controversial
- Majority recover completely
- A few develop chronic myocarditis ± CHF

Acute Pericarditis

- Fever
- Precordial pain (sharp, substernal; may radiate to neck)
- Pericardial friction rub
- Cardiomegaly, but quiet and hypodynamic heart
- ± Signs of tamponade: tachycardia, pulsus paradoxus
- Hepatomegaly
- Venous distension

Investigations
- ECG
  1. Low voltages
  2. Time-dependent changes secondary to myocardial involvement: initial ST elevation → return of ST to baseline with T inversion
- CXR: cardiomegaly and effusion, increased pulmonary venous markings if tamponade
- 2D-ECHO
- Pericardiocentesis

Treatment
- Medical: treat underlying condition
- Surgical: pericardiocentesis for relief of tamponade, or drainage of purulent pericarditis and 4-6 wk of IV antibiotics
- Digoxin contraindicated (blocks compensatory tachycardia). Low-dose ASA may be used for persistent effusion.

Cyanotic Spells in Tetralogy of Fallot

- Paroxysmal dyspnea with cyanosis; increased respiratory rate and depth of breathing (Kussmaul)
- Quieter and shorter ejection murmur (increased R → L shunting)
- Floppy
- Can lead to loss of consciousness, seizures, death

Investigations
- ABG: acidosis with hypoxia
- CXR: decreased pulmonary blood flow (*rarely* done during episode)
- ECG: increased P wave

Treatment
- Knee-chest position (decreases venous return, therefore decreases right-to-left shunt)
- O_2 by mask or hood (6-8 L/min or 100% O_2)
- Propranolol 0.05-0.1 mg/kg slow IV push (over 10 min)
- Morphine 0.1 mg/kg IV or SC (may depress respiration)
- $NaHCO_3$ 1-2 mEq/kg IV, for correction of metabolic acidosis
- Phenylephrine 0.10 mg/dose IM (vasoconstrictor—increases systemic vascular resistance and therefore decreases right-to-left shunt)
- Transfuse if anemic (Hb < 150 g/L [15 g/dl])
- Chronic treatment: propranolol

Cardiology

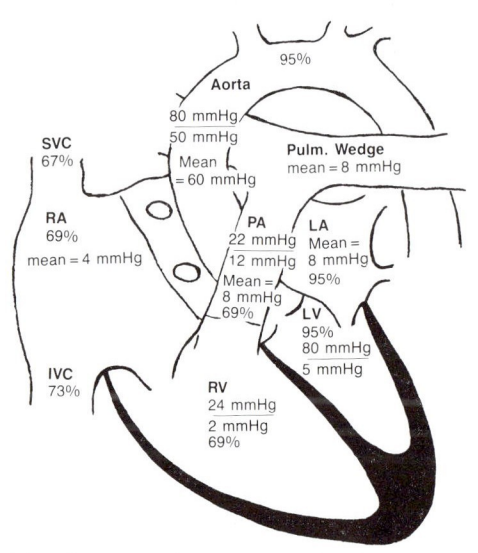

Figure 3-15 **Normal cardiac catheterization data in children older than 1 month of age. Catheterization values: oxygen saturation as % saturation. Pressure as mm Hg.**

FOUR

Dentistry

- Parent education and prevention most important—discourage bedtime bottle to prevent "nursing caries" or "baby bottle" syndrome
- Encourage parents to clean child's teeth as soon as they appear (initially with gauze swab and later with soft toothbrush)
- Recommend regular dental visits, beginning not later than 36 mo

Dental Pain

- Most dental pain requires referral to dentist
  1. Simple hyperemia due to trauma or large restorations
  2. Pulpitis due to dental caries
     - Serous pulpitis: tooth sensitive to cold; pain relieved by heat
     - Suppurative pulpitis: tooth sensitive to heat; cold may relieve pain
  3. Pulpal necrosis with abscess
     - May occur without facial swelling or systemic signs
     - Management: analgesics, antipyretics, antibiotics (Pen V), possible removal of offending tooth
  4. Periodontal abscess
     - Usually pain (localized or referred) with associated facial swelling and fever
     - Management: analgesics, antipyretics, surgical drainage

Dental Trauma

- Displacement of deciduous teeth interferes with development and eruption of adjacent permanent teeth
- Interference with blood supply may result in pulpal necrosis (indicated by blue-black discoloration of crown) and infection
- Space preservation is unnecessary in the anterior segment, but imperative in posterior segments of deciduous dental arch
- All cases require referral to dentist

Management

- Clean site of blood, debris for maximum visualization
- Determine time of accident; age of patient; whether tooth is deciduous or permanent; whether tooth is loose, out, intruded or fractured; and whether dental pulp is visible (pinkish coloration or direct visualization of blood)
- Therapy depends on type of injury and tooth affected
  1. Loosened or displaced anterior teeth
     - Deciduous: removal of injured tooth
     - Permanent
       a. Consult dentist immediately (the affected tooth will be immobilized with an acrylic splint)
       b. Every 6 wk observe the tooth for signs of pulpal necrosis due to interference with neurovascular supply (less likely in younger children and where dental trauma has been treated promptly)
  2. Fractured permanent anterior teeth
     - Early referral (especially if temperature sensitive)
     - Even small enamel fractures in teeth may have associated root fractures, which may require rigid stabilization for a minimum of 6 wk

3. Avulsed teeth
   - Deciduous
     a. No treatment required except roentgenographic search for remnants in the jaw, lips, or lungs, if indicated
     b. *Never* replant an avulsed primary tooth
   - Permanent
     a. Ask patient to bring tooth along ASAP!
     b. *Keep tooth moist in cold milk or ice water*
     c. Early referral for replanting and immobilization
     d. Prognosis dependent on length of time out of mouth (extra-alveolar period <30 min has ~ 90% chance of long-term retention), contamination of tooth (should avoid handling root surface), and age of patient

Dental Postoperative Hemorrhage

- Definition: bleeding longer than 4 hr, or delayed recurrent bleeding

Management

- Apply pressure: have patient bite firmly on a folded 2 × 2 gauze pack positioned over the extraction socket
- *Recheck in ~ 10 min for hemostasis*
- If above unsuccessful:
  1. Local infiltration of 2% Xylocaine with epinephrine 1:100,000 and curette socket
  2. Topical hemostatic agents (e.g., bovine thrombin)
  3. Further therapy (Gelfoam gauze pack or suturing) rarely needed

Acute Herpetic Gingivostomatitis

Management
- Mainly supportive: self-limiting disease lasting 10-14 days
  1. Topical analgesic mouthwash—e.g., benzydamine (Tantum)
  2. Topical antiseptics: antiseptic mouthwash—e.g., dequalinium (Dequadin)
  3. Topical anesthetics (e.g., benzocaine) not usually required; apply carefully with Q-tip to affected areas; may be used as oral rinse (risk of methemoglobinemia if swallowed)
  4. Acetaminophen for pain and fever
  5. Tantum oral rinse for pain
  6. Systemic antibiotic only for secondary bacterial infection
  7. Soft bland diet with extra fluids should be encouraged

FIVE

Dermatology

Acne

- Two types of lesions
  1. Noninflammatory: comedones (open, closed)
  2. Inflammatory: papules, pustules, cysts
- Neonatal acne—due to maternal hormones (usually self-limited)
- General measures
  1. Exclude androgenic causes
  2. Use drying soaps (benzoyl peroxide) if oily
  3. Do not use moisturizers, steaming, or saunas
  4. Use oil-free make-up
- Topical medication
  1. Benzoyl peroxide (2.5% to 20%)
     - Oxidizer; inhibits *Propionibacterium acnes*
     - Comedolytic
     - Apply qhs; start with 5-10%; then increase % PRN
  2. Vitamin A acid (0.01%, 0.025%, 0.05%) cream and gel
     - May worsen initially
     - Apply qhs; start at 0.01% for ½ hour; increase slowly
     - Use for a minimum of 6 wk
     - May be associated with photosensitivity—wear sun block
  3. Antibiotics
     - For inflammatory lesions; erythromycin (Staticin) or 2% clindamycin solution in Duonalc solution bid
- Oral medication (for inflammatory acne)
  1. Antibiotics
     - Bacteriostatic for *P. acnes*; inhibit lipases, which produce free fatty acids
     - Tetracycline (do not use if under 8 yr or pregnant), 1 g daily × 1 wk and then 500 mg daily; *or* minocy-

cline, 50-100 mg/day; *or* erythromycin, 500 mg – 1 g/day. Can be maintained long term on 250 mg daily until acne is cured
- With prolonged use of antibiotic (1½-2 yrs) and decreasing effect, may switch to another antibiotic, or discontinue. Patient may have quiescent disease at this point.
2. Isotretinoin (Accutane)
   - Anti-inflammatory; decreases sebaceous gland secretion; normalizes keratinization of follicular epithelium
   - Best used only by a dermatologist or physician familiar with this drug
   - For nodulo-cystic, scarring acne that is resistant to oral antibiotics
   - Discontinue antibiotics while patient is receiving Accutane
   - Four- to five-month course and laboratory tests every 4 wks (liver function tests, urinalysis, CBC, cholesterol, and triglycerides)
   - *Must avoid pregnancy* during and for 1 mo after treatment is finished (mandatory pregnancy test prior to starting Accutane)
   - Use oral contraceptives during course of treatment, where appropriate
   - Side effects: cheilitis (100%), xerostomia, xerosis, myalgia, facial dermatitis, headache (all reversible when drug is discontinued)
   - Rise in AST, cholesterol, and triglycerides
- If necessary, dermatology referral for
  1. Intralesional steroid injections of cysts and scars
  2. Acne surgery (comedone removal)

Alopecia

- The three most common causes of patchy nonscarring alopecia in children are alopecia areata (see below), trichotillomania, and tinea capitis
- Examine entire skin, mucosal surfaces, nails, and teeth

- Depending on the etiology, fungal or other microbiological studies, Wood's lamp examination of the scalp, light microscopic examination of hair, or scalp biopsy may be indicated

ALOPECIA AREATA

- Smooth bald areas; exclamation mark hairs
- Rarely may be associated with autoimmune disease
- For prolonged disease, potent topical steroids, e.g., fluocinonide 0.05% tid (Lidex or Topsyn Gel), or intralesional steroids if patient can tolerate injections and areas are small

Atopic Dermatitis

- General Measures
  1. Prevent overheating—wear cotton clothes, ensure adequate control of ambient temperature (air conditioning if necessary)
  2. Humidification—humidifier, daily bath (add oilated Aveeno, Alpha Keri, or baby oil to bath); pat dry
  3. Chemical—use mild soaps (e.g., Dove or baby soap); wash clothes in Ivory and rinse well, no bleach or fabric softener
- Topical agents
  1. Steroids (see p 70)—start with hydrocortisone, 1% ointment (may be used on face), tid to qid; if necessary, use more potent steroid (e.g., Betnovate 0.05% ointment) to body (NOT to face or groin)
  2. Emollients (see p 71)
- Antihistamines: diphenhydramine, hydroxyzine, or terfenadine may help (especially if child cannot sleep because of itchiness)
- Antibiotics: erythromycin or cloxacillin PO for impetigo
- Avoid systemic steroids

Furunculosis

- A furuncle is an acute infection (usually staphylococcal) arising in a hair follicle
- Erythematous, tender, often "points," then spontaneously drains
- Usually in a hairy area or area of friction (posterior neck, axillae, thighs, perineum)
- A carbuncle is a deeper infection of several adjacent hair follicles, with multiple draining sites

Management

- Hot compresses
- Incise and drain (when "pointing")
- Oral cloxacillin

Impetigo

- Contagious infection by *S. aureus* and rarely beta-hemolytic streptococcus
- Child not systemically ill
- Staphylococcal impetigo
  1. Bullous; often begins in folds (neck, groin)
  2. *Staphylococcus* reservoir: upper respiratory tract
- Streptococcal impetigo
  1. Honey-colored crusts ("classic impetigo")
  2. Poststreptococcal glomerulonephritis can occur after impetigo; rheumatic fever does not

Management

- Cool compresses to dry lesions
- Cloxacillin or erythromycin PO for 10 days
- If streptococcal impetigo, use penicillin or erythromycin PO
- Topical therapy unnecessary

Poison Ivy Contact Dermatitis

- Burow's compress 1:20 tid × 15 min
- Potent steroid cream (e.g., Betnovate 0.1% cream tid)
- Use prednisone if extensive (start at 1 mg/kg/day PO and taper over 2-3 wk period)

Diaper Dermatitis

Clinical Features and Differential Diagnosis

- Irritant dermatitis: due to urine, feces, and maceration. Creases may be spared. If severe, may be erosive. More common with cloth diapers that are washed at home
- Seborrheic dermatitis: greasy, scaly, and erythematous. Areas of involvement: cradle cap, ears, axillae, and groin. If seborrheic dermatitis fails to respond to treatment, consider the possibility of histiocytosis X.
- *Candida:* erythematous, satellite pustules or red papules with scaly border. May have associated oral thrush. Creases are involved.

Management

- Use diaper service or disposable diapers; change diaper frequently and expose buttocks to air
- Burow's 1:20 compresses for 10-15 min tid if macerated
- 1% hydrocortisone ointment for contact dermatitis, seborrheic dermatitis
- If *Candida,* 1% hydrocortisone in Canesten cream is best choice
- Apply barrier ointment (zinc oxide)

Erythema Multiforme

Etiology
- Infection: herpes simplex, mycoplasma
- Drugs: sulfa, phenytoin, and phenobarbital are most commonly implicated
- Idiopathic

Management
- Treat underlying cause
- In recurrent erythema multiforme minor with herpes, can often abort episode by use of acyclovir or prednisone for 2 wk
- Stevens-Johnson syndrome: generally treated as burn; ophthalmology consult mandatory; prednisone use controversial and generally not indicated

Hemangiomas

- Capillary (strawberry) hemangioma
  1. Immature capillaries—may be present at birth—usually appear within first 2 wk; increase in size for several months; usually start to involute by end of second year; 90% regress by age 9 yr
- Cavernous hemangioma
  1. Deeper and larger vessels than capillary type; may be present at birth
  2. Regress by age 9 yr—may leave redundant skin
- Nevus flammeus
  1. Dilated mature vessels; present at birth; grow with patient

Complications and Associated Syndromes
- May enlarge very quickly (bleeding into hemangioma)
- May develop Kasabach-Merritt syndrome (platelet sequestration by large hemangioma)

- May be in injury-prone location
- May affect important organs, especially eyes (amblyopia, glaucoma, strabismus)
- Klippel-Trenaunay syndrome: port wine stain with underlying soft tissue or bone hypertrophy of limb
- Neonatal hemangiomatosis: multiple cutaneous and visceral hemangiomas, which may lead to cardiac failure and GI hemorrhage
- Sturge-Weber syndrome: port wine stain in distribution of cranial nerve V_1 ($\pm V_2$, V_3)

Management of Capillary and Cavernous Hemangiomas

- Generally, no treatment is necessary
- Prednisone, 1-3 mg/kg/day (may require several months of treatment with careful follow-up) if:
  1. Enlarges very quickly
  2. Affects vital structures, respiratory tract, eye
  3. Kasabach-Merritt syndrome
- Cosmetic treatment: pulsed dye laser; makeup
- Embolization

Lice

- Pediculosis capitis (head louse): Adult louse is 3-4 mm long, the eggs (nits) are 1 mm, usually white, and firmly adherent to the hair shafts; usually <ten adults on an individual; postauricular and occipital regions are the most common sites.
- Pediculosis pubis (crab louse): Smaller than head and body louse; found on eyelashes and pubic hair; transmitted by sexual contact or, rarely, by shared clothing and bed linen

Management of Pediculosis Capitis and Pediculosis Pubis

- Gamma benzene hexachloride 1% (Kwellada) shampoo to affected hair-bearing site; lather for 10 min and rinse; repeat in 7 days

Dermatology

- Eyelash involvement with pediculosis pubis; apply petrolatum to eyelashes bid or tid for 10 days
- Nits can be removed with vinegar soaks (5% acetic acid) and a fine-toothed comb
- Soak combs, brushes, barrettes in Kwellada shampoo for 10 min
- Clothing and bed linen should be washed in hot water or dry cleaned; pillows and mattresses should be vacuumed
- For head lice, permethrin (Nix) can be used as follows: wash, rinse, and towel dry hair; apply Nix as cream rinse for 10 min, then rinse. *Nix is ovocidal; therefore, nits do not have to be combed out;* contraindicated in individuals with allergy to chrysanthemums.

Molluscum Contagiosum

- Occurs anywhere in children; mostly axillae and genital area
- Contagious and autoinoculable
- Usually asymptomatic; some develop a surrounding pruritic dermatitis
- Lesions last from a few weeks to 2 yr

Management

- Children: topical cantharidin (0.7%) applied by the physician to lesions (avoid surrounding skin); *warn patients to expect blistering*
- Older children: can use cantharidin (0.7%), or curettage
- Repeat treatment as new crops of lesions arise

Pityriasis Rosea

- Lasts 6-8 wk and resolves spontaneously
- If pruritic, use oilated baths and topical steroids

Scabies

- Incubation period: 3-6 wk; primary lesion is a burrow 2-10 mm in length, with the female mite at the end
- Sites of predilection: finger webs, axillae, genitalia, periumbilical area; palms, soles, nape of neck, and axillae in infants; face usually not involved except in infants and Norwegian (extensive) scabies
- Nodular lesions common in axillae and groin

Management

- Under age 2 yr: 10% precipitated sulfur in white petrolatum bid to entire body for 24 hours, × 2 consecutive days; repeat 1 week later
- Over age 2 yr: Kwellada (gamma benzene hexachloride) cream—apply from neck down, wash off after 8 hr (overnight ideal); repeat next day and 1 wk later
- Wash all bed and personal clothing used recently
- Advise that pruritus and rash may persist for several weeks after mite eradicated
- Nodular lesions may persist for months after active infection is controlled (topical steroids may be beneficial)
- Treat all household contacts as above, whether itchy or not

Seborrheic Dermatitis

- Scalp: daily tar shampoo; 1% hydrocortisone lotion or cream tid
- Body: 1% hydrocortisone cream tid

Staphylococcal Scalded Skin Syndrome (SSSS)

- Cloxacillin for 7-10 days; may require admission to hospital and IV therapy
- Emollients when dry

Tinea Capitis

- Most frequent organisms: anthropophilic *(Microsporum audouinii, Trichophyton tonsurans)* and zoophilic *(Microsporum canis)*
- Nonscarring alopecia with associated scale
- "Black dot alopecia" (hairs very short because they break at scalp level)
- Kerion (allergic inflammation) often causes scarring

Management
- Wood's lamp fluorescence of hair (green) if *M. audouinii* or *M. canis* (dandruff appears white), N.B.: *T. tonsurans* does not fluoresce.
- Potassium hydroxide (KOH) prep of scale and hair (see p 578)
- Fungal culture
- Griseofulvin for 3 mo

Urticaria

- Serious acute associated features are pharyngolaryngeal edema and anaphylaxis
- History and physical examination to eliminate obvious causes
- Symptomatic treatment: oral antihistamines
- If chronic, consider CBC, differential, ESR, urinalysis, stool for ova and parasites

Verrucae

- Common wart (verruca vulgaris)
  1. Apply 75% salicylic acid in petrolatum, cover with adhesive bandage and leave on for 1 wk; then debride in office
  2. Repeat until all warty tissue is removed
  3. Liquid nitrogen (if child over 5 yr old) weekly until tissue scabs and heals

- Plantar wart (verruca plantaris)
  1. Single warts: treat as above
  2. Multiple warts (mosaic): soak feet in 10% glutaraldehyde solution 15 min daily; then apply Soluver (20% salicylic acid in acrylic vehicle) to warts bid and cover with adhesive bandage
- Condyloma acuminata
  1. Apply (in office only) 25% podophyllin and leave on 6 hr (avoid contact with normal surrounding skin)
  2. Patient washes it off at home with soap and water
  3. Repeat weekly
  4. In children, suspect sexual abuse

Topical Steroids

- Use a lotion on the scalp (e.g., Betnovate 0.1%)
- Ointments are used more in the winter (to prevent drying) and on dry lesions
- Creams are used more during the summer and on moist lesions
- Use creams in flexural areas
- Avoid using fluorinated steroids on face and in flexural areas
- Rule of thumb: 30 g (1 oz) of medication will cover an entire adult body once
- Side effects of prolonged topical steroid use include local atrophy, striae, purpura, telangiectasia, hypertrichosis

TABLE 5-1 Examples of Topical Steroids

Potency	Brand Name	Generic Name
Nonfluorinated, lowest potency		Hydrocortisone (1%)
Nonfluorinated, low potency	Tridesilon Westcort	Desonide (0.05%) Hydrocortisone valerate (0.2%)
Intermediate potency	Betnovate (0.05%; 0.1%) Valisone scalp lotion Synalar (0.025%)	Betamethasone valerate (0.05%; 0.1%) Betamethasone valerate (0.1%) Fluocinolone acetonide (0.025%)

Emollients

- Use after bath and PRN for dry skin
- Some examples include 10% urea in hydrous eucerin (may sting) and proprietary preparations such as Complex 15 cream, Nutraplus, Lachydrin
- Vaseline and Nivea are inexpensive, safe, and effective
- 10% glycerine in Glaxal base

SIX

Endocrinology

Diabetes Mellitus

NEWLY DIAGNOSED DIABETES

- Diagnosis: random blood glucose >11 mmol/L

Management

Insulin:
- 0.1-0.25 U/kg subcutaneous Regular (crystalline) insulin for symptomatic relief on day of diagnosis
- Next day, start *before breakfast* NPH/Lente insulin, ~1 unit per year of age; *before supper* give second dose of insulin, usually ¼ to ⅓ of morning dose initially entirely as NPH/Lente
- Monitor blood glucose level before meals, before bed, and at specific additional times as indicated during periods of adjustment
- Adjust insulin daily to achieve target blood glucose level of 4-10 mmol/L
    1. Adjust insulin in 10-20% increments
    2. Add Regular insulin as required
- Most new patients are hospitalized for stabilization, family education, diet management
- Anticipate a decrease in insulin requirements in first few weeks postdischarge with increased activity and honeymoon period
- Clear-cut mechanism for communication with diabetes team must be established

Diet:
- To start, 1000 kcal + 100 kcal/yr of age; individualize according to age, appetite, activity
- Composition
  1. 50-55% CH_2O (¾ complex CH_2O)
  2. 30-35% fat (polyunsaturated to saturated ratio, 1.2:1)
  3. 15-20% protein

DIABETIC KETOACIDOSIS

Diagnosis

- Vomiting, abdominal pain, rapid or Kussmaul respiration, altered level of consciousness
- Measure blood glucose, pH, pCO_2, HCO_3, electrolytes, BUN, urine ketones
- Calculate anion gap [Na− (Cl +HCO_3)] and serum osmolality (2 × Na + glucose + BUN)

Management

Monitoring:
- NPO in severe acidosis
- Careful hourly documentation of vital signs, level of consciousness, accurate intake and output
- Blood glucose q2h, biochemistry as above q4h

Fluids:
- Initially: 0.9% saline at 15-20 ml/kg/hr × 2 hr, then 10-15 ml/kg/hr until acidosis corrected
- Potassium: Add KCl (20-40 mmol/L of IV solution) after patient voids (or immediately if K^+ < 4 mmol/L)
- Glucose: Add to IV fluids when blood glucose <15 mmol/L, by changing IV solution to 5% dextrose in 0.2% saline or 3.33% dextrose in 0.3% saline

Insulin:
- Start insulin infusion immediately. Dose: 0.1 U/kg/hr (dilute 25 U Regular insulin in 250 ml saline as second IV line or in Y tubing)
- Decrease dose to 0.02 U/kg/hr when blood glucose <15 mmol/L

Bicarbonate:
- Generally given as $NaHCO_3$, monitor Na
- Usually given when plasma HCO_3 < 12 mmol/L and pH < 7.2
- Dose = (12 − [HCO_3] plasma) × weight (kg) × 0.6
- Give ½ IV over 10-20 min and infuse remainder over 2 hr

Complications:
- Hypoglycemia
- Hypokalemia
- Persistent acidosis
- Cerebral edema

MANAGEMENT OF INTERCURRENT ILLNESS
(Table 6-1)

- Measure blood glucose and urine ketones immediately and q4h around the clock
- If child unable to eat, offer sugar-containing fluids such as regular soda pop or juice
- Antipyretic as indicated
- Should vomiting develop twice in a 4-6 hr period, the child should be assessed in the emergency department. If the child has been vomiting clear fluids and is nauseated, keep NPO and establish IV to provide maintenance fluids and glucose.

TABLE 6-1 Guidelines for Insulin Adjustment During Intercurrent Illness

Sickness Profile	A	B	C	D	E
Blood glucose in mmol/L	≥4.4 and <13.3	≥13.3 and <22.2	≥22.2	≥13.3	<4.4
Urine ketones	Neg. or pos.	Neg.	Neg.	Pos.	Neg. or pos.
Action	Wait; continue to monitor carefully	Wait; if the condition persists, increase insulin next day by 10-20%/day until aims are achieved	Give extra regular insulin q4h, equal to ~20% of total daily dose until urine ketones clear and/or blood sugar <13.3 mmol/L; then proceed as for regimen in columns A and B		Decrease daily insulin by 20%/day until blood glucose is between 4.4 and 13.3 mmol/L

HYPOGLYCEMIA IN DIABETES MELLITUS

- Early warning symptoms: tremors, diaphoresis, palpitations, hunger, pallor, dizziness, blurred vision
- Neuroglycopenia: confusion, coma, seizures
- All patients should have clear instructions regarding management of hypoglycemia, including use of glucagon

Treatment

Mild:
- Concentrated carbohydrate (juice, glucose tablets)
- If repeated, may need diet or insulin adjustment

Severe:
- Hospitalize if altered level of consciousness
- Treat initially at home with glucagon, 1 mg SC for age >5 yr, 0.5 mg SC for age <5 yr
- At hospital: if altered level of consciousness or history of seizure, give glucose, 0.5 g/kg (= 1 ml/kg 50% dextrose, 2ml/kg 25% dextrose)
- Continue dextrose solution (5% dextrose, 10% dextrose) for several hours
- Adjust diet and insulin; counsel regarding prevention methods

Management During Surgery

- May need several days in hospital to correct blood glucose level if in poor control. If in good control, admit day *prior* to surgery.

Minor procedures (<1 hr)
- Patients will be able to take fluids shortly after procedure
- IV 3.33% dextrose and 0.3% saline or 5% dextrose in 0.2% saline plus KCl at *maintenance* rates (start at 7:30 AM)
- *Insulin* ⅔ daily dose given as intermediate-acting insulin only (NPH/Lente) SC
- Blood glucose preoperatively and immediately postoperatively; monitor as necessary
- Regular insulin given postoperatively as necessary to maintain blood glucose at 5-15 mmol/L
- Usual dose of insulin is resumed when child is able to take a normal diet

Major procedures (>1 hr)
- Patient unlikely to drink shortly after procedure
- No SC insulin on day of surgery
- NPO postoperatively
- IV as above
- Insulin infusion, 0.02 U Regular insulin/kg/hr
- Adjust insulin infusion to maintain blood glucose at 5-15 mmol/L
- Monitor *blood glucose* hourly intraoperatively, q4h postoperatively, *urine ketones* bid
- When tolerating fluids PO (usually next day):
  1. Discontinue insulin infusion
  2. Start SC insulin (⅔ usual dose and increase as indicated, may use short- and long-acting; or long-acting alone, depending on intake)
- For emergency procedures, surgery should be delayed, if possible, until acidosis and dehydration are corrected

Hypoglycemia

- Ketotic hypoglycemia is the commonest cause of hypoglycemia in children aged 1-4 yr
- Critical blood sample for diagnosis: glucose, blood gas, electrolytes, insulin, growth hormone, lactate, ketones, cortisol, β-hydroxybutyrate
- Treat with glucose 0.5 g/kg (1 ml/kg 50% dextrose, 2 ml/kg 25% dextrose) IV bolus, plus continuous glucose infusion to maintain glucose level in normal range
- More detailed investigation may require admission for monitored starvation challenge
- Neonates: see p 321

TABLE 6-2 Major Differential Diagnoses of Hypoglycemia

	Hyperinsulinism	Substrate Deficiency	Ketotic Hypoglycemia (including GH & Cortisol Deficiency)
Glucose	Low	Low	Low
Insulin	High	Low	Low
Lactic acid	Normal to low	High	Normal
3-hydroxybutyric acid	Low	High	Very high

From Aynsley-Green A. Hypoglycemia in infancy and childhood. Clin Endocrinol Metab 1982; 11:159.

Hypocalcemia

Definition
- Term infant: Ca < 1.9 mmol/L
- Preterm infant: Ca < 1.75 mmol/L
- Older children: Ca < 2 mmol/L
- If hypoalbuminemia present, measured Ca may be falsely low:

    Adjusted Ca (mmol/L) = Ca (mmol/L) $- \frac{\text{albumin (g/L)}}{40} + 1$

- Measure ionized Ca if serum protein or pH is abnormal

Management
- Most mild hypocalcemia can be managed without IV calcium infusion
- If IV calcium infusion is required (Ca gluconate or Ca chloride), administer as diluted solution, e.g., 10% Ca gluconate diluted to 2% solution. For serious hypocalcemia (convulsions and arrythmias), give Ca, 0.1 mmol/kg/hr. For less severe cases (muscle cramps, paresthesiae) give Ca, 0.05 mmol/kg/hr.
- 10 ml of 10% Ca gluconate contains 90 mg of elemental Ca (2.25 mmol). Add 10 ml of 10% Ca gluconate to 40 ml of saline to obtain 2% solution. This dilution contains Ca, 0.04 mmol/ml.
- Adjust infusion rate q4h based on plasma Ca level. Aim for >2 mmol/L. Reduce infusion rate slowly once desired level reached.
- All patients receiving IV calcium should be on cardiac monitor
- Monitor IV site: high risk of extravasation burns and venous thrombosis
- Addition of 0.1 ml of heparin, 1000 U/ml, to each 100 ml of Ca gluconate reduces risk of thrombosis
- Do not administer calcium and $NaHCO_3$ in same IV tubing
- Never give Ca IM or SC

TABLE 6-3 Plasma Chemistry Findings in Conditions Associated with Hypocalcemia

	PO$_4$	ALP	PTH	25-(OH)vit D	1,25-(OH)$_2$vit D
Hypoparathyroidism	↑	↓ or N*	↓	N	↓
Pseudohypoparathyroidism					
Type 1	↑	N	↑ or N	N	↓
Type 2	↑	N	↑ or N	N	
Neonatal hypocalcemia	↑	N	Variable	N	
Hypomagnesemia	N or ↑	N	↓	N	
Vitamin D deficiency and malabsorption syndromes	↓	↑	↑	↓	N or ↓
Renal failure	↑	↑ or N	↑	N	N or ↓
Hereditary vitamin-D–dependency rickets					
Type 1	↓	↑	↑	N	↓
Type 2	↓	↑	↑	N	↑

*N = normal range.
From Fraser D, et al. Calcium and phosphate metabolism. In Tietz NW, editor: Fundamentals of clinical chemistry. 3rd ed. WB Saunders Co., Philadelphia, 1987:1329.

- Maintain oral Ca intake of 100 mg/kg/day; use supplement if needed, e.g., calcium lactate
- Consider starting vitamin D metabolites: 1,25 (OH)$_2$ vitamin D$_3$ or 1α(OH) vitamin D$_3$ if prolonged use of IV calcium is anticipated

Hypercalcemia

Definition

- Ca > 2.8 mmol/L

Management

- Low Ca, high fluid diet for all patients
- For emergency treatment give IV fluids to increase extracellular fluid volume (0.9% saline 2.5 × maintenance) ± furosemide ± steroids
- May require calcitonin in refractory cases
- Oral phosphate may be used if serum phosphate concentration is low

Ambiguous Genitalia (Table 6-4)

Investigations

- Serum 17-hydroxyprogesterone (after day 3)
- Chromosomes (sex chromatin NOT reliable)
- Testosterone, FSH, LH
- Abdominal and pelvic ultrasound
- May need cystogram

TABLE 6-4 Diagnostic Classification of Ambiguous Genitalia

Female pseudohermaphrodite (virilized female—46 XX)
  Congenital adrenal hyperplasia
  Maternal androgen ingestion
  Iatrogenic fetal virilization
  With associated congenital malformations (e.g., Seckel, Zellweger)

Male pseudohermaphrodite (testes present—46 XY)
  Impaired Leydig cell activity
    Inborn errors of testosterone biosynthesis
    Leydig cell hypoplasia
  Impaired peripheral metabolism of androgens
    5-α-reductase deficiency
    Androgen insensitivity (complete or incomplete)
  Other forms
    With associated congenital anomalies (e.g., Smith-Lemli-Opitz, Meckel)
    Iatrogenic male pseudohermaphroditism
    Persistent Mullerian structures

Abnormal gonadal differentiation
  Mixed gonadal dysgenesis (e.g., 46XY/45X mosaic)
  "Agonadism" and "micropenis with rudimentary testes"
  Dysmorphic syndromes associated with hypogonadism
  True hermaphroditism
  XX males

Modified from Savage MO. Ambiguous genitalia, small genitalia, and undescended testes. Clin Endocrinol Metab. 11:127-158, 1982.

Adrenal Insufficiency

- Major cause in neonatal period is congenital adrenal hyperplasia
- Addison's disease is rare; iatrogenic adrenal suppression may occur in children taking pharmacologic doses of adrenal steroids
- Children with diseases of the hypothalamic-pituitary axis (e.g., craniopharyngioma) are also at risk for adrenal insufficiency during an intercurrent illness
- Clinical: shock with dehydration, decreased Na, increased K, ± decreased glucose

Investigations

- Measure plasma cortisol, renin, aldosterone, electrolytes *before treatment*
- If newborn (especially with ambiguous genitalia), 17-hydroxyprogesterone most important investigation (done after 3 days of age)
- May need abdominal ultrasound, head CT, ACTH studies

Management

- Glucose for hypoglycemia; hyponatremia can be corrected with IV saline, but needs mineralocorticoid for maintenance in salt-losing states. Dose: 9-α-fluorohydrocortisone, 0.05-0.2 mg/day
- Solucortef 100 mg/m^2 stat and q4h IV

Antidiuretic Hormone

DEFICIENCY (DIABETES INSIPIDUS)

- Presence of urine SG $\leq$ 1.005, hypernatremia, increased serum osmolality
- Do water deprivation test to differentiate central diabetes insipidus from nephrogenic diabetes insipidus and psychogenic polydipsia

- Treat underlying cause; give DDAVP, 0.05-0.1 ml intranasally q12-24h for symptomatic control (monitor by urine output, specific gravity, thirst). Allow free access to water.

EXCESS (SIADH)

- Generally caused by CNS disorder (infection, trauma, tumor), but also caused by drugs (vincristine, vancomycin) and respiratory and paralytic diseases
- Hallmark is hyponatremia, with decreased serum osmolality in the face of urine SG $\geq$ 1.005; urine Na > 20 mmol/L; urine osmolality > plasma osmolality, i.e., urine Na and osmolality higher than expected for serum levels.
- Treatment: fluid restriction (50-60% maintenance) *or* insensible water losses (400 ml/m^2/day) + ½ to ¾ urine output. Rarely requires 3% NaCl + diuresis (furosemide) for symptomatic hyponatremia.

Short Stature

- After the age of 2.5 yr, growth rate should be $\geq$ 4 cm/yr
- Growth velocity should be calculated at intervals of not $\leq$6 mo
- Constitutional short stature in males is common
- Chromosomal analysis should be performed in any girl measuring less than the 3rd centile in height to exclude absence of an X chromosome (1:3000 live births) or mosaic forms of Turner's syndrome
- A disproportionate failure in weight gain should direct investigations to the gastrointestinal tract, "occult" anorexia nervosa, or to the possibility of parental deprivation
- The more retarded the bone age (accurately determined), the greater the likelihood of organic disease, particularly long-standing hypothyroidism, and the greater the potential for "catch up"
- Hormonal causes of short stature are relatively uncommon (<15% of cases) with the exception of acquired thyroiditis

Endocrinology

- Cortisol administration in excess of hydrocortisone, 25 mg/m^2 body surface area per day (prednisone, 5 mg/m^2/day) will retard normal somatic growth (a 10-yr-old child is approximately 1 m^2 in body size)
- A rough estimate of the final height of a normal child can be made by calculating the mid-parental height (MPH):

MPH
$$\text{for boys} = \frac{\text{father's Ht (cm)} + \text{mother's Ht (cm)} + 13 \text{ cm}}{2}$$

MPH
$$\text{for girls} = \frac{\text{father's Ht (cm)} - 13 \text{ cm} + \text{mother's Ht (cm)}}{2}$$

Note: 13 cm is the inherent mean difference in final height between men and women

Investigations

- Complete blood count and sedimentation rate
- Thyroid function tests: serum T4, TSH, T3 uptake
- BUN, creatinine
- Karyotype in girls or in any child with dysmorphic physical features
- Urinalysis (pH, protein, blood, glucose, WBC, RBC)
- Radiologic investigations: bone age; skull radiographs if CNS disorder is suspected

TABLE 6-5 Average Growth Rates During Early Childhood

Age	Growth Rate (cm/yr)
1-6 mo	18-22
6-12 mo	15-18
12 mo	11-12
2 yr	8.5
4-9 yr	5-6

Thyroid Disease (Fig. 6-1)

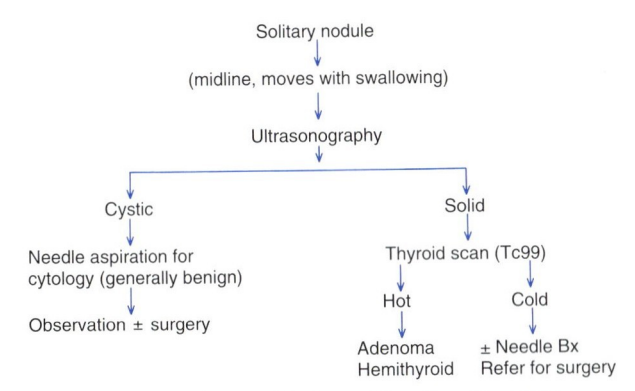

```
                        Solitary nodule
                              ↓
                (midline, moves with swallowing)
                              ↓
                       Ultrasonography
                              ↓
              ┌───────────────┴───────────────┐
              ↓                               ↓
            Cystic                          Solid
              ↓                               ↓
    Needle aspiration for            Thyroid scan (Tc99)
    cytology (generally benign)              ↓
              ↓                    ┌─────────┴─────────┐
    Observation ± surgery          ↓                   ↓
                                  Hot                 Cold
                                   ↓                   ↓
                                Adenoma         ± Needle Bx
                               Hemithyroid      Refer for surgery
```

Figure 6-1 **Approach to the solitary thyroid nodule.**

SEVEN

Fluids and Electrolytes

Conversions

- Millimole (mmol) to mg = number of mmol × molecular weight: e.g., 1 mmol NaCl = 23 + 35.5 = 58.5 mg; 2 mmol Ca = 2 × 40 mg = 80 mg
- Mmol to milliequivalent (mEq) = number of mmol × valence: e.g., 1 mmol Na^+ = 1 mEq; 1 mmol Ca^{2+} = 2 mEq
- Milliosmoles (mOsm) = mmol × number of particles produced by dissociation: e.g., 1 mmol $CaCl_2$ = 3 mOsm
- Osmolality (mOsm/kg) = number of mOsm/kg solvent: e.g., plasma osmolality is 275-295 mOsm/kg
- To calculate estimated serum osmolality: 2 × Na (mmol/L) + glucose (mmol/L) + urea (mmol/L)

Maintenance Fluid and Electrolyte Requirements (per 24 hr) (Table 7-1)

- Water: body weight
  1. 0-10 kg = 100 ml/kg
  2. 11-20 kg = 1000 ml + 50 ml/kg
  3. 21-70 kg = 1500 ml + 20 ml/kg *or* 1500 ml/m², see pp 640, 641
- Sodium: 2-3 mmol/kg
- Potassium: 2-3 mmol/kg
- Suggested maintenance solutions: 5% dextrose and 0.2% saline with 20 mmol/L of KC1, or 3.33% dextrose and 0.33% saline (⅔ : ⅓) with 20 mmol/L KCl
- These values assume normal renal function and average losses and need to be modified for certain disease states. For neonatal requirements, see p 315
- Fever: add 12% to total maintenance requirements per 1°C rise

TABLE 7-1 **Average Normal Values for Various Body Compartments (L/kg)**

	Newborn	Child	Adult Male	Adult Female
TBW*	0.75	0.65	0.60	0.55
ICF*	0.40	0.40	0.40	0.40
ECF*	0.35	0.25	0.20	0.15
Blood volume	0.07-0.09	0.07-0.08	0.07-0.08	0.07-0.08

*TBW = total body water; ICF = intracellular fluid; ECF = extracellular fluid.

Dehydration

- Most common cause in childhood is gastroenteritis

Investigations

- Serum electrolytes, venous gas, glucose (high in hypernatremia), calcium (low in hypernatremia, alkalemia, and hyperphosphatemia), BUN, creatinine, CBC
- Determine type of dehydration, based on serum Na level and calculated osmolality:
  1. Isotonic: [Na] = 130-150 mmol/L; osmolality = 280-300 mOsm/kg
  2. Hypertonic: [Na] > 150 mmol/L; osmolality > 300 mOsm/kg
  3. Hypotonic: [Na] < 130 mmol/L; osmolality < 280 mOsm/kg
- Determine acid-base status: acidosis (diabetic ketoacidosis, diarrhea) or alkalosis (pyloric stenosis).

TABLE 7-2 Composition of Some Common Parenteral Solutions (mmol or mEq/L)

Solution	Na$^+$	K$^+$	Cl$^-$	HCO$_3^-$*	Comments
Isotonic (0.9%) NaCl (**normal saline**)	154		154		
Hypertonic (3%) NaCl	513		513		
3.33% Dextrose and 0.33% NaCl ("2/3 : 1/3")	52		52		Contains 33.3g/L dextrose; useful maintenance fluid and replacement fluid for Na$^+$
5% Dextrose + 0.2% NaCl (**D^5 : 0.2 normal saline**)	34		34		Contains 50 g/L dextrose; useful Na$^+$ maintenance fluid
8.4% NaHCO$_3$ (**1 mmol[mEq]/ml**)	1000			1000	1 mmol of Na$^+$ and bicarbonate/ml
Lactated Ringer's	130	4	109	28	Ca^{2+} 3 mg/dl
0.5 normal saline (**0.45%**)	77		77		
5% Dextrose (**D$_5$W**)					50 g/L dextrose

*Bicarbonate or potential bicarbonate.

TABLE 7-3 **Approximate Electrolyte Composition of Gastrointestinal Fluids**

			mmol(mEq)/L		
Fluid	H^+	Na^+	K^+	Cl^-	HCO_3^-
Gastric	80	40 (20-80)	20 (5-20)	150 (100-150)	0
Small intestinal	0	130 (100-140)	20 (5-25)	120 (100-130)	30
Pancreatic	0	135 (120-140)	15 (5-15)	100 (90-120)	50
Diarrheal	0	40	40	40	40

TABLE 7-4 Clinical Features of Dehydration*

Severity	Age <1 Yr % Water Deficit†	Age <1 Yr Water Deficit†	Age >1 Yr % Water Deficit	Age >1 Yr Water Deficit	Clinical Signs
Minimal	<5		<3		Thirst, mild oliguria
Mild	5	50 ml/kg	3	30 ml/kg	Dry mucous membranes, axilla, groin
Moderate	10	100 ml/kg	6	60 ml/kg	Loss of skin turgor, severe thirst, sunken eyeballs and fontanelle
Severe	15	150 ml/kg	9	90 ml/kg	Low BP, poor circulation, CNS changes, fever

*In hypernatremic dehydration, neurologic features predominate early, whereas ECF volume is preserved.
†Refers to deficit requiring replacement.

Treatment

- Restore circulating volume
  1. Normal saline or Ringer's lactate* 20-40 ml/kg IV over 20-40 min
  2. Plasma, blood (if anemic) or 5% albumin 10-20 ml/kg over 1 hr
- If circulating volume is still inadequate after 40 ml/kg, consider CVP monitoring
- Calculate fluid and electrolyte requirements: *maintenance, deficit and ongoing losses* (Table 7-5)
- Subtract the resuscitation fluid volume from the calculated 24-hour fluid requirement
- Correct metabolic acidosis with $NaHCO_3$ if pH ≤7.1 or HCO_3^- <12 mEq/L. Rehydration alone may correct acidosis if pH >7.1.
- First 8 hr (repletion phase—replacement of extracellular deficits): give maintenance fluids plus 50% of calculated deficit plus replace ongoing losses. Correct sodium deficit in hyponatremia (see below)
- Next 16 hr (recovery phase—replacement of intracellular deficits): continue maintenance fluids and replacement of ongoing losses and replace the remaining 50% of the calculated deficit
- Potassium replacement should begin as soon as the patient voids, unless renal disease present
- Monitor fluid, electrolyte, and acid-base status frequently, especially in hypernatremia

---

*Metabolism of Ringer's lactate is limited in patient with hypovolemic shock.

TABLE 7-5 Practical Approach to Correction of Fluid and Electrolyte Deficits

Type	Electrolyte	Deficit* 5%	Deficit* 10%
Isotonic	Na	4-5 mmol/kg	8-10 mmol/kg
	K	2-3 mmol/kg	4-5 mmol/kg
	Suggested Solution†: 3.33% dextrose and 0.33% saline with 20 mmol KCl/L		
Hypotonic	Na	5-6 mmol/kg	10-12 mmol/kg
	K	3 mmol/kg	5 mmol/kg
	Suggested Solution†: 5% dextrose and 0.45% saline with 20 mmol KCl/L		
Hypertonic	Na	2-4 mmol/kg	2-4 mmol/kg
	K	2-4 mmol/kg	2-4 mmol/kg
	Suggested solution†: 5% dextrose and 0.2% saline with 40 mmol KCl/L, BUT usually start with 5% dextrose and 0.45% saline with 40 mmol/l KCl (once urine output established) and adjust based on serum sodium.		

*Fluid deficit in 5% dehydration = 50 ml/kg; 10% dehydration = 100 ml/kg.
†Suggested solutions most closely approximate ideal solution to correct both fluid and electrolyte deficits.

SPECIFIC APPROACH TO CORRECTION OF FLUID AND ELECTROLYTE DEFICIT (see Table 7-5)

Hypotonic Dehydration

- In addition to correction of volume deficit, correct hyponatremia to an isotonic state using Table 7-5 (estimate), or calculate exact deficit:
  1. [Na^+] (deficit = ([Na^+] desired $-$ [Na^+] actual) × body wt (kg) × total body water (L/kg)
  2. [Na] ≥105 mmol/L: correct to 125-130 mmol/L as "desired Na^+"
  3. [Na] <105 mmol/L: correct by 20 mmol/L maximum
- When deficit known, correct by ~50% over first 8 hr and remainder over next 16 hr. Knowing Na^+ deficit and fluid deficit, select appropriate Na^+-containing fluid (generally, 5% dextrose and 0.45% saline with 20 mmol KCl/L
- Rate of use of Na should not exceed 2-5 mmol/L/hr
- For symptomatic hyponatremia (seizures), correct serum sodium to 125 mmol/L over 0.5-4 hr, i.e., (125 $-$ measured [Na^+] × body wt × total body water to calculate deficit. Use hypertonic saline 3-5% (3% = 0.5 mmol/ml, 5% = 0.855 mmol/ml) (Fig. 7-1)

Hyponatremia
Assess Circulating Volume

Decreased

Urine [Na$^+$] <20 mEq/liter(mmol/L)
- Gastrointestinal losses
- Burns
- Diuretics (late)

Correction of shock
Saline replacement
Specific replacement therapy

Urine [Na$^+$] >20 mEq/liter(mmol/L)
- Diuretics (early)
- Adrenal insufficiency
- Salt wasting renal disease

Normal or Increased

Urine [Na$^+$] <20 mEq/liter(mmol/L)
- Nephrotic syndrome
- Cirrhosis
- Cardiac failure

Urine [Na$^+$] >20 mEq/liter(mmol/L)
- SIADH
- Renal failure
- Polydipsia

Water restriction
Specific therapy

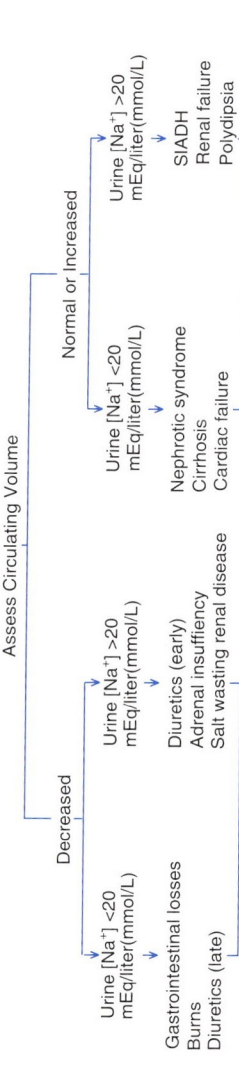

Figure 7-1 **Differential diagnosis of hyponatremia and approach to therapy.** (From Perkin RM, Lewin DL. Common fluid and electrolyte problems in the pediatric intensive care unit. Pediatr Clin North Am 1980; 27:573.)

Hypertonic Dehydration

- Doughy or velvety skin and CNS disturbances, especially irritability. Minimal signs of intravascular volume depletion. Occurs with high fever, boiled milk feeds, diabetes insipidus, or in infants or handicapped children who have no access to free water.
- Avoid rapid rehydration because of risk of cerebral edema and seizures (correct fluid deficit over 48 hr)
- Restore circulating volume and urinary output as a priority
- Use 75% of calculated value for maintenance fluids because of the risk of SIADH
- Lower serum sodium by 10-15 mmol/L/day maximum
- Calculate water deficit to be replaced in such a way as to lower serum sodium by a predictable amount:

$$H_2O = [(Na^+ \text{ actual} - Na^+ \text{ desired})/Na^+ \text{ desired}] \times \text{total body water (L/kg)}$$

- Fluids for 24 hr = 75% maintenance + water deficit + ongoing losses
- *Rule of thumb:* 4 ml/kg of free water lowers the serum sodium by 1 mmol/L
- Avoid use of insulin for hyperglycemia as this rapidly lowers the extracellular osmolality and may cause cerebral edema
- For jitteriness: monitor rate of fall of $[Na^+]$, check $[Ca^{+2}]$, monitor CNS status (e.g., subdural)
- Treat water intoxication with 3% NaCl 3-5 ml/kg over 30 min-1 hr

Salt Poisoning

- Serum [Na$^+$] >200 mmol/L may occur, with increase in total body load of sodium
- Treat with maintenance fluids. If [Na] >180 or renal function poor, peritoneal dialysis using 7-8% glucose electrolyte-free solution.
- Furosemide 1 mg/kg, while replacing urine output with 10% dextrose, can be used when renal function is good and electrolytes are properly monitored

Pseudohyponatremia

- Associated with hyperlipidemia (depending on measurement technique) or hyperglycemia
- [Na$^+$] decreases by 1.6 mmol/L for each rise in glucose of 5.5 mmol/L (i.e., a decrease in Na$^+$ is normal with hyperglycemia)

Hypokalemia

- Serum [K$^+$] < 3.0 mmol/L
- Causes include poor intake (e.g., TPN) or excess losses (vomiting, diarrhea, NG suction, diuretics, and renal tubular acidosis)
- Clinical features include weakness, hyporeflexia, paresthesias, ileus, polyuria, polydipsia, dysrhythmias, low amplitude T waves, S-T depression, and "U" waves
- Investigations should include ECG, electrolytes, urinalysis, and urine electrolytes
- Cardiac monitor if [K$^+$] < 3.0 or patient receiving digoxin
- Ensure intake of maintenance potassium; replace ongoing losses (e.g., prophylactic supplementation for patients receiving diuretic therapy)

- Replace potassium deficits (difficult to estimate, as potassium is an intracellular ion)
- Maximum potassium concentration in peripheral IVs = 40 mmol/L. For concentrations of 60-80 mmol/L or greater, use a CVL and ECG monitoring. Maximum rate = 0.5 mmol/kg/hr.

Hyperkalemia

- See p 348

Acid-Base Disorders

- Normal pH = 7.38-7.42
- Vital organ dysfunction occurs at pH < 7.1 or > 7.6
- Measure serum pH, pCO_2, HCO_3^- and electrolytes
- Calculate unmeasured anion gap: $Na^+ - (Cl^- + HCO_3^-)$. Normal value = 12 ± 4.

METABOLIC ACIDOSIS (Fig. 7-2)

- Treat if pH <7.2 or [HCO_3^-] <12 mmol/L
- Calculate the bicarbonate deficit:
  1. (desired HCO_3^- − actual HCO_3^-) × body wt (kg) × 0.6
  2. For desired [HCO_3^-] use 18-24 mmol/L depending on age
- Give HALF the calculated bicarbonate deficit over 2-4 hr then reassess (bolus with 1 mmol/kg bicarbonate IV over 15-30 min, then remainder over 1.5-3.5 hr)

TABLE 7-6 **Common Patterns of Blood Gas Abnormality**

Respiratory acidosis (acute): pH (↓), Pco_2 (↑), HCO_3^- (N) or slightly ↑

Respiratory acidosis (chronic): pH (↓ slightly), Pco_2 (↑), HCO_3^- (↑)

Respiratory alkalosis (acute): pH (↑), Pco_2 (↓), HCO_3^- (N) or slightly ↓

Respiratory alkalosis (chronic): pH (N or ↑), Pco_2 (↓), HCO_3^- (↓)

Metabolic acidosis: pH (↓), Pco_2 (↓), HCO_3^- (↓)

Metabolic alkalosis: pH (↑), Pco_2 (N or ↑), HCO_3^- (↑)

Rule of thumb:
1. For every 3 mm Hg ↑ in Pco_2 in chronic respiratory acidosis, bicarbonate will ↑ by ~1 mmol/L; i.e., 3:1 ratio.
2. For metabolic acidosis, every 1 mmol/L ↓ in bicarbonate [HCO_3] means Pco_2 will ↓ by 1 mm Hg; i.e., 1:1 ratio.

METABOLIC ACIDOSIS

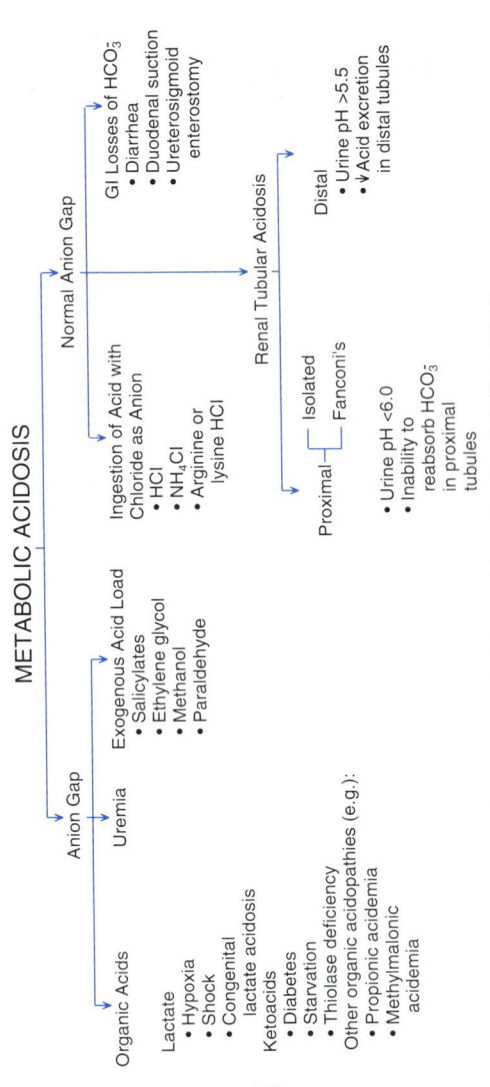

Anion Gap

- Organic Acids
  - Lactate
    - Hypoxia
    - Shock
    - Congenital lactate acidosis
  - Ketoacids
    - Diabetes
    - Starvation
    - Thiolase deficiency
  - Other organic acidopathies (e.g.):
    - Propionic acidemia
    - Methylmalonic acidemia
- Uremia
- Exogenous Acid Load
  - Salicylates
  - Ethylene glycol
  - Methanol
  - Paraldehyde

Normal Anion Gap

- Ingestion of Acid with Chloride as Anion
  - HCl
  - NH_4Cl
  - Arginine or lysine HCl
- Renal Tubular Acidosis
  - Proximal — Isolated / Fanconi's
    - Urine pH <6.0
    - Inability to reabsorb HCO_3^- in proximal tubules
  - Distal
    - Urine pH >5.5
    - ↓Acid excretion in distal tubules
- GI Losses of HCO_3^-
  - Diarrhea
  - Duodenal suction
  - Ureterosigmoid enterostomy

Figure 7-2 **Differential diagnosis of metabolic acidosis.**

Urinary Alkalinization

- Indications: prevention of uric acid stones (e.g., myeloproliferative disorders), dissolution of uric acid (desired pH 6.5-7.0) and cysteine stones (desired pH 7.5-9), enhancement of drug excretion (e.g., salicylate intoxication; desired pH 7.5)
- Keep urine pH >7.0 to enhance solubility but <8.0 to avoid precipitation of calcium salts. Monitor urinary pH q4-6h.
- Watch for systemic alkalosis
- Administer sodium bicarbonate 1-2 mmol/kg/day, via continuous infusion, or IV bolus q6h
- For chronic therapy, use potassium citrate (caution in renal failure) or sodium citrate 1-2 mmol/kg/day PO
- Maintain diuresis along with alkalinization
- N.B.: With salicylate intoxication, use of bicarbonate may be accompanied by severe alkalosis due to respiratory stimulation and resultant respiratory alkalosis. Therefore, acetazolamide may be used to alkalinize urine.

EIGHT

Gastroenterology

Diarrhea (Fig. 8-1)

ACUTE DIARRHEA

Investigations
- History and physical examination, assess degree of dehydration
- Rectal examination for stool consistency, fecal leukocytes (microscopy)
- Stool for bacterial cultures, virology (electron microscopy and cultures), ova and parasites. *Clostridium difficile* culture and toxin identification must be specifically requested.
- Blood tests (if severe): CBC, differential, electrolytes, BUN, creatinine, ± blood culture, urine culture, *Yersinia* titre

Management
- Antibiotic therapy for specific organisms and systemic infection when present
- Oral rehydration therapy (small frequent volumes if vomiting); Pedialyte approximates fecal losses in most common infections (Table 8-1)
- IV required for moderate to severe dehydration; must replace deficit as well as provide for ongoing losses (see p 88)

- *Early refeeding advisable*
  1. Continue breast feeding when possible
  2. Allow child to eat solids as soon as tolerated and appetite has returned. Most solids are acceptable; sugar-containing foods and drinks should be avoided initially.
  3. Avoidance lactose-containing formulas and foods may be required for 48-72 hr. Soy formulas are an option (Prosobee contains glucose, Isomil:sucrose).
- Antidiarrheal medications rarely indicated
- Specific therapy:

C. difficile	Vancomycin, metronidazole
Campylobacter	Erythromycin
Shigella	Amoxicillin, trimethoprim-sulfamethoxazole (sensitivities may vary)
Giardia lamblia	Metronidazole, furazolidone
Yersinia	Trimethoprim-sulfamethoxazole, chloramphenicol, tetracycline (>age 9 yr)

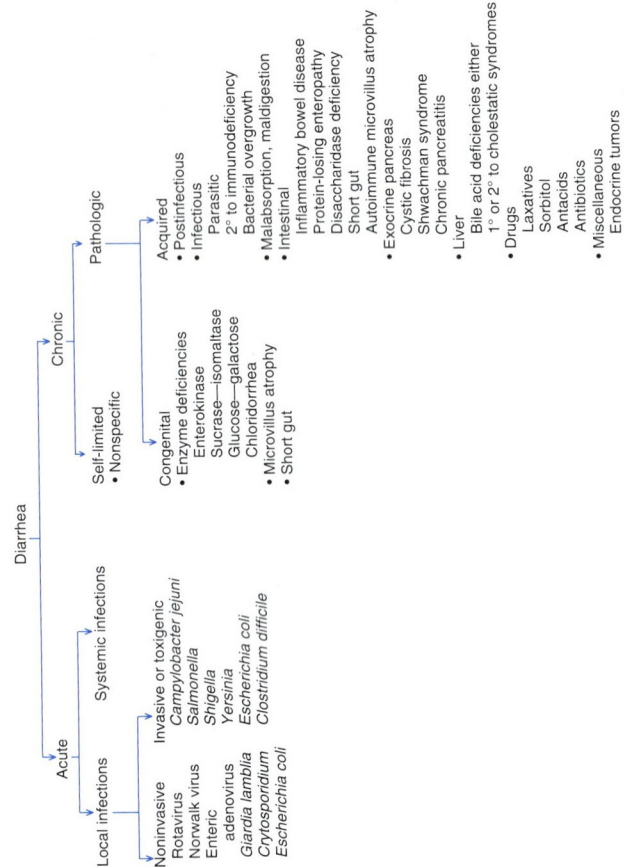

```
Diarrhea
├── Acute
│   ├── Local infections
│   │   Noninvasive
│   │   Rotavirus
│   │   Norwalk virus
│   │   Enteric
│   │     adenovirus
│   │   Giardia lamblia
│   │   Crytosporidium
│   │   Escherichia coli
│   └── Systemic infections
│       Invasive or toxigenic
│       Campylobacter jejuni
│       Salmonella
│       Shigella
│       Yersinia
│       Escherichia coli
│       Clostridium difficile
└── Chronic
    ├── Self-limited
    │   • Nonspecific
    │     Congenital
    │       • Enzyme deficiencies
    │         Enterokinase
    │         Sucrase—isomaltase
    │         Glucose—galactose
    │         Chloridorrhea
    │       • Microvillus atrophy
    │       • Short gut
    └── Pathologic
        Acquired
        • Postinfectious
        • Infectious
          Parasitic
          2° to immunodeficiency
          Bacterial overgrowth
        • Malabsorption, maldigestion
        • Intestinal
          Inflammatory bowel disease
          Protein-losing enteropathy
          Disaccharidase deficiency
          Short gut
          Autoimmune microvillus atrophy
        • Exocrine pancreas
          Cystic fibrosis
          Shwachman syndrome
          Chronic pancreatitis
        • Liver
          Bile acid deficiencies either
          1° or 2° to cholestatic syndromes
        • Drugs
          Laxatives
          Sorbitol
          Antacids
          Antibiotics
        • Miscellaneous
          Endocrine tumors
          Heavy metal poisoning
```

Figure 8-1 **Causes of diarrhea.**

TABLE 8-1 Composition of Oral Rehydration Fluids

	Glucose (g%)	Na (mmol/L)	K (mmol/L)	Cl (mmol/L)	Base (mmol/L)
WHO solution	2.0	90	20	80	30
Toronto Hospital for Sick Children, solution	2.0	50	20	40	30
Pedialyte	2.5	45	20	35	30
Gastrolyte	2.0	50	20	52	18
Ricelyte	3.0	50	25	45	34

CHRONIC DIARRHEA

Investigations
- Serial heights and weights, growth percentiles. Note that with nonspecific diarrhea of infancy, child is growing and thriving well
- Rectal examination for stool consistency, pH, reducing substances; microscopy for fecal leukocytes, fat crystals or globules, blood (visible or occult)
- Urinalysis
- Stool collection (multiple samples)
  1. Ova and parasites, cultures
  2. Fat malabsorption: 3-5-day fecal fat balance
  3. Protein malabsorption: α_1-antitrypsin clearance (requires 24-hr stool collection plus measurement of serum α_1-antitrypsin at start of collection)
  4. Electrolytes
  5. Alkalinization: pink color indicates phenolphthalein, present in some laxatives
- CBC, differential, ESR, smear, electrolytes, total protein, albumin, immunoglobulins
- Biochemical assessment of absorptive and nutritional status: Ca^{2+}, PO_4, Mg, Zn, iron, ferritin, folate, fat-soluble vitamins, PT, PTT, trypsinogen. If warranted, consider liver function tests, cholesterol, triglycerides
- If indicated, test thyroid function tests, urine VMA and HVA, HIV testing, lead levels
- Ancillary: sweat chloride, breath hydrogen tests
- Radiologic examinations: upper GI series ± follow through, double-contrast barium enema to evaluate for inflammatory lesions of the bowel
- Specialized tests
  1. Small bowel biopsy ± aspiration
  2. Upper and lower GI tract endoscopy and biopsy
  3. Quantitative exocrine pancreatic testing

Management

- Most otherwise healthy children require minimal diagnostic work-ups. Nonspecific diarrhea of infancy (Toddler's diarrhea) is the most common diagnosis in these children (6 mo to 3 yr) and often begins after an acute gastroenteritis; it requires no specific therapy (avoiding high sorbitol-containing fruit juices—e.g., apple juice—helps). *Avoid elimination diets.*
- Children with pathologic chronic diarrhea may require electrolyte and water replacement. Critical to consider protein, calorie, and other nutrient requirements, e.g., postinfectious diarrhea is commonest cause of this group of disorders and although requires no specific therapy, adequate protein and calorie replacement factors most in recovery.
- Specific therapy may be required (Table 8-2) for other etiologies

TABLE 8-2 Specific Therapeutic Modalities in Chronic Diarrhea

Condition	Therapy
Enterokinase deficiency	Protein hydrolysate formula (infants), pancreatic enzyme replacement
Short gut, microvillus atrophy	± Parenteral nutrition, consider somatostatin analogues, prednisone (autoimmune etiology)
Protein-losing enteropathy	Depends on underlying disorder
Bacterial overgrowth	Poorly absorbed antibiotics, e.g., metronidazole, gentamycin
Inflammatory bowel disease	See p 116
Exocrine pancreatic insufficiency	Titrated pancreatic enzyme replacement, fat-soluble vitamin supplements, ↑ calories (120-150% recommended daily intake)
Lactase deficiency	Lactase additives, avoid lactose-containing products
Celiac disease	Gluten-free diet

Protein-Losing Enteropathy

- General term that describes hypoproteinemia secondary to gastrointestinal plasma protein loss
- Common causes: milk-soy protein intolerance, celiac disease, inflammatory bowel disease, giardiasis, gastroenteritis
- Cow's milk protein intolerance most common. Fifty percent also reactive to soy protein. May present as proctitis or colitis with blood, loose stools, and eosinophils in stool smear (Wright's stain) in young infant. Older infant may present with edema, hypoalbuminemia, ± iron-deficiency anemia. Most children tolerate cow's milk by 2 yr.
- Investigations include urinalysis, α_1-antitrypsin clearance, CBC, smear, WBC and differential, ESR, total protein, albumin, globulins, carotene, Fe studies

Vomiting (Fig. 8-2)

Investigations

- Vomitus: evidence of bile or blood (visible, occult)
- Urinalysis, microscopy ± culture
- CBC, differential, ESR, electrolytes, blood gases, BUN, creatinine, ± blood cultures. Consider testing for iron, ferritin, folate, calcium, albumin, protein, specific drug screen.
- Radiologic investigations: plain abdominal radiographs (supine, upright), ultrasonography, upper GI series ± follow through (not reliable to document reflux); barium enema ± double contrast (anatomic or mucosal abnormalities)
- Specialized tests
  1. Upper and/or lower GI tract endoscopy with biopsy
  2. Small bowel biopsy ± aspiration
  3. 24-hr esophageal pH monitoring
  4. Esophageal motility testing
  5. Gastric emptying studies
  6. Milk scintiscan

Vomiting

Acute

Gastrointestinal
- Congenital anomalies
  - Atresias
  - Tracheoesophageal fistula
  - Malrotation and volvulus
- Meconium ileus
- Intussusception
- Infection
  - Gastroenteritis
  - Peritonitis
  - Appendicitis
  - Hepatitis

Nongastrointestinal
- CNS
  - ↑ICP
  - Drugs
  - Intoxicants
- Urinary infections
- Systemic infections

Chronic

Gastrointestinal
- Gastroesophageal reflux
- Mechanical obstruction
  - Congenital anomalies
  - Malrotation and volvulus
  - Intussusception
  - Foreign bodies, bezoars
  - Chronic granulomatous disease
- Primary motility disorders
  - Achalasia
  - Intestinal pseudo-obstruction
- Intestinal inflammation
  - Celiac disease
  - Crohn's disease
  - Eosinophilic enteritis
  - Infections
  - Duodenal ulcer
  - Gastric inflammation
    - 1°, 2°, gastritis
  - Gastric ulcer
- Other
  - Anorexia, bullimia
  - Cyclic vomiting
  - Fecal impaction

Nongastrointestinal
- CNS
  - ↑ICP
  - Drugs
- Urinary tract infections

Figure 8-2 **Causes of vomiting.**

110

Management

- Prevention and treatment of dehydration and electrolyte imbalance (see p 88)
- Antiemetic medications should be used with caution—rule out surgical cause of vomiting
- Bowel rest (depends on cause)
- Always consider mechanical obstruction (intermittent, persistent)

Gastroesophageal Reflux

- Indications for investigation and therapy
  1. Failure to thrive
  2. Recurrent pneumonia, bronchospasm
  3. GI blood loss
- Conservative therapy: small, frequent feeds, thickened feeds, positioning prone at 45° during sleep and post feeding
- Medical therapy: short-term enteral feedings to enhance weight gain; H_2 blockers indicated when esophagitis present. Role of prokinetics (domperidone, cisapride) uncertain but trial may be indicated.
- Surgical therapy: indicated for failure of medical therapy; may be indicated earlier in specific groups, e.g., severely neurologically impaired, or if there is evidence of aspiration

Gastrointestinal Bleeding (Fig. 8-3)

UPPER GI BLEEDING

Investigations

- Hemodynamic status, evidence of oropharyngeal bleed or chronic liver disease (splenomegaly, spider nevi, ascites, jaundice)
- Nasogastric aspirate: test for blood (note: gastric acid may interfere with hemoccult testing), pH, Apt test in newborn (distinguishes maternal from fetal RBC)
- CBC, hematocrit, smear, platelets, PT, PTT, BUN, creatinine, urinalysis; liver function tests if indicated. Follow CBC, reticulocytes.

Management

- Acute stabilization
  1. Stabilize airway, breathing, circulation
  2. Semi-sitting
  3. Vitamin K, 5-10 mg IV (slow)
  4. Volume and blood replacement (urgent cross-matching for adequate volumes)
  5. NG saline lavage (omit if source known to be esophageal varices)
  6. IV H_2 blocker (cimetidine, ranitidine)
  7. ± NG antacids
- If continues unstable:
  1. IV vasopressin (generally requires intensive care setting)
  2. ± Intervention endoscopy, balloon tamponade, angiography with embolization, surgery
- Once stabilized: diagnostic endoscopy ± biopsy (*Helicobacter pylori* found on antral biopsy samples, not cultures); radiologic examinations of little benefit

DUODENAL ULCER

- *Helicobacter pylori* positive: Consider amoxicillin plus bismuth subsalicylate × 6 weeks plus Flagyl × 10 days
- *H. pylori* negative: ranitidine × 10 wk

Gastroenterology

LOWER GI BLEEDING

Investigations

- Hemodynamic status, evidence of growth failure, fevers. Differential diagnosis of black stools: iron, bismuth, spinach. Tumors and hemorrhoids presenting with lower GI bleeding are very rare.
- Nasogastric aspirate: upper GI bleed may present as melena or hematochezia
- Anal and rectal examination: tags, fissures, anal fistulas, polyps, trauma, foreign bodies, long patulous canal, blood (visible, occult), stool appearance (gross blood, streaking) and microscopy for leucocytes.
- Stool cultures, *C. difficile* culture toxin, urinalysis and microscopy
- CBC, smear, differential, platelets, ESR, electrolytes, BUN, creatinine, PT, PTT, Apt test (newborn), albumin, total protein, iron studies, *Yersinia* titers, *Amoeba* titers, carotene
- Radiologic investigations: plain abdominal x-rays to rule out obstruction, barium enema (single contrast: obstructive causes; double contrast: mucosal abnormalities), upper GI ± follow through
- Specialized tests
  1. Diagnostic endoscopy ± biopsy
  2. Meckel's scan
  3. Angiography
  4. ^{99}Tc RBC scan, ^{99}Tc sulfur colloid scan

Management

- Acute stabilization
  1. Volume and blood replacement
  2. Bowel rest: NPO, NG to suction
- If continues unstable
  1. Consider IV broad-spectrum antibiotics
  2. Angiography with embolization
  3. Surgery

Gastrointestinal bleeding

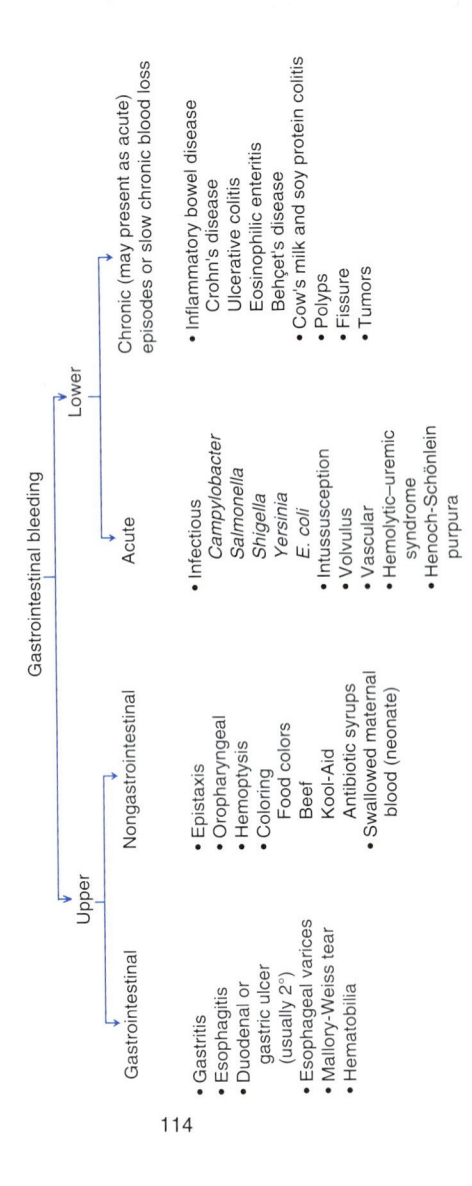

Upper

Gastrointestinal
- Gastritis
- Esophagitis
- Duodenal or gastric ulcer (usually 2°)
- Esophageal varices
- Mallory-Weiss tear
- Hematobilia

Nongastrointestinal
- Epistaxis
- Oropharyngeal
- Hemoptysis
- Coloring
  - Food colors
  - Beef
  - Kool-Aid
  - Antibiotic syrups
- Swallowed maternal blood (neonate)

Lower

Acute
- Infectious
  - *Campylobacter*
  - *Salmonella*
  - *Shigella*
  - *Yersinia*
  - *E. coli*
- Intussusception
- Volvulus
- Vascular
- Hemolytic–uremic syndrome
- Henoch-Schönlein purpura

Chronic (may present as acute episodes or slow chronic blood loss)
- Inflammatory bowel disease
  - Crohn's disease
  - Ulcerative colitis
  - Eosinophilic enteritis
  - Behçet's disease
- Cow's milk and soy protein colitis
- Polyps
- Fissure
- Tumors

- Collagen vascular
- Thrombosis/Embolus
- Ectopic gastric mucosa-Meckel's
  - Duplications
- Antibiotic associated
- AV malformation
- Foreign body
- Trauma
- Neonatal
  Necrotizing enterocolitis
  Hirschsprung's colitis
  Vitamin K deficiency
  Swallowed maternal blood

Figure 8-3 **Causes of GI bleeding.**

Inflammatory Bowel Disease

ULCERATIVE COLITIS

- Mild
  1. Oral: salazopyrine, 5-aminosalicylate (Asacol, Pentasa, Dipentum)
  2. Rectal: steroid enemas (Cortenema, Cortifoam), 5-ASA enemas; rectal therapy may be used alone (when distal disease) or in combination with oral therapy
- Moderate
  1. Prednisone 1 mg/kg/day (max, 40-60 mg) × 6 wk and then taper
- Severe
  1. Hospitalize, NPO
  2. IV steroids ± steroid and 5-ASA enemas
  3. Consider IV broad-spectrum antibiotics
  4. Blood products as required
  5. Colectomy if not settled within 5-7 days (curative procedure) N.B. In severe colitis, monitor for toxic megacolon (physical exam, electrolytes, plain abdominal x-rays). *If toxic megacolon suspected, barium enema studies and morphine-derivative analgesics are contraindicated.*
- Maintenance
  1. Salazopyrin (Asacol) proven to reduce exacerbations
  2. Continue for 2 yr after asymptomatic

CROHN'S DISEASE

- Small bowel disease: 5-ASA preparations (Asacol, Pentasa)
- Small bowel + colonic: salazopyrine, Asacol
- Colonic disease: salazopyrine, metronidazole
- Prednisone 1 mg/kg/day (maximum 40-60 mg) PO × 6 wk, then taper. Usually for severe disease, though may not be superior to elemental NG feeds.

- Metronidazole of benefit in perianal disease, fistulas; role in colonic disease uncertain
- Other drugs: 6-mercaptopurine (to reduce steroid dependency); may take 3-6 mo until effects seen. Role of cyclosporin unclear.
- Nutritional: elemental diet via nighttime NG feeds, TPN
- Surgery: symptomatic treatment, *not* curative
- Maintenance: no therapy proven to prevent exacerbations

Acute Abdominal Distension (Fig. 8-4)

Investigations
- CBC, differential, ESR, blood gases, electrolytes, BUN, creatinine, amylase, blood cultures, liver function tests
- Radiologic investigations
  1. Double bubble: duodenal obstruction
  2. Plain abdominal x-ray: small bowel obstruction (plicae circulares occupy entire transverse diameter). Large bowel obstruction (colonic haustral markings occupy a small portion of bowel diameter).
  3. Air enema: intussusception
  4. Barium enema: malrotation
  5. Upper GI and follow through
  6. Ultrasonography: may be useful in pyloric stenosis
  7. Angiography

Management
- Treat underlying systemic cause, electrolyte disturbances
- Bowel rest: IV fluids, NPO, NG to suction for most situations
- Surgery as required

Acute Abdominal Distension

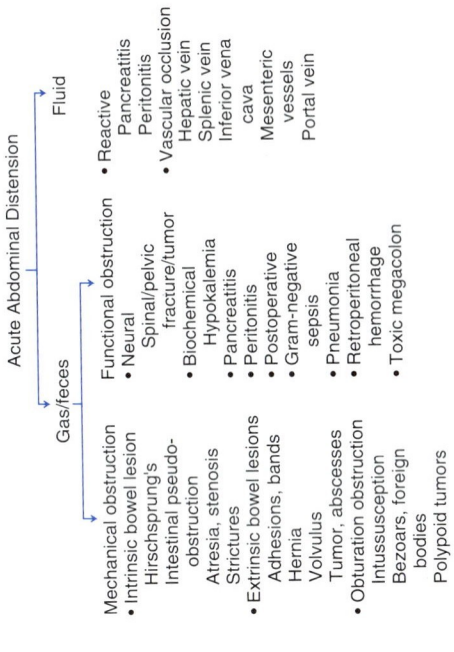

Gas/feces

Mechanical obstruction
- Intrinsic bowel lesion
  Hirschsprung's
  Intestinal pseudo-obstruction
  Atresia, stenosis
  Strictures
- Extrinsic bowel lesions
  Adhesions, bands
  Hernia
  Volvulus
  Tumor, abscesses
- Obturation obstruction
  Intussusception
  Bezoars, foreign bodies
  Polypoid tumors

Functional obstruction
- Neural
  Spinal/pelvic fracture/tumor
- Biochemical
  Hypokalemia
- Pancreatitis
- Peritonitis
- Postoperative
- Gram-negative sepsis
- Pneumonia
- Retroperitoneal hemorrhage
- Toxic megacolon

Fluid
- Reactive
  Pancreatitis
  Peritonitis
- Vascular occlusion
  Hepatic vein
  Splenic vein
  Inferior vena cava
  Mesenteric vessels
  Portal vein

Figure 8-4 **Causes of acute abdominal distension.**

Chronic Abdominal Distension (Fig. 8-5)

Investigations
- CBC, differential, smear, ESR, albumin, urinalysis. As indicated: total protein, carotene, liver function tests, iron studies, electrolytes, BUN, creatinine, thyroid function, calcium, parathyroid hormone, sweat chloride, lead, folate.

Radiologic investigations:
- Initial: abdominal flat plate: feces, caliber of intestinal lumen, calcifications, organomegaly
- U/S abdomen: masses, organomegaly
- Motility studies: gastric emptying study (solid meal)
- Upper GI and follow through: structure, intestinal transit time
- Barium enema: single, unprepared: Hirschsprung's
- Angiography: occlusions

Specialized tests:
- Breath hydrogen studies
- Rectal suction biopsies, surgical full-thickness biopsies
- Endoscopy and biopsy
- Duodenal aspirate and biopsy

Management

- Treat underlying disorder; antiflatulence agents generally do not work
- Prokinetic agents may be of benefit in primary motility disorders (domperidone, cisapride, metoclopramide) and selected secondary motility disorders
- Constipation: Most children have voluntary retention-type constipation and require minimal investigation. Consider further investigation in patients with onset at <3 mo of age, those with encopresis, and nonresponders to conventional treatment.
  1. Education: toilet training, regular attempts just after meals, proper position (hips flexed, feet flat; may need support for feet)
  2. Diet: increased fiber and fluids
  3. Initial evacuation: suppositories (irritative, e.g., bisacodyl), enemas (saline, hypertonic phosphate, 10 ml/kg), GI lavage—Golytely electrolyte solution
  4. Maintenance: mineral oil, 15 ml/15 kg, increase by 1 tsp every 3 days if not effective until oil is leaking from anus. Continue 4-6 mo prior to weaning. Avoid use in small infants and neurologically impaired due to risk of aspiration. Lactulose, prune juice are alternatives.
  5. No role for irritative suppositories or prokinetic agents for voluntary retention.

Chronic Abdominal Distension

Gas
- Altered transport: primary
  Chronic idiopathic
  intestinal pseudo-obstruction
- Altered transport: secondary
  Intestinal smooth muscle
  Endocrine
  Intestinal nervous system
  Drugs
- Increased production
  Disaccharidase deficiencies
  Bacterial overgrowth
  Malabsorption syndromes

Fluid
- Normal albumin
  Portal vein thrombosis
  Hepatic vein thrombosis
  Cardiovascular disorders
   constrictive pericarditis
   congestive heart failure
  Lymphatic obstruction
  Reactive (inflammatory)
- Hypoalbuminemia
  Nephrosis
  Protein-losing enteropathy
  Hepatic failure
  Nutritional (severe)

Stool
- Hirschsprung's
- Motility disorders (see "Gas")
- Voluntary retention
- Chronic dehydration

Masses
- Liver
- Kidney
- Adrenal
- Tumors
- Urinary bladders
- Spleen
- Uterus
  Hydrometrocolpos
  Fetus
- Cysts

Figure 8-5 **Causes of chronic abdominal distension.**

Recurrent Abdominal Pain (Table 8-3)

Definition
- Three or more attacks of abdominal pain severe enough to affect the normal activities over at least a 3-mo period

Management
- CBC, differential, ESR, urinalysis, stool for occult blood, further tests as indicated
- Radiologic investigations: ultrasonography, plain abdominal x-ray; further tests as indicated

TABLE 8-3 Features of Recurrent Abdominal Pain

Organic	Functional
Crampy, colicky pain Wakens from sleep Consistent description Radiation to back, groin Age < 4 yr Associated features: vomiting, diarrhea, weight loss, fever, distension, bleeding, joint problems, skin rashes	Variation of description Complains on awakening Other somatic complaints: headaches, limb pain Otherwise well

NINE

Genetics

Approach to a Child with Multiple Congenital Abnormalities or Mental Retardation and Dysmorphism

DIAGNOSTIC CATEGORIES

- Malformation syndromes caused by single gene defects (Mendelian inheritance)
  1. 0.3 to 1.2% of live births (estimates vary)
  2. Autosomal dominant, e.g., tuberous sclerosis
  3. Autosomal recessive, e.g., cystic fibrosis, β-thalassemia
  4. X-linked recessive, e.g., Duchenne muscular dystrophy
  5. X-linked dominant, e.g., X-linked hypophosphatemic rickets
- Malformation syndromes caused by chromosomal abnormalities
  1. 0.6% of live births
  2. 50% of all spontaneous abortions
  3. 5% of stillbirths
  4. Aneuploidy (abnormal number of chromosomes): all trisomies, e.g., 21, 13, 18, Klinefelter syndrome 47,XXY; monosomy X, i.e., Turner syndrome 45,X; tetraploidy
  5. Structural rearrangement
     - Visible deletion, e.g., 5p −: Cri du chat syndrome
     - Minor deletion, e.g., 13q −: retinoblastoma (this is an example of a contiguous gene defect that involves one definite gene locus that accounts for the tumor, and other, probably adjacent, loci, which account for the associated mental retardation and dysmorphism)

- Chromosomal breakage syndromes, e.g., Fanconi's anemia
- Fragile X syndrome
- Non-Mendelian malformation syndromes
  1. This category probably accounts for most of the common birth defects
  2. Multifactorial inheritance, i.e., genetic and possible environmental factors involved
  3. Examples include neural tube defect, club foot, VSD
  4. Genetic predisposition is probably related to multiple gene loci (polygenic)
  5. Empiric recurrence risk to first-degree relatives is 3-5%
- Environmentally induced abnormalities
  1. History of teratogen exposure
  2. Congenital infections (TORCH); drugs, e.g., thalidomide, anticonvulsants (phenytoin), retinoic acid, warfarin, alcohol, antineoplastics (methotrexate); metabolic diseases, e.g., uncontrolled or undiagnosed maternal phenylketonuria, which causes microcephaly and mental retardation in offspring

CHROMOSOME ANALYSIS

- Indicated for confirmation of a clinical diagnosis or when a new chromosomal abnormality is suspected. Usual karyotyping examines chromosomes in metaphase; can be done in 3-4 days on heparinized peripheral blood leukocytes or in 6 hr on bone marrow aspiration samples (lower success rate; life or death decisions). For additional information, or where mosaicism suspected, fibroblasts (cultured from skin biopsy tissue) or other tissue can be used. Prenatal diagnosis by chromosomal analysis of amniocytes (amniocentesis) or chorionic villi (chorionic villous sample) possible.
- Small deletions may be missed on metaphase banding; if a high index of suspicion exists for specific deletion syndromes, prophase banding is superior. Similarly, fragile X and chromosome breakage studies require special requisition.

BIOCHEMICAL TESTS

- In dysmorphic syndromes characterized by biochemical abnormalities or enzyme deficiencies, specific diagnostic metabolic tests are recommended (see Chapter 15)

PHOTOGRAPHS

- Photographs of facial features, full body, and specific birth defects are recommended where indicated; these are useful for second opinion referrals, as well as for retrospective assessment.
- Radiographs

Approach to a Dying Child or Stillbirth with a Suspected Genetic Syndrome or Inborn Error of Metabolism (IEM)

- Every attempt should be made to make an accurate diagnosis to enable accurate counseling. Remember IEM even in cases of so-called SIDS.
- Contact local genetics or metabolic disease consultant as soon as possible
- Whenever possible, obtain consent after death for full postmortem examination or at least a limited examination or biopsy of the organs of interest as soon as possible
- Photographs are essential to document abnormalities
- Radiologic investigations: full skeletal survey for any suspected or obvious skeletal dysplasia. May be useful for metabolic diseases (e.g., storage) as well. Ultrasonography of heart and kidneys, especially if full autopsy not performed.
- Collect the following samples:
  1. Sterile skin biopsy for fibroblast culture for metabolic work-up, chromosome analysis, and possible future DNA analysis. About 0.5 cm^2 of full-depth skin is required and should be stored in fresh tissue culture medium at 4° C until processed. Biopsy is preferable prior to death to avoid bacterial contamination.

2. Sterile blood—peripheral or by cardiac puncture. 5-10 ml clotted blood for serum and 5-10 ml heparinized blood for plasma should be centrifuged, and separated and stored at $-20°$ C for enzyme and biochemical work-up as indicated. Also, 5 ml heparinized blood for lymphoblast line and karyotype analysis—may keep at room temperature but should be processed as soon as possible.
3. Urine—as large a volume as possible (± 30 ml) and store at $-20°$ C for metabolic screen, organic acids, mucopolysaccharide and oligosaccharide screening, and other tests as indicated by clinical findings
4. Skeletal muscle, e.g., gastrocnemius 0.5–1 g in three pieces
    - Rapid freeze sample in liquid nitrogen (available from pathology or histology) and store at $-70°$ C for enzyme activity and histochemistry. If not available, wrap small pieces of tissue (± 1.5 cm^3) in aluminum foil, freeze on dry ice for 10 min, and then store at $-70°$ C (preferably not at $-20°$ C).
    - Place sample in universal fixative for electron microscopy (available from pathology)
    - Place sample in 10% formalin (available in operating room or pathology) and keep at room temperature or $+4°$ C
5. Liver: three to four needle core samples
    - One to two cores in universal fixative for electron microscopy
    - One to two cores rapid frozen for histochemistry
    - One to two in 10% formalin
    - Without an open biopsy, there is usually too little tissue available for enzyme assays
6. Vitreous humor from needle aspiration of the orbit. Many biochemical assays can be performed on this sample and it is especially useful if urine cannot be obtained. Freeze at $-20°$ C.
7. Tissue biopsies, e.g., skin, spleen, and lung, can be cultured for chromosome analysis (see above).

TEN

Genitourinary Disease

Vaginal Bleeding

NEONATAL

- Usually occurs between 5-10 days of age
- Difficult to distinguish from hematuria
- Must do thorough search for other signs of a bleeding diathesis
- Look for other evidence of estrogen effect (e.g., breast buds)
- Major differential diagnoses include maternal estrogen effects (most common), gynecologic disease (infection, tumor), and bleeding diathesis
- Investigations include CBC, PT, PTT, and bleeding time, platelets; swab for culture; vaginal cytology for hormonal effect; urinalysis and culture

Treatment

- If physical and laboratory data consistent, diagnosis is likely maternal estrogen effects and withdrawal bleeding. Observe; follow-up in 6-8 wks.
- In the absence of a bleeding diathesis, all other causes need a gynecology referral and assessment

PREMENARCHAL: EARLY AND LATE CHILDHOOD

- Differential Diagnosis
  1. Trauma: careful perineal examination for trauma or discharge. Generally limited to external examination of vagina and vulva. *Always do a rectal examination.*
  2. Foreign body
  3. Sexual abuse: observe patient's behavior (suggestive of sexual abuse)

4. Precocious puberty: assess height, weight, signs of pubertal change
5. Hormone withdrawal: history of hormone ingestion or vaginal cream (must ask if mother or adolescent in the home is using these medications)
6. Vaginitis (uncommon): group A β-streptococci, *Shigella;* consider sexual abuse and sexually transmitted disease, nonspecific vaginitis
7. Uterine, vaginal, urethral pathology (uncommon): assess for evidence of systemic illness
8. Bleeding diathesis (rare)

Investigations
- CBC
- Vaginal culture
- Vaginal cell maturation index

Treatment
- Gynecology referral for vaginoscopy and therapy unless only superficial trauma, foreign body can be easily removed, or vaginitis with positive culture

PERIMENARCHAL

- Similar in pattern to those of premenarchal group
- Always consider pregnancy, as it is possible to become pregnant prior to first menses

Differential Diagnosis
- Menarche
- Trauma
- Sexual abuse
- Bleeding diathesis (would present as heavy flow at menarche)
- Uterine, vaginal disease (uncommon)
- Pregnancy complication

Genitourinary Disease

Investigations
- CBC
- Platelets, PT, PTT, and bleeding time (if bleeding considered excessive for normal menarche)
- Urine or plasma β-hCG

Treatment
- Gynecology referral if trauma requiring examination under anesthesia (EUA) or sutures, pregnancy complication, or uterine and vaginal disease suspected; bleeding disorder may also require hematologic consultation
- Child protection services referral if sexual abuse (see page 149)

POSTMENARCHAL

- Always consider patient sexually active until proven otherwise, i.e., pregnancy or complication thereof a strong possibility
- Dysfunctional uterine bleeding (DUB) is a diagnosis of exclusion
- A complete menstrual and sexual history is mandatory, but may not be completely reliable
- Determine contraceptive use, compliance, and need
- Do as complete a pelvic examination as possible

Differential Diagnosis
- DUB (75%): anovulatory cycles, common in first 2 yr post menarche
- Bleeding diathesis (5-20%)
- Gynecologic disease
  1. Infections: PID, endometritis
  2. IUD-related
  3. Oral contraceptive misuse

Investigations
- CBC, differential, platelets
- PT, PTT, bleeding time
- Thyroid function, prolactin

- Cervical swabs for gonorrhea and *Chlamydia*
- Pap smear
- β-hCG
- Urinalysis
- Blood glucose

Treatment

- Mild bleeding (DUB)
  1. Usually chronic erratic menses with normal hemoglobin
  2. Explain to patient and arrange close follow-up after two cycles (8 wk) with menstrual calendars
- Moderate bleeding (DUB)
  1. Usually Hb ≥100 g/L and stable
  2. Birth control pill (BCP)
     - Ovral: two tabs initially and then one tab qid until bleeding stops (5 days maximum)
     - When bleeding stops, continue one to two tabs PO daily for a total of 21 days; then withdraw for 7 days
     - Pre-empt next two cycles with daily BCP
  3. Alternatively: medroxyprogesterone chemical curettage with 5 mg bid PO × 7 days every 35-60 days
- Grossly irregular menses with profuse or prolonged bleeding (DUB)
  1. Gynecology referral
  2. BCP therapy as in moderate bleeding
- Severe acute bleeding (DUB ± coagulation disorder)
  1. Hb <100 g/L
  2. Admit to hospital: urgent gynecology referral
  3. IV fluid resuscitation and blood transfusion as necessary
  4. Premarin (conjugated estrogens), 25 mg IV q4h PRN, for a maximum of 24 hr to stop bleeding
  5. Simultaneously Ovral, 2 tabs initially and then 1 tab qid and continue as for "moderate bleeding"
  6. Replace clotting factors as needed (fresh frozen plasma, cryoprecipitate, or platelets)
  7. Give antinauseants with the IV Premarin
  8. Hematology referral for bleeding problems

Vulvovaginitis

- Infection with gonorrhea, herpes, *Chlamydia,* condylomata, and *Trichomonas* generally means venereal transmission (nonvenereal possible but rare). Must rule out sexual assault.

PREPUBERTAL

- Nonbloody discharge and pruritus are common in children because of poor hygiene, proximity to anus, and susceptibility of thin vaginal mucosa to infection

Differential Diagnosis

- Noninfectious
  1. Poor hygiene
  2. Foreign body
  3. Chemical irritant
  4. Trauma or sexual abuse
  5. Generalized skin disease
- Infectious
  1. Nonspecific bacterial (usually coliforms from bowel, *not Gardnerella* as in adults)
  2. Pinworms
  3. Group A β-hemolytic streptococcus
  4. STD, e.g., *Trichomonas,* gonorrhea. Latter causes vaginitis in prepubertal, *not* in postpubertal children; prepubertal girls do not develop cervicitis
  5. *Candida* uncommon before hormonal changes of perimenarchal stage

Investigations

- Perineal examination
- Culture vagina (use soft plastic eyedropper or moistened urethral swab to collect specimen if needed) for gonorrhea and β-hemolytic streptococci if discharge present
- Wet prep for *Trichomonas* if profuse purulent discharge or sexual assault suspected)

- Referral to gynecology for vaginoscopy if
  1. Bloody discharge
  2. Foreign body suspected and unable to remove by gentle irrigation with normal saline and Foley catheter (one attempt)
  3. Symptoms recurrent or not resolving

Treatment
- Hygiene education
- Sitz baths tid
- Skin hydration (Aveeno)
- Avoid soaps
- Remove foreign bodies (see above)
- Treat specific organisms

POSTPUBERTAL

Differential Diagnosis
- Physiologic leukorrhea
- Noninfectious—generalized dermatitis, poor hygiene, retained tampon
- Infectious
  1. Nonspecific vaginitis ("*Gardnerella* vaginitis")
     - Synergistic infection caused by *Gardnerella* and anaerobes together
     - *Gardnerella* may be normal vaginal flora
     - Grey malodorous discharge with "clue cells"
  2. *Candidiasis* ("yeast"): cheesy white discharge, pruritic; common after antibiotics, in diabetics, pregnancy
  3. *Trichomonas:* green frothy foul discharge, often pruritic
  4. Gonorrhea: often asymptomatic; may have cervicitis with purulent cervical discharge
  5. *Chlamydia:* often asymptomatic; may be cervicitis; may be concomitant with or present after treatment of gonorrhea
  6. Herpes: history of recurrence, usually painful, vesicles ulcerate, inguinal adenopathy
  7. Condylomata accuminata: nonplanar perineal warts

8. Parasites: scabies, pediculosis pubis
9. Mycoplasma: role unclear; may grow in association with other organisms or in asymptomatic patients

Investigation

- Perineal examination
- Vaginal swab: KOH prep for *Candida;* wet prep for *Trichomonas* + "clue cells" (*Gardnerella:* organisms on epithelial cell surface)
- Cervical swabs for gonorrhea (Gram stain, culture) and *Chlamydia* (immunofluorescent Ab to detect Ag, cultures), if sexually active
- Herpes: electron microscopy to demonstrate viral particles; viral culture of lesion; scrapings with Wright stain: multinucleated giant cells
- Maturation index helpful in physiologic leukorrhea
- Bimanual pelvic examination is necessary in all sexually active girls

Treatment

- No treatment for physiologic leukorrhea
- Hygiene education
- Nonspecific *(Gardnerella)* vaginitis: metronidazole, 500 mg bid × 7 days
- *Trichomonas:* metronidazole 500 mg bid × 7 days or 2 g PO × one dose (adult); must treat partner; advise to avoid alcohol
- *Candida:* miconazole (Monistat) cream or ovules intravaginally × 3 nights
- Gonorrhea: see p 138
- *Chlamydia:* see p 137
- Herpes: symptomatic treatment
- Condylomata: gynecology referral for chemical treatment, cryotherapy, cautery, or laser
- Scabies, pediculosis: see p 68

Labial Fusion

- Generally an asymptomatic benign condition, seen from age 2 mo to menarche; presents due to maternal concern; resolves when endogenous estrogen is produced. May be corrected by application of exogenous estrogen (Premarin, bid × 14 days to vulva) if
  1. Urethral meatus (and urinary output) obstructed (uncommon)
  2. Strong parental anxiety
  3. Confusion with other diagnoses, e.g., vaginal agenesis, excessive virilization
- No indication for surgical revision or forcing labia apart

Sexually Transmitted Diseases

- Always include in differential diagnosis of abdominal pain and urethral and/or vaginal discharge in adolescent
- Upper genitourinary tract infection in females often associated with pain and systemic symptoms
- *Chlamydia* and *N. gonorrheoa* often occur together (20-30%) and, along with genital herpes may be asymptomatic at any age
- Suspect child abuse in all prepubescent and nonsexually active postpubescent children with these infections
- Important management tasks
  1. Contact tracing and treatment
  2. Reporting to Public Health Department
  3. Optimizing compliance
  4. Follow-up *essential* but may be difficult in some social situations
  5. Counseling regarding HIV, birth control, safe sex
  6. Screening of high-risk groups for HIV, with consent
  7. Awareness of long-term risks for infertility, ectopic pregnancy

Clinical Features of Pelvic Inflammatory Disease (PID) in Females

- Fever, abdominal pain, anorexia, diarrhea
- Vaginal discharge or bleeding
- Usually occurs following menses
- Pain worse with walking, intercourse
- Acute and subacute clinical courses
- Physical signs include lower quadrant tenderness, cervical excitation pain and adnexal tenderness, perihepatic pain (Fitz-Hugh-Curtis syndrome), elevated WBC and ESR
- Consider ectopic pregnancy, ovarian cyst or torsion, and appendicitis in the differential diagnosis of PID

Chlamydia Trachomatis

- Inclusion conjunctivitis (neonates), pneumonia (1-4 mo), urethritis, cervicitis, epididymitis, lymphogranuloma venereum
- Often asymptomatic. May coexist with gonorrhea (must rule out) or present after gonorrhea treated.
- Swab for *Chlamydia* Ag (immunofluorescent antibody); cultures
- Treatment shown in Table 10-2

Neisseria Gonorrhoeae

- Urethritis, epididymitis, vaginitis (prepubertal); cervicitis, salpingitis (post pubertal)
- Gram stain and culture: In females—endocervical, vaginal, rectal ± pharyngeal swabs. In heterosexual males—urethral; homosexual males—urethral, pharyngeal, rectal. Other: neonates—conjunctiva; joint, blood as indicated.
- Swabs should be plated promptly onto Thayer-Martin agar plates or placed in transport medium
- Include urethral (male), vaginal, and cervical cultures or immunofluorescent antibodies for *Chlamydia*
- Baseline VDRL with follow-up at 8 wk

TABLE 10-1 Causes of the Major STD Syndromes*

Syndrome	Sexually Transmitted	Other
Urethritis and PID	Chlamydia trachomatis Neisseria gonorrhoeae	
Cervicitis	C. trachomatis N. gonorrhoeae Herpes simplex virus (HSV)	
Epididymitis	C. trachomatis N. gonorrhoeae	Urinary tract pathogens
Prepubertal vaginitis	C. trachomatis N. gonorrhoeae	Group A streptococci Nonspecific
Postpubertal vaginitis	Trichomonas vaginalis Bacterial vaginosis (Gardnerella vaginalis) Yeast	Yeasts
Genital ulcer disease	Treponema pallidum (painless) Herpes simplex Haemophilus ducreyi	
Genital and anal warts	Human papillomavirus	
Proctitis	C. trachomatis N. gonorrhoeae Herpes simplex T. pallidum	E. histolytica Campylobacter Shigella C. difficile

N.B.: Vaginitis rather than cervicitis occurs in prepubertal girls.
*See Canada Diseases Weekly Reports, 1988 Canadian guidelines for the treatment of sexually transmitted diseases in neonates, children, adolescents, and adults. Health and Welfare Canada. Vol. 14 S2(April 1988) and vol. 15 S1(March 1989) for detailed diagnosis and treatment guidelines.

TABLE 10-2 Treatment of Genital *Chlamydia trachomatis**

Uncomplicated urethritis, cervicitis, proctitis
Tetracycline 500 mg PO 4 times daily for 7 days
or
Erythromycin 500 mg PO 4 times daily for 7 days
or
Doxycycline 100 mg twice daily for 7 days

Epididymo-orchitis
Tetracycline 500 mg PO 4 times daily for 10 days
or
Doxycycline 100 mg twice daily for 10 days

---

*Children < 9 yr: Erythromycin, 10 mg/kg PO 4 times daily for 7 days (10 days for epididymitis)
Children > 9 yr: Tetracycline, 10 mg/kg PO 4 times daily for 7 days (10 days for epididymitis)

Treatment (Table 10-3)

- Asymptomatic infant born to mother with gonorrhea
  1. Gastric and rectal cultures (for gonorrhea and *Chlamydia*)
  2. Routine eye prophylaxis
  3. Penicillin G, 100,000 U IM/IV × one dose
  4. If resistance is suspected, use ceftriaxone, 125 mg IM × one dose
- Gonococcal ophthalmitis: ceftriaxone or penicillin IV
- Uncomplicated gonorrhea: see Table 10-3
- In penicillin allergy or if organism is penicillin resistant or sensitivity unknown, use ceftriaxone (N.B.: 15% to cross-reactivity between penicillin and cephalosporins) IM × one dose or spectinomycin IM × one dose
- Pharyngeal or anorectal gonorrhea: amoxicillin and spectinomycin are not effective. All females should have rectal cultures if gonorrhea is suspected. (See Table 10-3.)

TABLE 10-3 Antibiotic Therapy for *Neisseria Gonorrhoeae*

Uncomplicated urethritis, cervicitis in adults
Aqueous procaine penicillin G 4.8 million U injected IM at 2 separate sites, with probenecid 1.0 g PO

or

Ampicillin 3.5 g or amoxicillin 3.0 g with probenecid 1.0 g PO in a single dose

or

Ceftriaxone 250 mg IM in a single dose

ALL FOLLOWED BY

Tetracycline* 500 mg PO 4 times daily for 7 days

or

Doxycycline* 100 mg PO twice daily for 7 days

Pharyngeal gonococcal infection
Aqueous procaine penicillin G with probenecid plus tetracycline or doxycycline, as above, is the preferred regimen

Anorectal gonococcal infection
Females: Treat as above for uncomplicated gonococcal disease

Males: Aqueous procaine penicillin G with probenecid plus tetracycline* or doxycycline,* as above, is the preferred regimen

Penicillin-resistant gonorrhoea
Ceftriaxone 250 mg IM in a single dose

or

Spectinomycin hydrochloride 2.0 g IM

Both followed by

Tetracycline* or doxycycline* as above

---

*In children age < 9 yr, replace tetracycline and doxycycline with erythromycin, 10 mg/kg PO qid.

TABLE 10-3 Antibiotic Therapy for *Neisseria Gonorrhoeae* (Cont'd)

Penicillin-allergic patients
Spectinomycin 2.0 g IM in a single dose
or
Ceftriaxone 250 mg IM in a single dose
Both followed by
Tetracycline* or doxycycline* as above

Pregnancy
All of the above regimens are safe during pregnancy except tetracycline and doxycycline, which should be replaced by
Erythromycin 500 mg PO 4 times daily for 7 days
or
Erythromycin 250 mg PO 4 times daily for 14 days

Children <45 kg
Recommended Dosages
Amoxicillin 50 mg/kg PO in a single dose
Probenecid 25 mg/kg PO in a single dose
Aqueous procaine penicillin G, 100,000 IU/kg IM in a single dose
Erythromycin 10 mg/kg PO 4 times daily
Ceftriaxone 125 mg IM in a single dose
Spectinomycin 40 mg/kg IM in a single dose

- N.B. Everyone should receive *in addition* to above treatment simultaneous treatment for *C. trachomatis* with either tetracycline, doxycycline, or erythromycin
- Treat sexual partners
- Disseminated infection (sepsis, arthritis): penicillin G IV × 7-10 days; ceftriaxone IV may be used for penicillin-resistant organisms
- All patients should return 3-7 days after completion of therapy for clinical evaluation and follow-up cultures
- Pelvic inflammatory disease (PID) (see Table 10-4)

TABLE 10-4 Treatment of PID

Whenever possible, patients should be admitted and treated in hospital. When hospitalization is not possible, the following regimens may be used on an ambulatory basis:

    Aqueous procaine penicillin G 4.8 million U IM at 2 separate sites with probenecid 1.0 g PO

or

    Amoxicillin 3.0 g or ampicillin 3.5 g with probenecid 1.0 g PO in a single dose

or

    Cefoxitin 2.0 g IM with probenecid 1.0 g PO

or

    Ceftriaxone 250 mg IM in a single dose*

All followed by

    Doxycycline 100 mg PO, twice daily for † 10-14 days

---

*Ceftriaxone is the only regimen effective against PID associated with resistant *N. gonorrhoeae*. It should be used if resistant strain is cultured, or if sensitivity is unknown. Chlamydia needs to be treated as well.

†Tetracycline hydrochloride, 500 mg PO 4 times a day for 10-14 days may also be used but is less active against certain infections.

N.B. Follow-up: Clinical re-evaluation of ambulatory patients treated for PID must be done in 48-72 hours. Nonresponders should be hospitalized.

EPIDIDYMITIS

- Must be differentiated from testicular torsion (see p 150)
- Etiology: *N. gonorrhoeae, C. trachomatis,* viruses, gram-negative organisms (associated with UTI), and TB
- Treat gonorrheal epididymitis as for uncomplicated gonorrhea (see above). Must treat for *Chlamydia* (with 10 days of tetracycline, doxycycline, or erythromycin) in addition.
- Follow-up cultures 3-7 days after therapy

Treponema Pallidum (Syphilis)

- Microscopic darkfield examination to identify spirochetes in material obtained from primary chancre, and skin and mucocutaneous lesions
- Serology
  1. Screening test: VDRL; if negative, repeat in 8 wk
  2. Serology may be negative early, i.e., in contacts or in patients with primary lesion
- Confirmatory specific tests: FTA-ABS (fluorescent treponemal antibody absorption), MHA-TP (microhemagglutination test for *T. pallidum*)
- Antibiotic therapy (treat contacts of positive cases as if they have the disease) (Table 10-5)
- Follow-up
  1. Report to Public Health Department for contact tracing
  2. Repeat VDRL at 3, 6, and 12 mo to follow response to treatment

TABLE 10-5 Antibiotic Therapy for Syphilis

	Without Penicillin Allergy	With Penicillin Allergy
Congenital: proven or suspected (VDRL-positive baby with inadequate or unknown history of treatment in mother)		
Symptomatic or asymptomatic (regardless of baseline CSF)	Penicillin G 50,000 U/kg/day IM/IV ÷ q12h for a minimum of 10 days, or procaine penicillin G 50,000 U/kg/day IM once daily for a minimum of 10 days	
Acquired*		
1. Primary, secondary, or early latent (duration < 1 yr)	Benzathine penicillin G 50,000 U/kg IM (maximum 2.4 million U—1.2 million U in each buttock)	Tetracycline (if > 8 yr) or erythromycin† 40 mg/kg/day PO ÷ q6h (maximum 2 g/day) × 15 days
2. Latent (duration > 1 yr) Normal CSF	Benzathine penicillin G 50,000 U/kg (maximum 2.4 million units) IM once weekly × 3 wk	Tetracycline (if > 8 yr) or erythromycin,† 40 mg/kg/day PO ÷ q6h (maximum 2 g/day) × 30 days

Abnormal CSF	Penicillin G 200,000 U/kg/day (maximum 12-18 million U/day) IV ÷ q4h × 10 days; then benzathine penicillin G 50,000 U/kg (maximum 2.4 million U) IM once weekly × 3 doses
	or
	Procaine penicillin G 50,000 U/kg (maximum 2.4 million U) IM daily + probenecid 500 mg PO qid × 10 days; then benzathine penicillin G 50,000 U/kg (maximum 2.4 million U) IM once weekly × 3 doses

*CSF should be examined for cells, protein, and VDRL if neurosyphilis is suspected or if the patient is symptomatic. Also, the CSF should be examined in any case of syphilis of > 1 year's duration when the patient has not been treated with penicillin G.
†Erythromycin has not been proved to be effective; careful follow-up is required.
N.B.: Jarisch-Herxheimer reaction: A febrile reaction may occur 8-12 hr post Rx—most commonly in early syphilis. The reaction is often accompanied by malaise and is not related to drug allergy. It usually lasts a few hours and can be treated with antipyretics.

Contraception

- IUDs are not recommended in nulliparous women, but may be the method of choice in individualized cases (Table 10-6)

BIRTH CONTROL PILLS (Tables 10-7 and 10-8)

- Work up prior to use of birth control pills
  1. Complete history including menstrual and sexual history and physical examination with blood pressure and pelvic examination if sexually active
  2. History of smoking
  3. Pap smear and cultures for gonorrhea and *Chlamydia*
  4. Pregnancy test
  5. Urinalysis
  6. Blood smear
  7. VDRL and rubella immune status
- N.B.: In the healthy adolescent, the risks to health from pregnancy outweigh those of low-dose birth control pills
- Major side effects
  1. Estrogen excess: nausea, vomiting, diarrhea, edema, chloasma, hypertension, breast tenderness
  2. Progesterone excess: acne, hirsutism, alopecia, depression, increased appetite, amenorrhea
- Begin with low-dose estrogen pill, i.e., <50 μg/pill (e.g., Ortho 1/35, Min-Ovral)

TABLE 10-6 Contraceptive Methods and Efficacy with Full Compliance

Method	Efficacy* (per 100 woman-years)
Oral contraceptives	98+
Intrauterine devices	96-98
Diaphragm and spermicide†	82-85
Condom and spermicide†	85-95
Condom alone†	70-95
Spermicide alone†	70-75
Rhythm†	65-70
Withdrawal	< 65-70
Postcoital interception (Ovral, 2 tabs q12h × 2 doses)	~98
Abstinence†	100

*Efficacy is lower in adolescents.
†N.B.: These methods are notoriously poorly used in adolescents.
From Special Advisory Committee on Reproductive Physiology to the Health Protection Branch, Health and Welfare, Canada. Report on oral contraceptives, 1985:12-13.

TABLE 10-7 Oral Contraceptives Available in Canada*

Product	Manufacturer	Estrogen	μg/Tablet†	Progestogen	μg/Tablet†
Estrogen, 20, 30, and 35 μg					
Minestrin 1/20	Parke-Davis	Ethinyl estradiol	20	Norethindrone acetate	1000
Min-Ovral	Wyeth	Ethinyl estradiol	30	d-Norgestrel‡	150
Loestrin 1.5/30	Parke-Davis	Ethinyl estradiol	30	Norethindrone acetate	1500
Demulen 30	Searle	Ethinyl estradiol	30	Ethynodiol diacetate	2000
Ortho 1/35	Ortho	Ethinyl estradiol	35	Norethindrone	1000
Ortho 0.5/35	Ortho	Ethinyl estradiol	35	Norethindrone	500
Brevicon 0.5/35	Syntex	Ethinyl estradiol	35	Norethindrone	500
Brevicon 1/35	Syntex	Ethinyl estradiol	35	Norethindrone	1000
Ortho 10/11[S,¶]	Ortho	Ethinyl estradiol	35(21)	Norethindrone	500(10) 1000(11)
Ortho 7/7/7[∥,¶]	Ortho	Ethinyl estradiol	35(21)	Norethindrone	500 (7) 750 (7) 1000 (7)

Triphasil‖,¶	Wyeth	Ethinyl estradiol	30 (6) 40 (5) 30(10)	d-Norgestrel‡	50 (6) 75 (5) 125(10)
Triquilar	Berlex	Ethinyl estradiol	30 (6) 40 (5) 30(10)	d-Norgestrel	50 (6) 75 (5) 125(10)

Estrogen, 50 μg: For contraception only when lower-dose formulations prove unsatisfactory**

Ovral	Wyeth	Ethinyl estradiol	50	d-Norgestrel‡	250
Norlestrin 1/50	Parke-Davis	Ethinyl estradiol	50	Norethindrone acetate	1000
Norlestrin 2.5/50	Parke-Davis	Ethinyl estradiol	50	Norethindrone acetate	2500
Demulen 50	Searle	Ethinyl estradiol	50	Ethynodiol diacetate	1000
Ortho-Novum 1/50	Ortho	Mestranol	50	Norethindrone	1000
Norinyl 1/50	Syntex	Mestranol	50	Norethindrone	1000

*Most of the estrogen–progestogen combination products listed in this table are also available with inert tablets that permit uninterrupted 28-day cycles of therapy.
†Days in parentheses for biphasics and triphasics.
‡Supplied as the dl – racemate in double the amount shown.
§Biphasic product.
‖Triphasic product.
¶The number of days each dosage of estrogen and progestogen is to be taken is shown in brackets in the dosage columns.
**Prolonged use of products with ≥ 50 μg of estrogen should be used only under the supervision of a gynecologist.
Modified from Special Advisory Committee on Reproductive Physiology to the Health Protection Branch, Health and Welfare, Canada. Report on oral contraceptives, 1985:16-17.

TABLE 10-8 Contraindications to Use of Birth Control Pill

Absolute contraindications
  Thromboembolic disorders
  Cerebrovascular accident
  Coronary artery disease
  Hepatic adenoma
  Breast or gynecologic estrogen-dependent malignancy
  Pregnancy
  Undiagnosed vaginal bleeding
  Active liver disease

Relative contraindications
  Hypertension
  Diabetes mellitus
  Acute phase mononucleosis
  Sickle cell disease
  Impaired liver function within last year
  Cardiac or renal disease
  Depression
  Epilepsy (pill may not be as effective if patient is taking anticonvulsants concurrently)
  Lipid disorders
  Migraine
  Smoking

Sexual Assault

- If the assault occurred within 24 hr, then a complete examination should be done immediately; otherwise examination can be done at the physician's and patient's convenience
- Contact local child protection services and the police (if patient <16 yr).
- Adolescent ≥16 years, contact police if they wish to press charges
- Obtain a brief history from the parents or guardians and then a full history from the patient. Record specific data and use the patient's own words.
- Obtain written consent prior to the examination from patient or guardian
- Use a sexual assault kit to collect appropriate specimens, and label them carefully. Follow enclosed guidelines (i.e., label slides with a diamond pencil; put clothing into paper bags), and give the evidence directly to the police officer. Obtain a signed receipt for the evidence.
- Perform a full physical and record all pertinent data carefully. Where possible, illustrate with diagrams and obtain medical photographs.
- Assess and record the patient's emotional state
- Examine the following specimens immediately: urine for hemoglobin, RBCs, and sperm; wet mount of vaginal swab for motile sperm
- Take appropriate samples for STDs
  1. Gonococcal swabs—endocervix, vaginal, urethral, rectal, and oral
  2. *Chlamydia*—endocervix, oral, rectal
  3. VDRL and follow-up in 8 wk with repeat VDRL
- Gynecology referral if a surgical problem is found—e.g., cervical or vaginal tear
- Prevent pregnancy ("morning after" pill)
  1. Treatment applies to all peri- and postmenarchal women regardless of the timing in the cycle; given within 72 hours of coitus
  2. Ovral, 2 tabs PO q12h × 2 doses
  3. N.B.: Serum β-hCG is positive at 29 days after last menstrual period

- STD prophylaxis
  1. Ceftriaxone, 250 mg IM
  2. Treat for *Chlamydia* as well (see p 137)
- Follow-up essential: psychologic/emotional counseling, as well as medical
- Refer to a rape crisis center if desired by patient or family
- Consider hepatitis B prophylaxis

Acute Scrotum

- Keep patient NPO: requires urgent referral to urologist in all cases
- Major differential diagnosis is epididymitis vs. torsion of appendix vs. torsion of testis + spermatic cord vs inguinal hernia
- History important: acute torsion of testis more likely with history of precipitating factor (e.g., stepping out of bathtub), cryptorchidism, peripubertal child. Torsion of appendix more common in ~ 6-7 yr old, less painful, more localized to upper pole (may have small palpable mass)
- With epididymitis and orchitis: investigate genitourinary tract with ultrasonography; occurs in older and/or sexually active boys ± urethritis
- Doppler studies: standard Doppler unreliable (may pick up signals from surrounding tissues and give false-negative results: i.e., torsion present in spite of signal pick-up). Color Doppler more reliable.
- Nuclear scan for torsion within first 12 hr after age 8. After 1-2 days, inflammation or even infarction may show increased uptake (i.e., difficult to differentiate epididymitis from torsion).
- Even if manual detorsion performed, patient must undergo bilateral orchiopexy as soon as possible
- Neonatal testicular torsion: generally involves entire scrotal contents (vs. cord only in older children where processus vaginalis obliterated). Virtually no chance of salvaging functional testicular tissue. Generally explored electively at age 6 mo with contralateral orchiopexy done at that time.

Neurogenic Bladder

- Refers to dyssynergy between bladder detrusor muscle tone and sphincter tone, most common in spinal cord injury or congenital anomaly (neural tube defects)
- Intravesical storage pressure is major predictor of upper urinary tract damage secondary to reflux; generally occurs if pressure > 35 cm H_2O
- Low sphincter tone may be managed with α-adrenergics (e.g., ephedrine) or surgical "tightening" (artificial sphincter)
- Spastic sphincter and unstable detrusor usually managed with antispasmodic (oxybutynin) $\pm$ surgery in conjunction with intermittent catheterization protocols
- Prophylactic antibiotics (trimethoprim-sulfamethoxazole)
- Concomitant constipation may contribute to high intravesical pressures

ELEVEN

Growth and Development

TABLE 11-1 Emerging Patterns of Behavior, from Birth Through Five Years*†

Neonatal period (first 4 weeks)

- **Prone:** Lies in flexed attitude; turns head from side to side; head sags on ventral suspension
- **Supine:** Generally flexed and a little stiff
- **Visual:** May fixate face or light in line of vision; "doll's-eye" movement of eyes on turning of the body
- **Reflex:** Moro response active; stepping and placing reflexes; grasp reflex active
- **Social:** Visual preference for human face

At 4 weeks

- **Prone:** Legs more extended; holds chin up; turns head; head lifted momentarily to plane of body on ventral suspension
- **Supine:** Tonic neck posture predominates; supple and relaxed; head lags on pull to sitting position
- **Visual:** Watches person; follows moving object
- **Social:** Body movements in cadence with voice of other in social contact; beginning to smile

At 8 weeks

- **Prone:** Raises head slightly farther; head sustained in plane of body on ventral suspension
- **Supine:** Tonic neck posture predominates; head lags on pull to sitting position
- **Visual:** Follows moving object 180 degrees
- **Social:** Smiles on social contact; listens to voice and coos

Continued.

---

*From Behrman RE, Vaughan VC, eds. Nelson textbook of pediatrics. 13th ed. Philadelphia: WB Saunders, 1987.
†Data are derived from those of Gesell, Shirley, Provence, Wolf, Bailey, and others. After 5 years the Stanford-Binet, Wechsler-Bellevue, and other scales offer the most precise estimates of developmental level. In order to have their greatest value, they should be administered only by an experienced and qualified person.

TABLE 11-1 Emerging Patterns of Behavior, from Birth Through Five Years (Cont'd)

At 12 weeks
- Prone: Lifts head and chest, arms extended; head above plane of body on ventral suspension
- Supine: Tonic neck posture predominates; reaches toward and misses objects; waves at toy
- Sitting: Head lag partially compensated on pull to sitting position; early head control with bobbing motion; back rounded
- Reflex: Typical Moro response has not persisted; makes defense movements or selective withdrawal reactions
- Social: Sustained social contact; listens to music; says "aah, ngah"

At 16 weeks
- Prone: Lifts head and chest, head in approximately vertical axis; legs extended
- Supine: Symmetrical posture predominates, hands in midline; reaches and grasps objects and brings them to mouth
- Sitting: No head lag on pull to sitting position; head steady, held forward; enjoys sitting with full truncal support
- Standing: When held erect, pushes with feet
- Adaptive: Sees pellet, but makes no move to it
- Social: Laughs out loud; may show displeasure if social contact is broken; excited at sight of food

At 28 weeks
- Prone: Rolls over; may pivot
- Supine: Lifts head; rolls over; squirming movements

Sitting:	Sits briefly, with support of pelvis; leans forward on hands; back rounded
Standing:	May support most of weight; bounces actively
Adaptive:	Reaches out for and grasps large object; *transfers* objects from hand to hand; grasps using radial palm; rakes at pellet
Language:	Polysyllabic vowel sounds formed
Social:	Prefers mother; babbles; enjoys mirror; responds to changes in emotional content of social contact

At 40 weeks

Sitting:	Sits up alone and indefinitely without support, back straight
Standing:	Pulls to standing position
Motor:	Creeps or crawls
Adaptive:	Grasps objects with *thumb and forefinger;* pokes at things with forefinger; picks up pellet with assisted pincer movement; uncovers hidden toy; attempts to retrieve dropped object; releases object grasped by other person
Language:	Repetitive consonant sounds (mamma, dada)
Social:	Responds to sound of name; plays peek-a-boo or pat-a-cake; waves bye-bye

At 52 weeks (1 year)

Motor:	Walks with one hand held; "cruises" or walks holding on to furniture
Adaptive:	Picks up pellet with unassisted pincer movement of forefinger and thumb; releases object to other person on request or gesture
Language:	A few words besides mama, dada
Social:	Plays simple ball game; makes postural adjustment to dressing

Continued.

TABLE 11-1 Emerging Patterns of Behavior, from Birth Through Five Years (Cont'd)

15 months
- Motor: Walks alone; crawls up stairs
- Adaptive: Makes tower of 2 cubes; makes a line with crayon; inserts pellet in bottle
- Language: Jargon; follows simple commands; may name a familiar object (ball)
- Social: Indicates some desires or needs by pointing; hugs parents

18 months
- Motor: Runs stiffly; sits on small chair; walks up stairs with one hand held; explores drawers and waste baskets
- Adaptive: Piles 3 cubes; imitates scribbling; imitates vertical stroke; dumps pellet from bottle
- Language: 10 words (average); names pictures; identifies one or more parts of body
- Social: Feeds self; seeks help when in trouble; may complain when wet or soiled; kisses parent with pucker

24 months
- Motor: Runs well; walks up and down stairs, one step at a time; opens doors; climbs on furniture
- Adaptive: Tower of 6 cubes; circular scribbling; imitates horizontal stroke; folds paper once imitatively
- Language: Puts 3 words together (subject, verb, object)
- Social: Handles spoon well; often tells immediate experiences; helps to undress; listens to stories with pictures

30 months
- Motor: Jumps

Adaptive:	Tower of 8 cubes; makes vertical and horizontal strokes, but generally will not join them to make a cross; imitates circular stroke, forming closed figure
Language:	Refers to self by pronoun "I"; knows full name
Social:	Helps put things away; pretends in play

36 months

Motor:	Goes up stairs alternating feet; rides tricycle; stands momentarily on one foot
Adaptive:	Tower of 9 cubes; imitates construction of "bridge" of 3 cubes; copies a circle; imitates a cross
Language:	Knows age and sex; counts 3 objects correctly; repeats 3 numbers or a sentence of 6 syllables
Social:	Plays simple games (in "parallel" with other children); helps in dressing (unbuttons clothing and puts on shoes); washes hands

48 months

Motor:	Hops on one foot; throws ball overhand; uses scissors to cut out pictures; climbs well
Adaptive:	Copies bridge from model; imitates construction of "gate" of 5 cubes; copies cross and square; draws a man with 2 to 4 parts besides head; names longer of 2 lines
Language:	Counts 4 pennies accurately; tells a story
Social:	Plays with several children with beginning of social interaction and role-playing; goes to toilet alone

60 months

Motor:	Skips
Adaptive:	Draws triangle from copy; names heavier of 2 weights
Language:	Names 4 colors; repeats sentence of 10 syllables; counts 10 pennies correctly
Social:	Dresses and undresses; asks questions about meaning of words; domestic role-playing

TABLE 11-2 Physician's Speech and Language Checklist: Birth to Five Years

Birth to 6 months
Startles to loud, sudden noises
Sometimes stirs or awakens when sleeping quietly and someone makes a loud noise
(3 to 6 months) stops moving when called

6 to 12 months
Turns toward a sound or when his name is called
Babbles, laughs, or makes sounds like "ga-ga," "ma-ma," or "ba-ba"

12 to 15 months
Repeats sounds
Understands some simple phrases like "Come here," "Don't touch"
Recognizes telephone or doorbell ringing

15 to 18 months
Says four to six words
Tells what he wants by pointing and saying a word
Understands phrases like "Give me that" when gestures are used
Recognizes names of common objects like ball, table, bed, car
Uses names of familiar things like water, cup, cookie, clock

18 to 24 months
Uses two word combinations
Says about 20 or more words
Uses words to express physical needs

Follows simple directions like "Sit down," "Give me that ball"
Points to appropriate picture when you say "Show me the dog (hat, man, etc.)"

2 to 3 years

Uses three word sentences
Tells a story or expresses his feelings in words
Remembers some recent past events
Counts to 3
Tells his first and last names
Is understood in 40 to 50% of what he says by people outside the family

3 to 4 years

Uses four to five word sentences
Tells a story
Asks a lot of questions
Repeats a sentence of eight to nine syllables, e.g., "We are going to buy some candy"
Names three colors
Uses plurals like "toys," "balls"
Can repeat three or four numbers

4 to 5 years

Can define four or more common words or tell how the objects are used (e.g., hat, dish, apples)
Can name a penny, a nickel, and a dime
Is understood in 80 to 90% of what he says by people outside the family
Likes to look at books and have someone read to him
Uses I, me, you, he, and him properly

Adapted from Speech and hearing checklist for the family physician. Toronto, Ontario: The Ontario Association Speech-Language Pathologists and Audiologists.

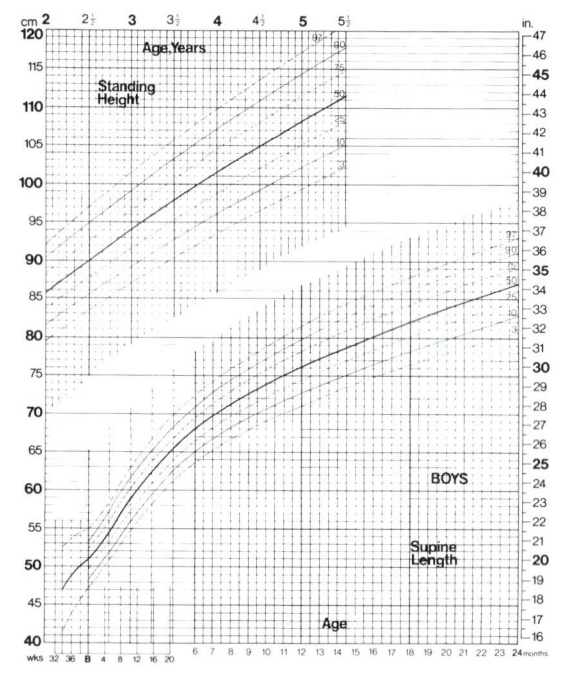

Figure 11-1 **Boys: birth through 5 years: height. Note: Age scale is divided into months.** (From Tanner JM, Whitehouse RH. Growth and development record. Swains Mill, Herts, England: Castlemead Publications, Ward's Publishing Services, 1984.)

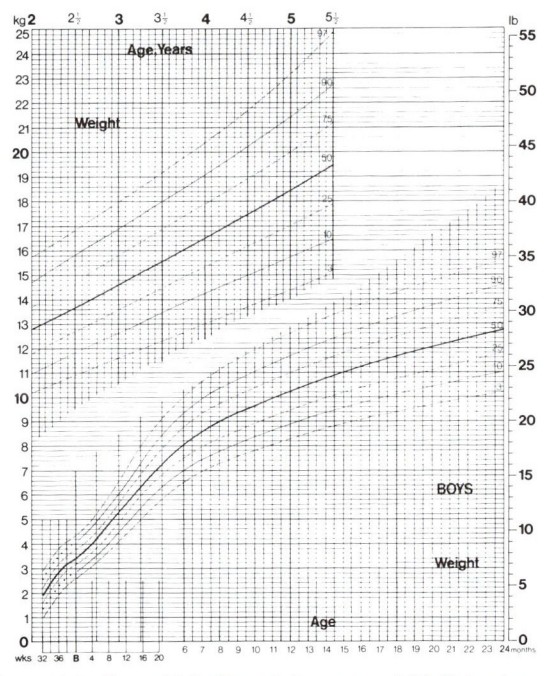

Figure 11-2 **Boys: birth through 5 years: weight. Note: Age scale is divided into months.** (From Tanner JM, Whitehouse RH. Growth and development record. Swains Hill, Herts, England: Castlemead Publications, Ward's Publishing Services, 1984.)

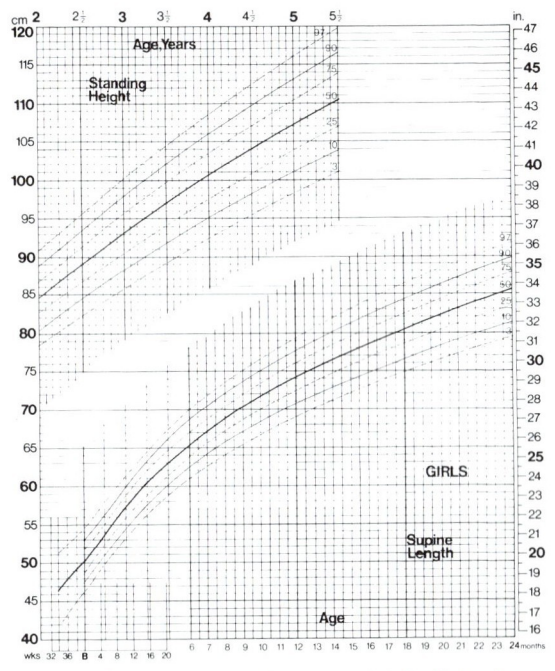

Figure 11-3 **Girls: birth through 5 years: height. Note: Age scale is divided into months.** (From Tanner JM, Whitehouse RH. Growth and development record. Swains Mill, Herts, England: Castlemead Publications, Ward's Publishing Services, 1984.)

Growth and Development 163

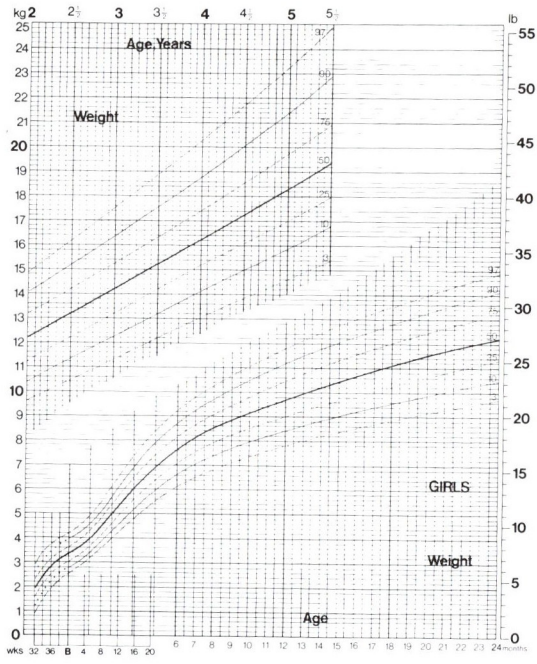

Figure 11-4 **Girls: birth through 5 years: weight. Note: Age scale is divided into months.** (From Tanner JM, Whitehouse RH. Growth and development record. Swains Mill, Herts, England: Castlemead Publications, Ward's Publishing Services, 1984.)

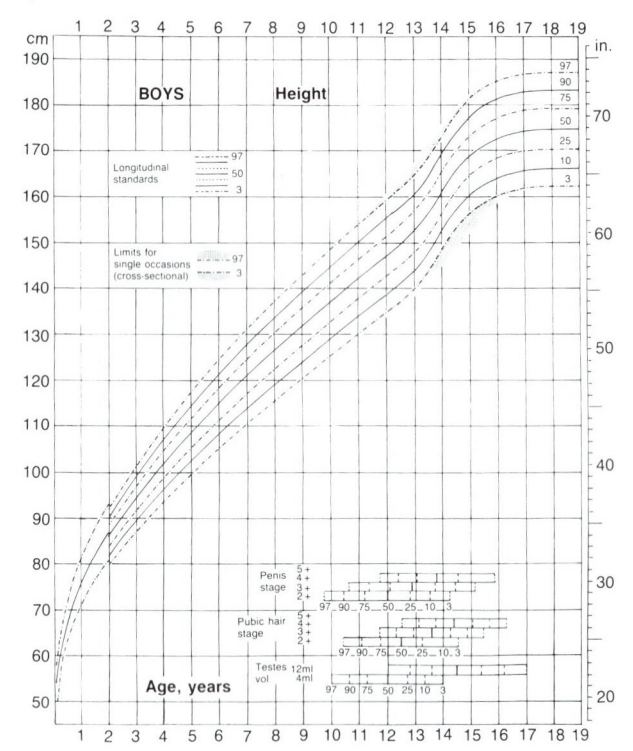

Figure 11-5 **Boys: birth through 19 years: height.** (From Tanner JM, Whitehouse RH. Growth and development record. London: University of London, Institute of Child Health, 1966.)

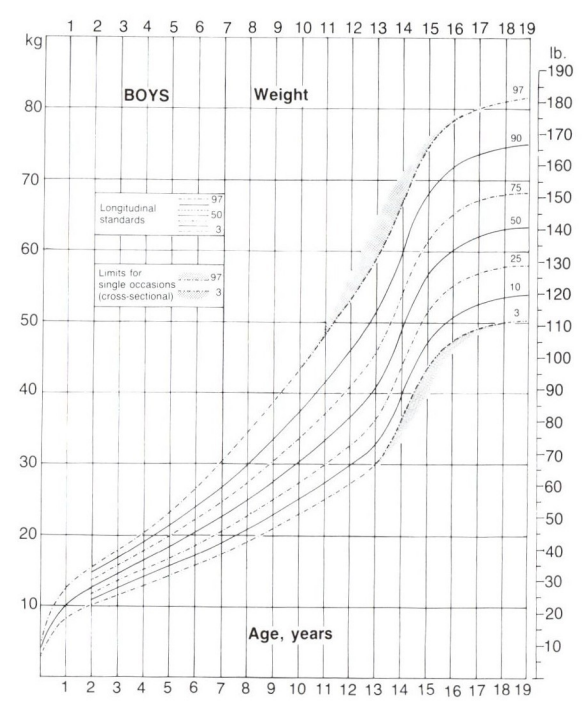

Figure 11-6 **Boys: birth through 19 years: weight.** (From Tanner JM, Whitehouse RH. Growth and development record. London: University of London, Institute of Child Health, 1966.)

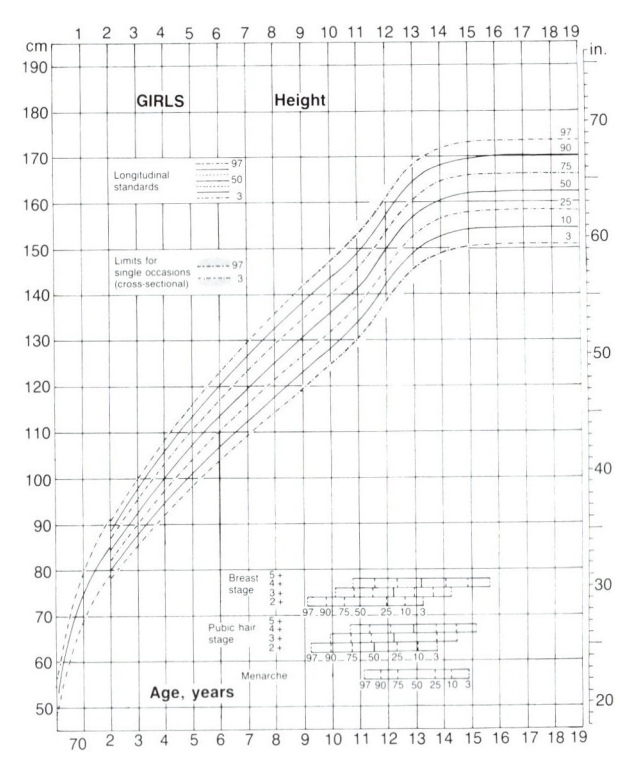

Figure 11-7 **Girls: birth through 19 years: height.** (From Tanner JM, Whitehouse RH. Growth and development record. London: University of London, Institute of Child Health, 1966.)

Growth and Development

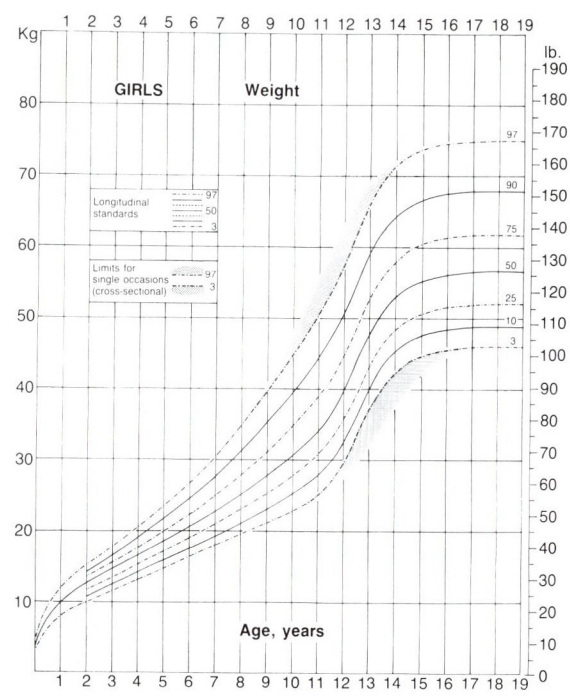

Figure 11-8 **Girls: birth through 19 years: weight.** (From Tanner JM, Whitehouse RH. Growth and development record. London: University of London, Institute of Child Health, 1966.)

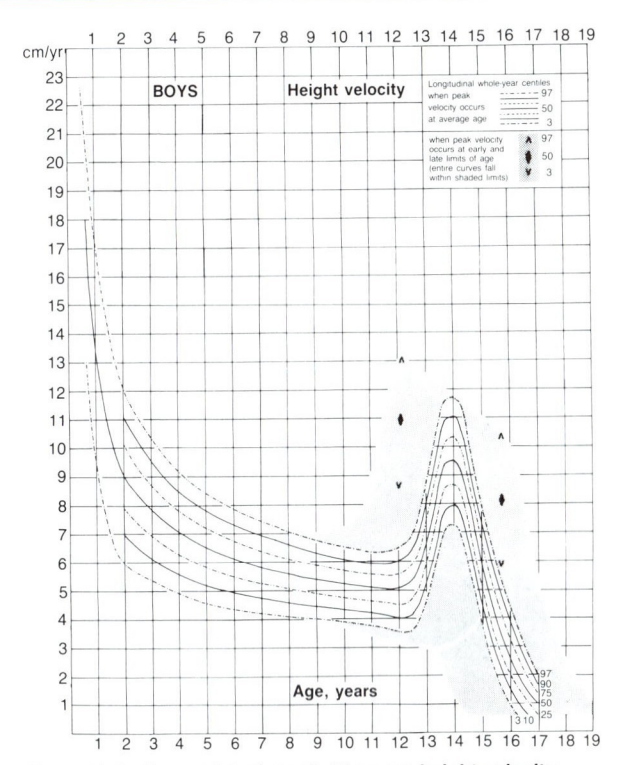

Figure 11-9 **Boys: birth through 19 years: height velocity.** (From Tanner JM, Whitehouse RH. Growth and development record. London: University of London, Institute of Child Health, 1966.)

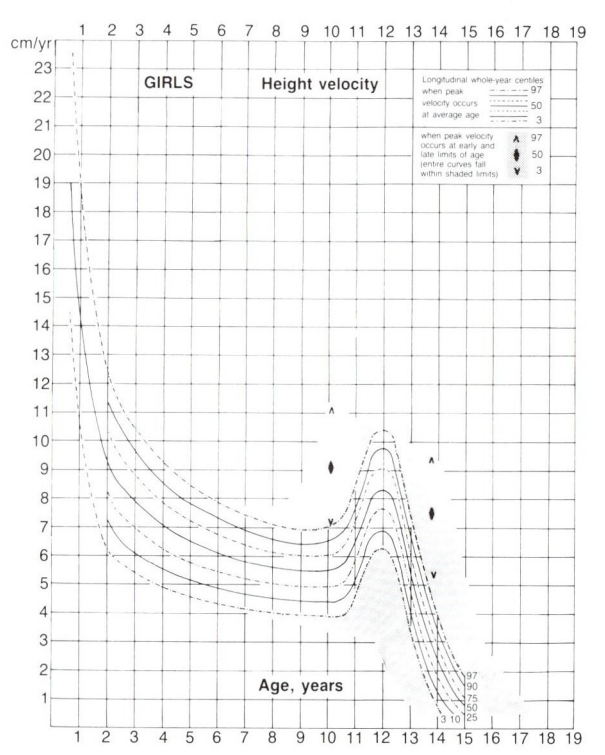

Figure 11-10 **Girls: birth through 19 years: height velocity.** (From Tanner JM, Whitehouse RH. Growth and development record. London: University of London, Institute of Child Health, 1966.)

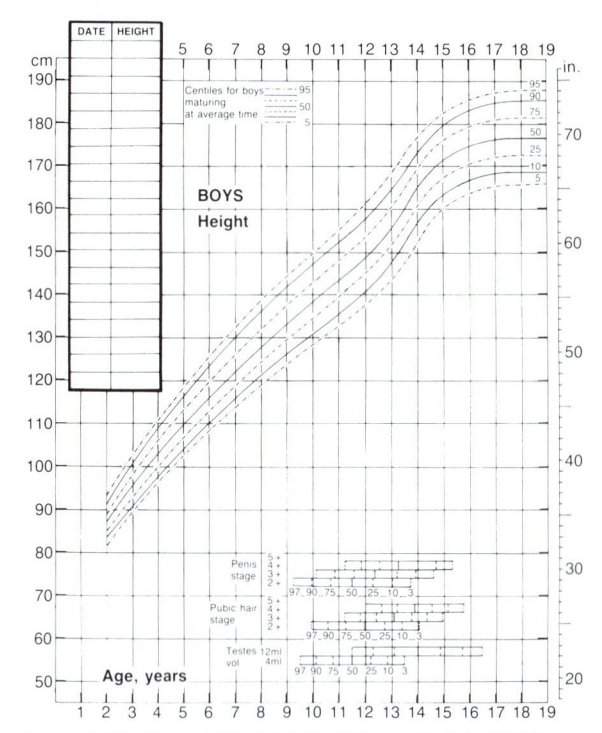

Figure 11-11 **Boys: birth through 19 years: height (North American standards).** (Modified from Tanner JM, Davies PSW. Clinical longitudinal standards for height and height velocity for North American children. J Pediatr 1985; 107:320.)

Growth and Development

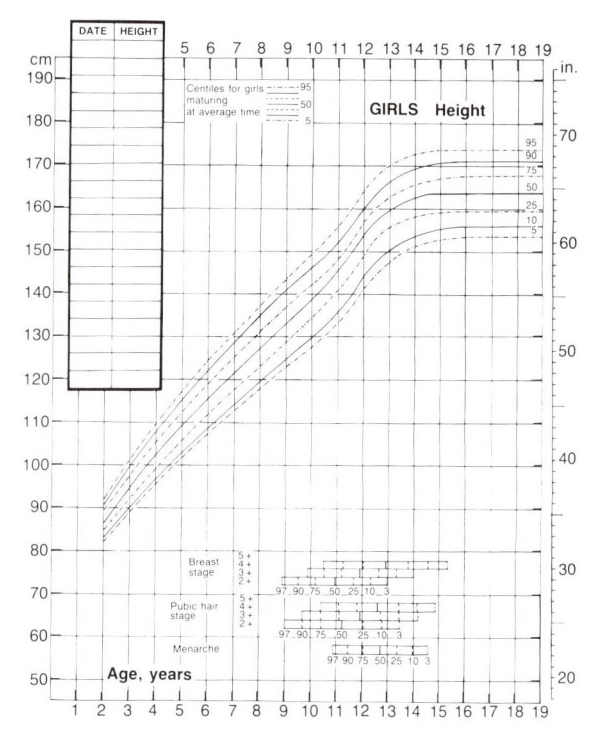

Figure 11-12 **Girls: birth through 19 years: height (North American standards).** (Modified from Tanner JM, Davies PSW. Clinical longitudinal standards for height and height velocity for North American children. J Pediatr 1985; 107:322.)

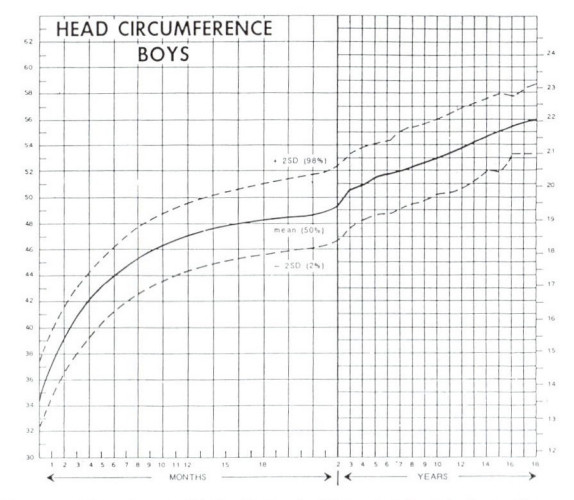

Figure 11-13 **Boys: birth through 18 years: head circumference.** (From G. Neihaus. Pediatrics 1968; 41:106. Reproduced with permission of Pediatrics.)

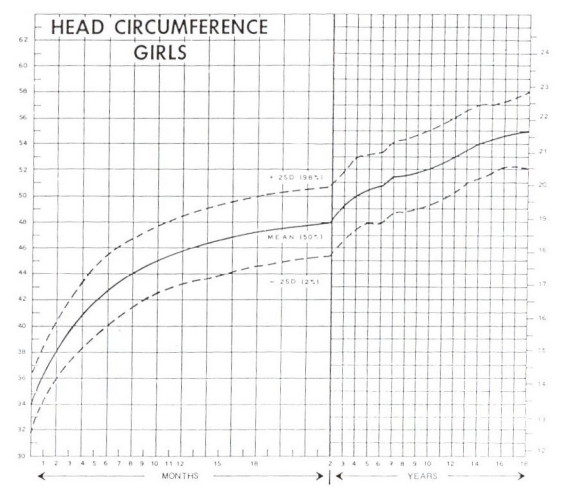

Figure 11-14 **Girls: birth through 18 years: head circumference.** (From G. Nelhaus. Pediatrics 1968; 41:106. Reproduced with permission of Pediatrics.)

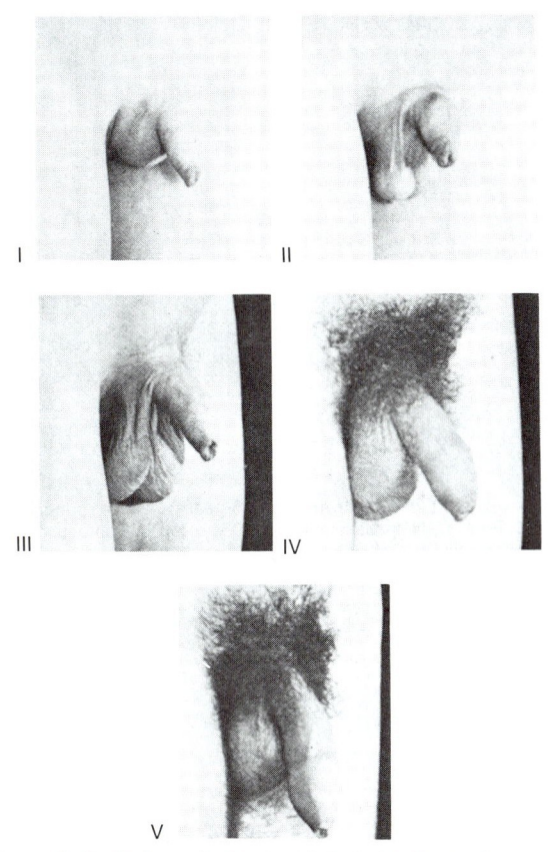

Figure 11-15 **Male genital and pubic hair development.** *Stage I:* prepubertal. *Stage II:* enlargement of testes, appearance of scrotal reddening, and increase in scrotal rugations. *Stage III:* increase in length and, to a lesser extent, breadth of penis, with further growth of testes. *Stage IV:* further increase in size of penis and testes and darkening of scrotal skin. **Stage V:** adult. (Modified from Van Wieringen, Wafelbakker F, Verbrugge HP. et al. Growth diagrams, 1965. Netherlands: Wolters-Noordhoff, 1971.)

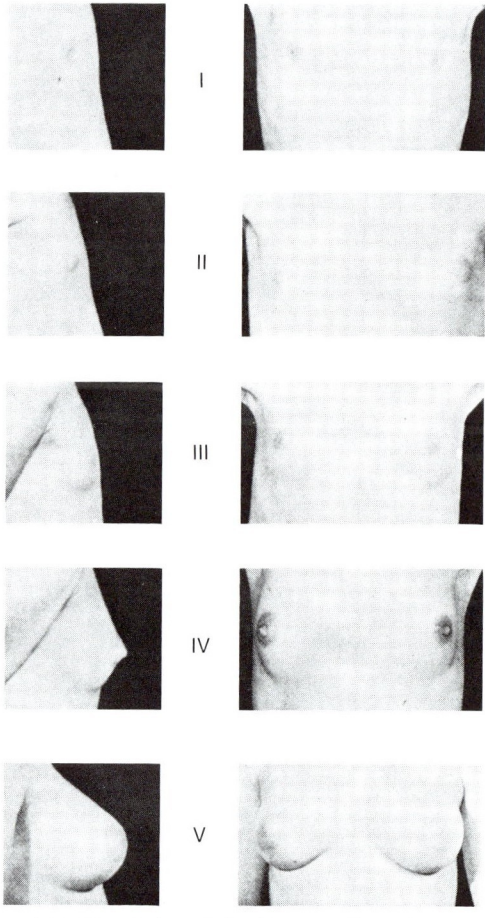

Figure 11-16 **Female breast development. *Stage I:* prepubertal. *Stage II:* budding. *Stage III:* appearance of small adult breast. *Stage IV:* areola and papilla form a secondary mound. *Stage V:* adult** (Modified from Van Wieringen, Wafelbakker F, Verbrugge HP. et al. Growth diagrams, 1965. Netherlands: Wolters-Noordhoff, 1971.)

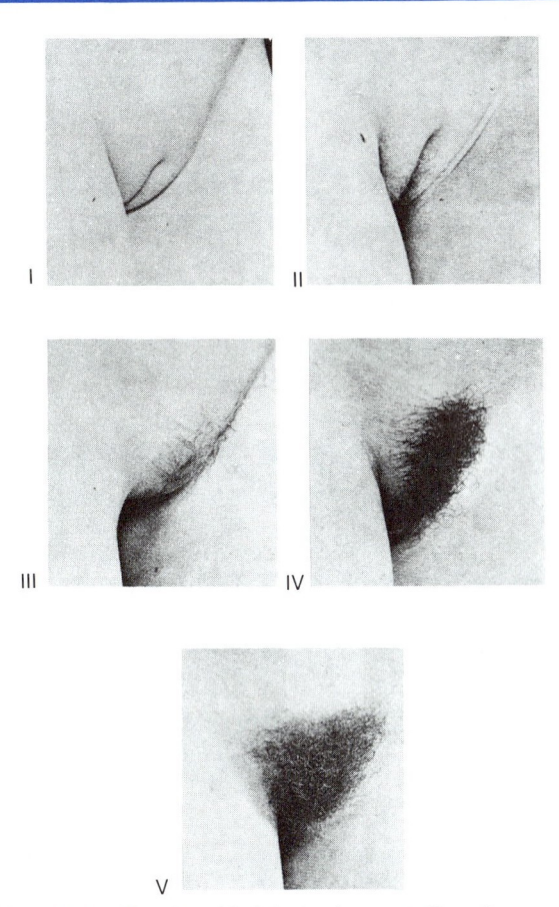

Figure 11-17 **Female pubic hair development. *Stage I:* prepubertal. *Stage II:* sparse growth of long, slightly pigmented hair. *Stage III:* hair darker, coarser, and curlier, and beginning to spread over symphysis pubis. *Stage IV:* hair is adult in character but not distribution, without spread to medial surface of thigh. *Stage V:* adult** (From Van Wieringen, Wafelbakker F, Verbrugge HP. et al. Growth diagrams, 1965. Netherlands: Wolters-Noordhoff, 1971.)

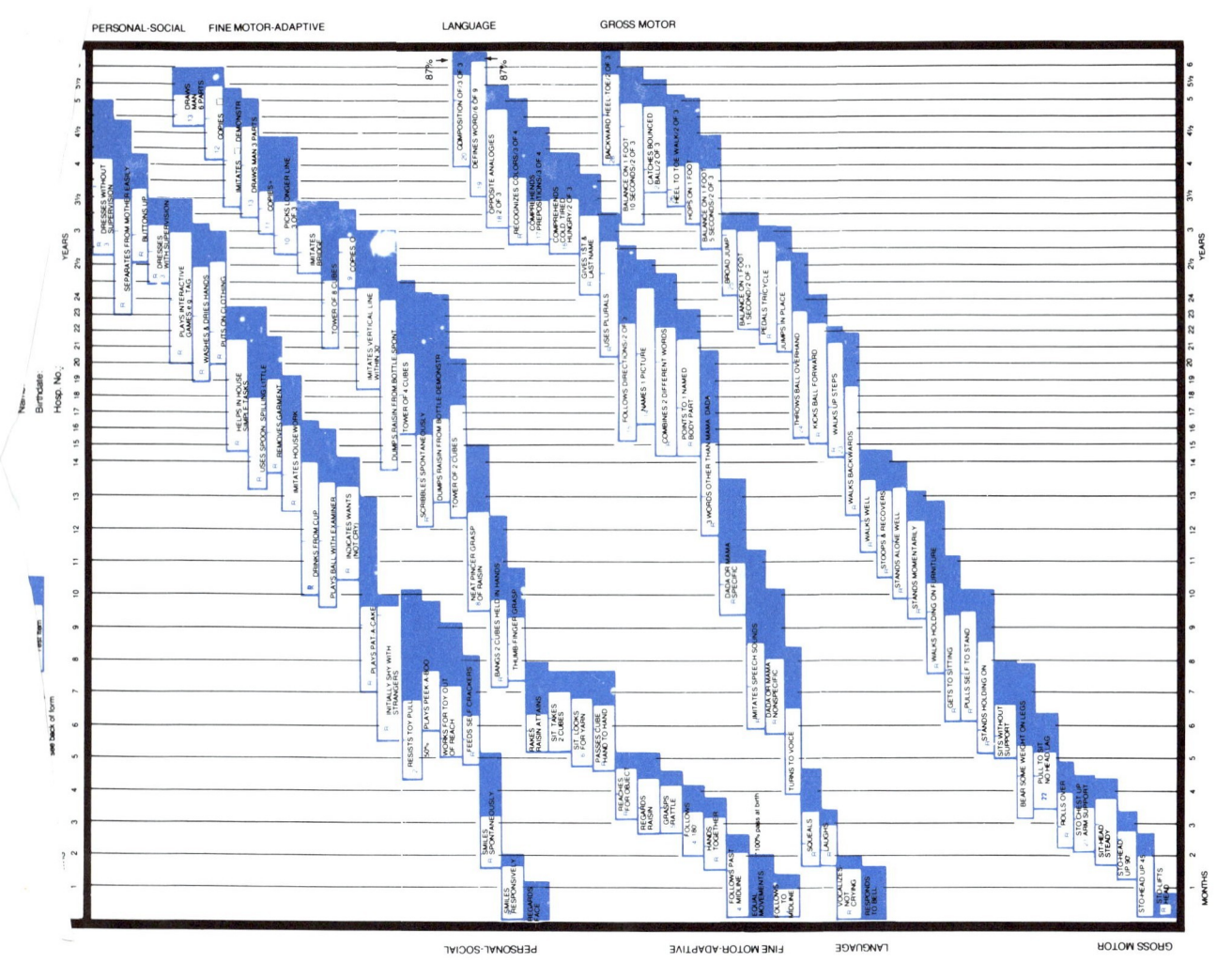

18 **Denver developmental screening test.** (From Frankenburg WK, Dodds JB. Denver: University of Colorado Medical Center, 1978.)

TABLE 11-3 Stretched Penile Length

	Mean ± S.D.*	Mean − 2½ S.D.*
Newborn: 30 wk	2.5±0.4	1.5
34 wk	3.0±0.4	2.0
term	3.5±0.4	2.5-2.4
0-5 mo	3.9±0.8	1.9
6-12 mo	4.3±0.8	2.3
1-2 yr	4.7±0.8	2.6
2-3 yr	5.1±0.9	2.9
3-4 yr	5.5±0.9	3.3
4-5 yr	5.7±0.9	3.5
5-6 yr	6.0±0.9	3.8
6-7 yr	6.1±0.9	3.9
7-8 yr	6.2±1.0	3.7
8-9 yr	6.3±1.0	3.8
9-10 yr	6.3±1.0	3.8
10-11	6.4±1.1	3.7
Adult	13.3±1.6	9.3

*Stretched penile length (cm) in normal males.
Adapted from Lee PA, Mazur T, Danish R, et al. Micropenis I. Criteria, etiologies and classification. Johns Hopkins Med J 1980;146:158.

TABLE 11-4 Chronology of Human Dentition

	Calcification		Eruption		Shedding	
	Begins At	Complete At	Maxillary	Mandibular	Maxillary	Mandibular
Primary or deciduous teeth						
Central incisors	5th fetal mo	18-24 mo	6-8 mo	5-7 mo	7-8 yr	6-7 yr
Lateral incisors	5th fetal mo	18-24 mo	8-11 mo	7-10 mo	8-9 yr	7-8 yr
Cuspids (canines)	6th fetal mo	30-36 mo	16-20 mo	16-20 mo	11-12 yr	9-11 yr
First molars	5th fetal mo	24-30 mo	10-16 mo	10-16 mo	10-11 yr	10-12 yr
Second molars	6th fetal mo	36 mo	20-30 mo	20-30 mo	10-12 yr	11-13 yr

Secondary or permanent teeth

Central incisors	3-4 mo	7-8 yr	6-7 yr
Lateral incisors	Max., 10-12 mo	8-9 yr	7-8 yr
	Mand., 3-4 mo		
Cuspids (canines)	4-5 mo	11-12 yr	9-11 yr
First premolars (bicuspids)	18-21 mo	10-11 yr	10-12 yr
Second premolars (bicuspids)	24-30 mo	10-12 yr	11-13 yr
First molars	Birth	6-7 yr	6-7 yr
Second molars	30-36 mo	12-13 yr	12-13 yr
Third molars	Max., 7-9 yr	17-22 yr	17-22 yr
	Mand., 8-10 yr		

From Behrman RE, Vaughan VC, eds. Nelson textbook of pediatrics. 13th ed. Philadelphia: WB Saunders, 1987:25.

TWELVE

Hematology and Oncology

Anemia

- Definition: Hb or hematocrit less than age-appropriate values (see laboratory values section, p 582)
- Volume overload may cause falsely low Hb; dehydration, heel prick may cause falsely high Hb
- If patient must receive transfusion before diagnosis is made, obtain blood for Hb electrophoresis, Hb H prep., Heinz body prep., red cell enzymes, vitamin B_{12}, folate

TABLE 12-1 Hematologic Parameters in Various Types of Anemia

Test	Aplastic Anemia	Thalassemia Major	Thalassemia Minor	Iron Deficiency	Anemia of Chronic Disease
Hemoglobin	↓*	↓	↓	↓	↓
MCV	N*	↓	↓	↓	N or ↓
MCH	N*	↓	↓	↓	N
Iron	N	↑	N or ↑	↓	N or ↓
TIBC	N	↑	N	↑	↓
Ferritin	N	↑	N or ↑	↓	↑
Transferrin	N	↑	N	↑	N or ↑
Bone marrow stainable iron	N	N	N	Absent	N
Reticulocyte count	↓	N	N	↓	N

*N = normal; ↑ = increased; ↓ = decreased. Additional parameters may be helpful, i.e., ↑ RBC count in thalassemia, ↑ free erythrocyte protoporphyrins in iron-deficiency anemia and lead poisoning.

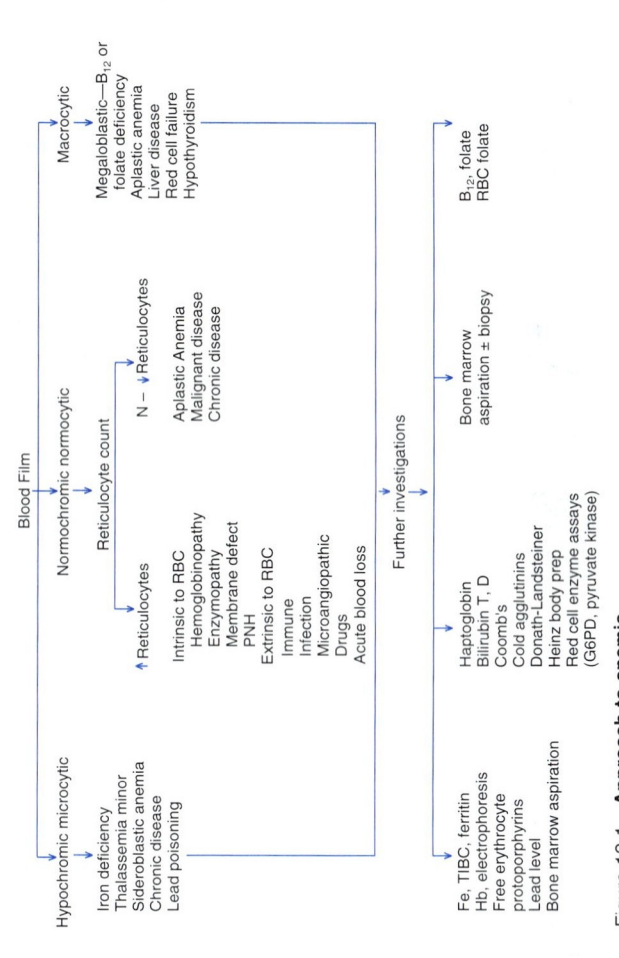

Figure 12-1 **Approach to anemia.**

IRON-DEFICIENCY ANEMIA

Investigations
- Serum Fe decreases, TIBC increases, ferritin decreases
- Free erythrocyte protoporphyrin increases
- Bone marrow stainable iron stores absent

Treatment
- Treat underlying cause, e.g., diet, identify source of blood loss (e.g., milk-induced microscopic blood loss)
- 6 mg elemental iron/kg/day PO divided into three doses on empty stomach ½ hr before meals (ferrous sulfate, ferrous fumarate, ferrous gluconate can be used equally)
- Expect reticulocyte response at 7-10 days
- After Hb becomes normal, treat for 2-3 mo to replenish iron stores
- Therapeutic trial of iron: In an infant 12-24 mo old with hypochromic microcytic anemia, a therapeutic trial of iron may be given for 4 wk without further investigation. If the anemia responds, continue iron therapy. If the anemia fails to respond, further investigation is required.

THALASSEMIA SYNDROMES

α-Thalassemia Minor
- Asymptomatic
- Peripheral smear: hypochromic microcytic red cells
- Hb H (a tetramer of β chains; i.e., $β_4$) prep positive
- *No* treatment required; if present in both parents, prenatal screening may be offered

β-Thalassemia Minor
- Peripheral smear shows microcytic, hypochromic red cells
- Increased HbA_2 on electrophoresis
- No therapy required

β-Thalassemia Major

Usually diagnosed in first year of life (as γ chain synthesis decreases): pallor, fatigue, failure to thrive, hepatosplenomegaly

- Investigations (see Table 12-1)
  1. CBC (decreased Hb, severe hypochromia, microcytosis, target cells, bizarre poikilocytosis)
  2. Hb electrophoresis: decreased or absent Hb A, increased Hb F
- Treatment
  1. Mainstay is *blood transfusion,* either high transfusion regimen (maintain Hb > 100 g/L) or supertransfusion (Hb > 120 g/L) with washed packed cells
  2. Chelation therapy: deferoxamine (desferrioxamine) infused subcutaneously overnight (12 hr) or through central venous line via indwelling subcutaneous port if chronic noncompliance with subcutaneous infusion. Chelation generally begun > age 3 yr due to potential effects on growth in younger children. Monitor neurotoxicity (audio and visual).
  3. Vitamin C: enhances iron excretion, but may be associated with cardiac toxicity; maximum daily dosage 100 mg
  4. Splenectomy when transfusion requirements exceed 220 ml packed RBCs/kg/yr

Hematology and Oncology

HEMOLYTIC ANEMIA

History
- Jaundice (especially neonatal and with infections)
- Anemia
- Painful crises
- Gallstones
- Transfusions
- Splenectomy
- Positive family history
- Acute vs. chronic
- Medications

Symptoms
- Acute
  - Fatigue
  - Headache
  - Dizziness, fainting
  - Fever
  - Abdominal or back pain
- Chronic
  - Gallbladder symptoms

Signs
- Tachycardia
- Dyspnea
- Pallor
- Jaundice
- Splenomegaly
- Dark or red urine
- Growth retardation
- Thalassemic facies
- Leg ulcers

↓

Haptoglobin
Indirect bilirubin
Reticulocytes, polychromasia

↓

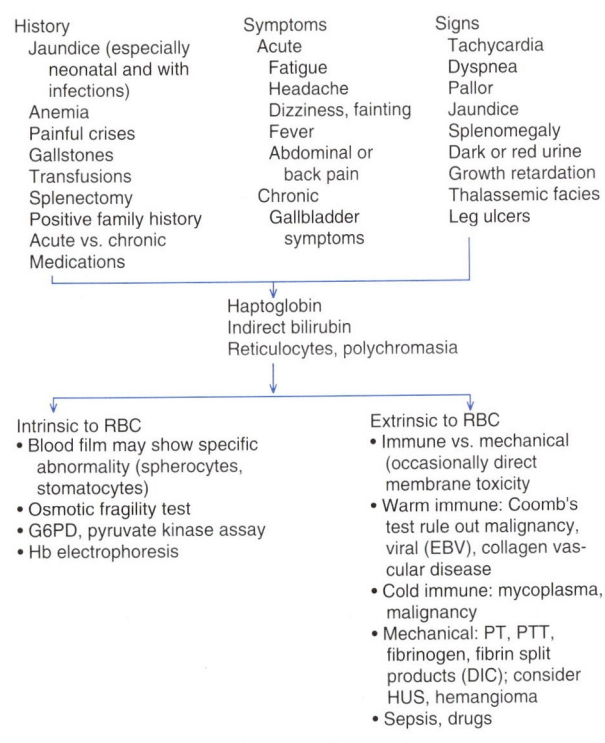

Intrinsic to RBC
- Blood film may show specific abnormality (spherocytes, stomatocytes)
- Osmotic fragility test
- G6PD, pyruvate kinase assay
- Hb electrophoresis

Extrinsic to RBC
- Immune vs. mechanical (occasionally direct membrane toxicity)
- Warm immune: Coomb's test rule out malignancy, viral (EBV), collagen vascular disease
- Cold immune: mycoplasma, malignancy
- Mechanical: PT, PTT, fibrinogen, fibrin split products (DIC); consider HUS, hemangioma
- Sepsis, drugs

Figure 12-2 **Approach to hemolytic anemia.**

SICKLE CELL DISEASE

Vaso-occlusive Crises

- General
  1. Pain management, often parenteral to start
  2. Fluids, 1.5 × maintenance
  3. O_2 (variable)
  4. After 24-48 hr, decrease fluids to maintenance levels
  5. Taper narcotics (10-20% decrements in dose, maintain frequency, change to PO when dose reaches ~ 50% of starting dose)
  6. Analgesia for discharge
- Pulmonary (Table 12-3): Treatment consists of supplemental O_2, broad-spectrum antibiotic coverage, packed RBC transfusion
- Bone (Table 12-4): Treatment same as for general management
- Abdominal
  1. High incidence of cholelithiasis (30% of children >10 yrs)
  2. Rule out surgical abdomen, check ALP, liver function tests, supportive care as above
  3. Elective cholecystectomy for recurrent episodes of pain and gallstones
- Central Nervous System
  1. 5% incidence of cerebral infarction, ⅔ repeat, usually within 3 yr
  2. O_2 therapy indicated in acute situation
  3. Transfusion program to maintain Hb S < 30%
- Priapism: early surgical consultation, sedation, analgesia, fluids as above

TABLE 12-2 Hemoglobin Electrophoresis Patterns in Sickle Cell Disorders

	Major Hemoglobins				
	S	A	F	C	A_2
SA	30-40%	60%	< 2%	0	2%-3.2%
SS	80-90%	0	2-20%	0	2%-3.2%
SC	50%	0	2%	< 50%	...*
SB$^+$thal	55-75%	10-30%	1-13%	0	> 3.2%
SB°thal	80-95%	0	1-15%	0	> 3.2%

*Not available because of difficulty in determining HbA$_2$ in presence of HbC.

TABLE 12-3 Differentiation Between Pneumonia and Pulmonary Infarction

Common features
- Chest pain
- Cough
- Fever
- CXR infiltrates
- Leukocytosis
- Hypoxemia
- Pleural effusion

Features favoring pneumonia
- Age ≤ 5 yr
- Shaking chills
- Upper lobe disease
- Bands > 1000 cells/mm^3
- Sputum Gram stain ⎫
- Cultures   ⎬ Positive
- Cold agglutinins   ⎭

Features favoring infarction
- Associated painful bone crisis
- Clear CXR at onset
- Lower lobe disease

Modified from Platt OS, Nathan DG. Sickle cell disease. In: Nathan DG, Oski FA, eds. Hematology of infancy and childhood. 2nd ed. Philadelphia: WB Saunders, 1981:703.

TABLE 12-4 Differentiation Between Osteomyelitis and Bone Infarction

Common features
Local pain, tenderness, swelling, and erythema
Fever
Leukocytosis

Features favoring osteomyelitis	Features favoring infarction
Single site	Multiple sites
Bands >1000 cells/mm^3	Patient description of "crisis"
Positive cultures	History of predisposing factor
	Negative cultures
	Response without antibiotics

Modified from Platt OS, Nathan DG. Sickle cell disease. In: Nathan DG, Oski FA, eds. Hematology of infancy and childhood. 2nd ed. Philadelphia: WB Saunders, 1981:702.

Anemic Crises

- Aplastic anemia
  1. Usually associated with acute infection (parvovirus)
  2. Supportive care and transfusion
- Acute splenic sequestration
  1. Rapid fall in hemoglobin, decrease in reticulocyte count, and enlarging spleen; may proceed very rapidly to shock
  2. Requires urgent transfusion, supportive care; predictive of subsequent episodes; consider splenectomy

Infection

- Bacterial sepsis *(Streptococcus pneumoniae, Haemophilus influenzae)* is a leading cause of death in SS patients with sickle cell anemia (secondary to RES blockade and impaired splenic function secondary to autoinfarction of the spleen; usually lost completely by age 4-7 yr)
- Other pathogens include *Escherichia coli, Salmonella* (75% of osteomyelitis in sickle cell disease), *Shigella,* and *Mycoplasma*
- May follow a rapidly fulminant course with shock and death within a few hours
- Prevention
  1. Pneumococcal vaccination (initially at 2 yr and booster 5 yr later)
  2. *H. influenzae* vaccine—give at 2 yr of age
  3. Influenza virus vaccination—for those > 6 mo old, given yearly in autumn
  4. Antibiotic prophylaxis
     < 35 mo—Pen-VK 125 mg PO bid
     > 35 mo—Pen-VK 250 mg PO bid
- Management
  1. Compliance with prophylaxis and response to vaccination cannot be assumed
  2. Usually hospitalize if < 3 yr, appears toxic, fever and pain present, infection of lesion or CSF suspected, decreased reticulocyte count below steady state values
  3. Temperature < 38.5° C orally: assess, culture, usually hospitalize; if not admitted, reassess within 24 hr
  4. Temperature > 38.5° C orally: culture, hospitalize, and cover with IV cefuroxime until culture results available

Surgery

- In black children a sickle test and if this is positive, a hemoglobin electrophoresis, should be done on an elective basis prior to any surgery
- Hb SA (sickle trait): no specific preparation
- Hb SS, SC, S thal: routine quantitation of Hb S unnecessary; transfuse to a Hb >100 g/L for routine or emergency surgery or radiologic procedures using contrast materials. For high-risk conditions (cardiovascular, neurosurgical, tourniquets in orthopedic procedures, eye sur-

gery, history of previous stroke), reduce Hb S to < 30% preoperatively.
- Unknown status: elective procedures should be postponed. Emergency procedures may be done following consultation with a hematologist.

Long-Term Management

- Folate supplementation
- Ophthalmology follow-up (proliferative and nonproliferative retinopathy)
- Renal function: tubular function, nephrotic syndrome, hematuria secondary to papillary necrosis
- Hepatobiliary: gallstones in 11-12%; 50% by adulthood
- Pulmonary: multiple chest crises lead to V/Q mismatch; restrictive lung disease as early as age 12 yr

Thrombocytopenia

Investigations

- Hb, platelet count, WBC count and differential, blood film
- Coagulation screen (bleeding time meaningless in the face of thrombocytopenia)
- Sepsis work-up (exclude LP if platelet count < 50,000), to be considered
- PL[A1] antigen and antibody
- Bone marrow examination
- Collagen vascular disease (complement, immunoglobulins, specific autoantibodies—e.g., ANA)

IDIOPATHIC THROMBOCYTOPENIC PURPURA (ITP)

Investigations

- Hb, platelet count, WBC count, differential
- Coombs test
- Blood group
- Collagen vascular disease (complement, immunoglobulins, specific autoantibodies—e.g., ANA)
- Quantitative immunoglobulins
- Bone marrow examination

Treatment

- High dose steroids—prednisone 4 mg/kg/day with rapid taper
- IV gamma globulin, 1g/kg × 2 doses, infused over 12 hr each
- Anti D globulin 25 µg/kg IV push × 2 days—*only* if Rh positive (research protocol)
- If life-threatening bleeding, IV gamma globulin or emergency splenectomy is treatment of choice
- May observe if platelet count > 20,000
- Long-term therapy usually consists of combinations of steroids, intermittent gamma globulin, ± splenectomy

NEONATAL THROMBOCYTOPENIA

If Maternal History of ITP, SLE, or Previously Affected Infant

- Monitor maternal platelet count during pregnancy
- At time of delivery, measure fetal platelet count by fetal scalp sampling
- If fetal platelet count > 50,000 proceed to deliver normally, but if < 50,000, perform cesarean section
- Measure platelet count in cord blood at birth; if normal, monitor for 1 wk, as it may fall
- Measure infant and maternal PL^{A1} antigen and antibody
- Steroid administration to mother in final 2 wk of pregnancy is controversial

Treatment

- Platelet count normal: no therapy
- Maternal PL^{A1}Ag negative: infuse maternal platelets into baby if thrombocytopenic. If mother's platelets or PL^{A1}– negative donor platelets are not available, use random donor platelets.
- Mother PL^{A1} positive, give IV gamma globulin or use steroids. (Platelet infusion may be effective.)

Hematology and Oncology

Coagulation Disorders

```
                    ┌─────────────────────┐
                    │ Coagulation cascade │
                    └─────────────────────┘
    Intrinsic (aPTT)           │           Extrinsic (PT)
                               │
         HMWK                  │
                               │
  Kallikrein ←──── Prekallrein │
                               │
         HMWK                  │
           ↓                   │
   XII ──→ XIIa                │
                               │
         HMWK                  │
           ↓                   │
    XI ──→ XIa                 │
              Ca++             │
    IX ──→ IXa                 │   VIIa ←── VII
                               │
         PL  VIIIa             │     TF
             Ca++              │     Ca++
```

Common Pathway

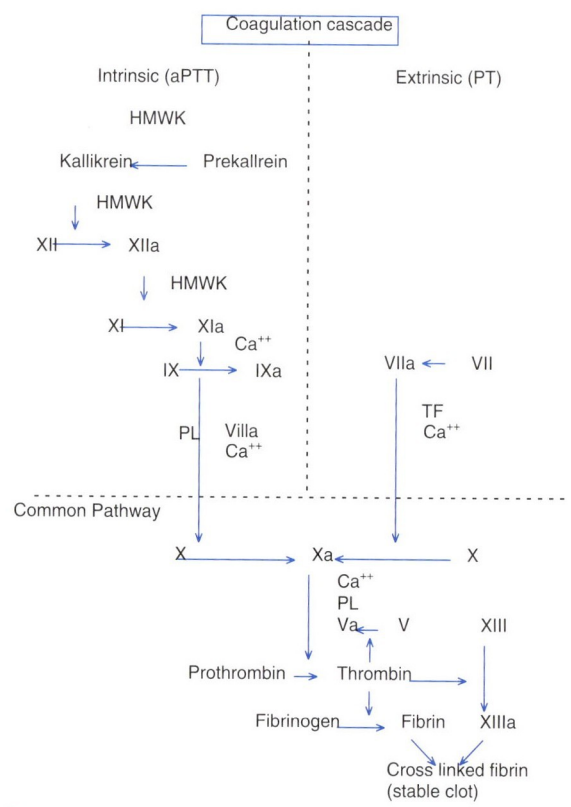

```
    X ─────────→ Xa ←───────── X
                 Ca++
                 PL
                 Va ←── V        XIII
                  ↓
  Prothrombin ──→ Thrombin ────→
                    ↓
   Fibrinogen ──→ Fibrin       XIIIa
                        ↘       ↓
                   Cross linked fibrin
                     (stable clot)
```

Figure 12-3 **Coagulation cascade.** Defects in either intrinsic or extrinsic pathways lead to prolongation of indicated tests. Defects in common pathway prolong both tests. Deficiency of XIII does not prolong either aPTT or PT. TT measures conversion of fibrinogen to fibrin. HMWK, high molecular weight kininogen. PL, phospholipid. TF, tissue factor.

TABLE 12-5 Investigation of Inherited Coagulation Disorders

Inherited Deficiency	Factor VIII	vWD*	Factor IX
Type of bleeding	Muscle, joint	Skin bruising, mucosal (e.g., epistaxis, menorrhagia)	Muscle, joint
Inheritance	Sex-linked	Autosomal (dominant and recessive)	Sex-linked
Laboratory			
PT	N	N	N
PTT	↑	N or ↑	↑
BT	N	↑	N
IX	N	N	↓
VIII:C	↓	↓	N
vWf	N	↓	N
VIIIR:RCo	N	↓	N

*Subtypes of vWD can be differentiated by multimer analysis and ristocetin-induced platelet aggregation (RIPA). N = normal; ↑ = increased; ↓ = decreased.

TABLE 12-6 Investigation of Acquired Coagulation Disorders

Acquired Disorder	DIC	Sepsis	Liver Dysfunction	Vitamin K Deficiency
History	Shock	Sepsis	Jaundice	Diet, diarrhea, antibiotics, malabsorption obstructive jaundice
Bleeding	Generalized*		Generalized	Generalized
Laboratory				
PT	↑	↑ or ↑	↑ or ↑	↑
PTT	↑	N or ↑	N or ↑	N
Platelets	N or ↓	↓	N or ↓	N
Fibrinogen	↓	N or ↓	N or ↓	N
FDP	↑	↑	N or ↑	N
Factors				
V	↓	N or ↓	↓	N
VII	N	N or ↓	↓	↓
VIII	↓	N or ↓	↑	N
IX	N or ↓	N or ↓	↓	↓
X	↓	N or ↓	↓	↓

*Particularly in the newborn infant, clinical bleeding is much more severe in the infant with DIC secondary to shock. N = normal; ↑ = increased; ↓ = decreased.

FACTOR VIII DEFICIENCY (CLASSIC HEMOPHILIA OR HEMOPHILIA A)

- Supportive measures (physiotherapy, patient education, home care programs)
- Early treatment of bleeds with either cryoprecipitate (one bag contains 80-100 U of Factor VIII activity) or factor VIII concentrates (1 U factor VIII/kg increases factor VIIIc concentrate activity by 2%, with a half-life of between 8-12 hr)
- All patients should be tested for HIV

VON WILLEBRAND DISEASE (VWD)

- Minor bleeding may require only supportive measures
- 1-Deamino-8-D-arginine-vasopressin (DDAVP, 0.3 μg/kg intravenously in normal saline at a concentration of 0.5 μg/ml to a maximum of 24 μg over 20 min) may be used in selected cases
- Replace with cryoprecipitate (20-40 U factor VIII activity/kg daily)

FACTOR IX DEFICIENCY (CHRISTMAS DISEASE OR HEMOPHILIA B)

- Supportive measures as per factor VIII deficiency
- Bleeds can be treated with factor IX concentrates (1 U/kg increases activity by 0.8-1.2% with a half-life of 18-24 hr)—usual dose is 15-40 U/kg daily (see Tables 12-7 and 12-8)
- Avoid giving antifibrinolytic agents (epsilon-aminocaproic acid [EACA] tranexamic acid) concurrently with Factor IX concentrates—due to risk of thromboembolic complications

TABLE 12-7 Initial Doses of Factor Replacement in Hemophilia

Indication for Replacement	Amount of Factor VIII Required	Amount of Factor IX Required
Hemarthrosis	15-20 U/kg once daily	15 U/kg once daily
Mucous membrane*	40 U/kg once	30 U/kg once
Hematuria†	40 U/kg daily or bid × 3-5 days	40 U/kg daily × 3-5 days
Major bleeding (CNS, surgery, retroperitoneal)	40 U/kg q12h as long as indicated	40 U/kg q12h as long as indicated

*EACA, 100 mg/kg q6h × 3-5 days may also be of value.
†Prednisone 2 mg/kg/day (maximum of 60 mg) may also be considered.

TABLE 12-8 Clinical Use of Blood Products

Blood Component	Indications for Use	Dose
Platelet concentrate (30-50 ml/U)	Bleeding due to thrombocytopenia	Platelets 1 U/5 kg; ↑ platelet count by 50,000-100,000
Fresh frozen plasma (200-250 ml/U)	Treatment of coagulation disorders	10 ml/kg
Cryoprecipitate (an average of 80 U of factor VIII activity per 5-10 ml bag)	Hemophilia A, vWD, and fibrinogen deficiency	1 bag/5 kg (1 U/kg ↑ factor VIII activity in plasma by ~ 2%)
Pooled factor VIII concentrate (~ 300 U/10-30 ml [varies from ~ 250-1000 U])	Hemophilia A	10-40 U/kg; t½ 8-12 hr; (1 U/kg ↑ activity by 2%)
Factor IX complex	Hemophilia B	15-40 U/kg; t½ 18-24 hr; (1 U/kg ↑ activity by 0.8-1.2%)
Packed RBCs (250-300 ml/U)	Severe anemia	10 ml/kg ↑ Hb by 20-30 g/L

DISSEMINATED INTRAVASCULAR COAGULATION (DIC)

- Supportive care; treat underlying cause
- Blood product support, e.g., packed RBCs and platelets as needed; fresh frozen plasma, 10 ml/kg every 8 hr; and cryoprecipitate (~1 bag/5 kg) for hypofibrinogenemia

HEPATIC FAILURE

- See pp 214-215
- Supportive care; treat underlying liver disease
- Blood product support as needed (see DIC for guidelines)
- Vitamin K_1 1 mg SC or by slow IV push

VITAMIN K DEFICIENCY

- Rule out malabsorption
- For urgent reversal, use FFP 10 ml/kg in addition to vitamin K_1
- Treat with vitamin K_1 1 mg SC or by slow IV push
- To reverse therapeutic anticoagulation, larger doses of vitamin K_1 may be required (2.5-5 mg)
- For oral supplementation, vitamin K_3 is better absorbed

DEEP VENOUS THROMBOSIS

- Uncommon in children
- Consider underlying thrombotic state

Investigations

- Imaging gold standard: venogram
- Other imaging techniques: ultrasonography, radionuclide scans
- Impedance plethysmography: not standardized for children

- Thrombotic work-up (if no clearly identified precipitant): protein C, protein S, reptilase time, thrombin time, fibrinogen, plasminogen, antithrombin III, lupus anticoagulant
- Baseline measurement of PT and PTT for monitoring of anticoagulant therapy
- CXR and ventilation/perfusion scan if pulmonary embolism suspected

Management

- Ensure adequacy of cardiorespiratory status if pulmonary embolism suspected
- Start anticoagulation if clinical suspicion of thrombosis is high, then therapy can be started prior to performance of imaging tests
- Initial anticoagulation with continuous IV infusion of heparin (see p 665)
- Oral anticoagulants (coumadin) can be started on the first day of anticoagulant therapy. Maintain INR of 2.0 to 3.0 (INR = international normalized ratio; compares PT result to a defined international standard and allows comparison of PT results from different labs). For coumadin guidelines, see p 697.
- In specific circumstances, consider either inferior vena caval ligation or the use of fibrinolytic agents

Transfusion Reactions

Immediate Reactions

- Fever
- Allergic manifestations: urticaria, anaphylaxis
- Bacteremia from infected blood
- Hemolysis
- Hemorrhagic state
- Circulatory overload

Delayed Reactions (up to days to months)

- Hemolysis
- Sensitization to red cell antigens
- Infectious diseases—e.g., CMV, hepatitis, HIV

Management of Acute Febrile Reactions
- Treat immediate reactions with acetaminophen/antihistamines (diphenhydramine), steroids as necessary
- May continue transfusion if reaction mild
- Prevention: leukocyte-poor (washed) red cells in patients requiring multiple transfusions

Hemolytic Transfusion Reaction
- Less common
- Medical emergency
- Symptoms—fever, dyspnea, chest pain, flank or infusion site, shock, bleeding
- Stop infusion, keep IV running
- Treat shock; monitor closely
- Notify blood bank
- Return offending blood product to blood bank with 5 ml of patient's blood carefully drawn without anticoagulant and the first post-transfusion urine specimen

Oncology

TUMOR LYSIS SYNDROME

- Hyperkalemia—rapid cell turnover may be rapidly progressive, accentuated by chemotherapy. May cause cardiac dysrhythmia and arrest.
- Hyperphosphatemia and hypocalcemia may cause tetany and cardiac dysrhythmia
- Hyperuricemia
- Metabolic acidosis
- Increased urea from protein catabolism
- Renal dysfunction secondary to urate, phosphate deposition in renal tubules

TABLE 12-9 Side Effects of Some Common Chemotherapy Agents*

Drug	Nausea and vomiting	Myelosuppression	Alopecia	Mucositis	Neuropathy	Pulmonary	Cardiac	Renal	Tissue Necrosis	Skin	Liver	Diarrhea	Other
Actinomycin D	++	++	++	++					++	++		++	Radiation reaction, abdo. pain
Adriamycin	++	++	++	+			++	±	++	+			Radiation reaction, red urine, fever, pigmentation
BCNU	++	+++†	+	±		++		±	+	+			Pigmentation, dizziness, ataxia
Bleomycin	+	±	+	++		++		+		++			Fever, hypotension, systemic sclerosis
Busulphan	+	+++†				++							Pigmentation, cataracts, gynecomastia
CCNU/methyl CCNU	++	+++†	±	±		+		+			+		CNS dysfunction
Chlorambucil	+	++				±	±				±		
Cyclophosphamide	++	++	++	+		+	±						Hemorrhagic cystitis, H_2O retention

202

Cytosine arabinoside	++	++	+	+		±	Fever
Daunorubicin	++	++	++	+			Fever
DTIC	++	++	+		++	+	Flu-like illness, facial paresthesia
5-Fluorouracil	+	++	+	++	±	+	Conjunctivitis, ataxia, and drowsiness
Melphalan	+	++†			±		
Methotrexate	+	++	+	+	+	++	Conjunctivitis
Mithramycin	++	++			+	+	Bleeding, fever, hypocalcemia, CNS dysfunction
Mitomycin C	+	++†	+	+	±	±	Hemolytic anemia
6MP	+	++		±	+	++	Fever
Nitrogen mustard	++	++	+			+	Encephalopathy
Cis-platinum	++	+		±	++		Ototoxic, hypersensitivity
Procarbazine	++	++		+	±	+	CNS dysfunction, MAOI, Antabuse, allergy

Continued.

*From Acronyms in cancer chemotherapy, Eli Lilly Canada, Inc., 1985 revised edition pamphlet, pp 54-55.
†Delayed myelosuppression.
++ = Major toxicity; + = less frequent or less severe; ± = infrequent, mild or uncertain.

TABLE 12-9 Side Effects of Some Common Chemotherapy Agents (Cont'd)

Drug	Nausea and vomiting	Myelosuppression	Alopecia	Mucositis	Neuropathy	Pulmonary	Cardiac	Renal	Tissue Necrosis	Skin	Liver	Diarrhea	Other
Streptozotocin	++	+				±		++			+	+	Hyperglycemia, ataxia, dizziness
Thioguanine	+	++		+							+	+	Abdo. pain
Vinblastine	+	++	+	+	±				++	+			Constipation, ataxia, inappropriate ADH, abdo. pain
Vincristine	±	+	+		++				+	+			Abdo. pain, constipation, fever
Vindesine	±	+	+		++					±		+	Fever, hypotension
VP16-213	+	++	+		±		+			±	±	+	Phlebitis, correct serum electrolyte imbalances prior to administration to avoid enhanced cardiotoxicity
M-AMSA	+	++		++	±					±	±		
Mitoxantrone	+	++	±	±	±		+				±	±	Phlebitis, blue/green urine discoloration, blue streaking of vein

Management

- Prevention
  1. Must have large-bore peripheral or preferably central venous line inserted
  2. Monitor electrolytes, calcium, BUN, creatinine, phosphate, uric acid q3-4h
  3. Accurate fluid balance and daily weight; assess urine output q2h
  4. Hydrate with fluids at 3-4 L/m^2/day, ensuring adequate urine output. If urine output drops to less than 60% of input give intravenous furosemide; may require mannitol.
  5. Withhold potassium supplementation during initiation of chemotherapy
  6. Allopurinol 400 mg/m^2/day in 3-4 divided doses (10-12.5 mg/kg/day)
  7. Alkalinize the urine to maintain a urine pH of 6.5-7.5. Commence with 50 mEq (mmol) sodium bicarbonate/L and adjust up or down in increments of 12.5 mEq/L according to urine pH. Do not allow pH to exceed 7.5, as phosphates precipitate in alkaline urine. Reassess bicarbonate dose after each void.
  8. Requires continuous cardiac monitoring, frequent BP monitoring
  9. Hemodialysis may be required prior to the institution of chemotherapy if diuresis is inadequate or biochemical tests are abnormal
- Treatment
  1. Hyperkalemia (see p 348), hyperphosphatemia (see p 348). Discontinue alkalinization when hyperphosphatemic.
  2. Do not treat hypocalcemia with calcium supplements unless symptomatic (risk of precipitation with phosphate) (see p 19)
  3. Dialysis as indicated

MASS EFFECT

- Major concerns are airway and spinal cord compression
- Requires dexamethasone, urgent surgical consultation, ± local radiation

INFECTION

See p 279

HYPERCALCEMIA

See p 81

AIRWAY COMPRESSION

Investigations
- CXR shows mediastinal mass with widening of the superior mediastinum
- CT scan of chest shows compression of vena cava, trachea, and bronchi

Treatment
- Urgent attention to airway status is mandatory. Alert anesthetist, radiotherapist, and surgeon, since intubation beyond the block may be necessary. *Do not attempt intubation yourself.*
- Steroids: IV dexamethasone 10 mg/m^2/day in three divided doses
- Do not delay making a specific diagnosis (e.g., lymph node biopsy, bone marrow aspiration, pleural tap), as not all masses will shrink dramatically with steroid therapy
- In acute impending respiratory failure, radiotherapy to the mediastinum may have to be considered
- No sedation or spinal taps until airway is secure

SPINAL CORD COMPRESSION

Investigations
- X-ray of chest, abdomen, and relevant spine
- CT scan of relevant area and urgent CT myelogram (the latter after neurosurgical consultation)
- Lumbar puncture may precipitate or worsen paralysis
- Establish tissue diagnosis (lymph node biopsy, bone marrow aspirate-biopsy, or laminectomy specimen)

Treatment
- Dexamethasone to reduce edema (see formulary)
- Urgent neurosurgical consult for consideration of decompression laminectomy
- Radiation or chemotherapy

THIRTEEN

Hepatology

Symptoms and Signs of Liver Disorder

Symptoms	Signs

Right upper quadrant pain
Pruritus
Systemic complaints:
  Anorexia
  Nausea
  Vomiting
  Diarrhea
  Fever
	Jaundice
	Hepatomegaly
	Splenomegaly
	Spider angiomata
	Palmar erythema
	Clubbing
	Collateral abdominal circulation
	Failure to thrive
	Hepatic bruits
	Ascites

- Normal values for liver spans (Fig. 13-1)

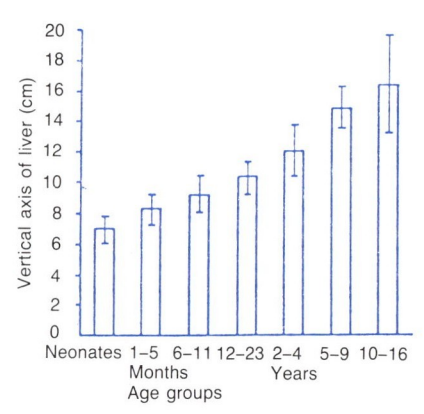

Figure 13-1 **Normal (average) values for liver spans in various age groups.** (Adapted from Deligeorgis D, Yannakos D, Doxiadis S. et al. Normal size of liver in infancy and childhood. Arch Dis Child 1973; 48:792).

Laboratory Tests

SERUM MARKERS OF HEPATOBILIARY DISEASE

- Hepatocellular necrosis
  1. Aminotransferases
     - Aspartate aminotransferase (AST)—present in heart, skeletal muscle, kidney, brain, liver
     - Alanine aminotransferase (ALT)—localized primarily in the liver
- Cholestasis
  1. Alkaline phosphatase (ALP)
     - Normal values vary with age
     - High levels in cholestasis, hepatic carcinoma
     - Low levels in Wilson's disease with hemolysis, zinc deficiency, hypothyroidism, pernicious anemia, congenital hypophosphatasia
     - Present in liver, bone, intestine, placenta, kidney, leukocytes

2. Gammaglutamyl transpeptidase (GGT)
   - Present in kidney, seminal vesicles, pancreas, liver, spleen, heart, brain—but not bone, unlike ALP
   - Normal values vary with age, sex
   - Most sensitive indicator of biliary tract disease
   - May be increased by enzyme-inducing drugs
3. 5'-Nucleotidase (5NT)
   - Present in intestine, brain, heart, blood vessels, liver, pancreas
   - Elevated only in hepatobiliary disease
   - Used to confirm liver disease when ALP is raised

TESTS OF LIVER FUNCTION

- Serum bilirubin
- Serum bile acids: major organic anions excreted by the liver
- Clotting factors: liver synthesizes factors I, II, V, VII, IX, X
- Albumin: not a good indicator of hepatic protein synthesis in *acute* liver disease
- Lipoproteins: increased triglycerides, decreased levels of cholesterol esters
- Globulins: gamma globulins increased in viral hepatitis, autoimmune chronic active hepatitis, cirrhosis

OTHER TESTS

- Ammonia
  1. Major source is bacterial production in the large bowel
  2. Elevated in liver disease, hemodialysis, valproic acid therapy, Reye's syndrome, urea cycle enzyme deficiencies, organic acidemias, carnitine deficiency
- Alpha fetoprotein: Elevated in hepatoma, hepatoblastoma, hepatocellular carcinoma, tyrosinemia

Reye's Syndrome

- Acute sporadic encephalopathy of unknown cause, characterized by a reversible abnormality of mitochondrial structure with decreased mitochondrial enzymatic activity
- Predominantly in patients aged 6 mo to 15 yr (range, 4 days-29 yr)
- 0.2-4.0 per 100,000 children
- 3-4 day prodromal viral illness—e.g., respiratory tract infection, gastroenteritis, varicella, influenza A and B
- Vomiting—profuse, persistent
- Rapid appearance of neurologic changes, seizures in 30%
- Encephalopathy: five stages leading brain death (Table 13-1)
- Etiology unknown, associated with ASA, aflatoxin

TABLE 13-1 Stages of Encephalopathy in Reye's Syndrome

	I	II	III	IV	V
Mental state	Quiet, responds to verbal commands	Lethargic, difficulty counting	Agitated, delerium, responds to pain	Coma, decerebrate posturing	Coma, spinal reflexes preserved
Muscle activity	Normal	Clumsy	Poorly controlled gross movements $\pm$ clonus	Opisthotonus, extensor spasms of arms, legs	Flaccid paralysis
Respiratory rate	Normal	Normal–increased	Normal–increased	Increased	None
Pupillary response	Normal	Normal	Dilated, responds rapidly	Dilated, responds slowly	Dilated, unresponsive
Fundi	Normal	Normal	Venous engorgement	Papilledema	Variable

Biochemistry

- Serum aminotransferases elevated 2-100 times normal
- Hyperammonemia—may be transient
- Mildly prolonged prothrombin time, bilirubin usually normal
- Hypoglycemia in severe cases
- CSF normal, but glucose concentration may be low

Treatment

- Intravenous glucose (10%), fluid restriction (60%)
- See management of ↑ICP (p 539) and acute fulminant hepatic failure (Fig. 13-2)

Mortality

- 30-60%

Text continued on p 226.

Definition: syndrome of severe impairment of hepatic function associated with progressive mental changes. Encephalopathy must develop within 8 wk of onset of liver disease, with no evidence of previous liver disease.

Signs and symptoms
Jaundice
Hepatic encephalopathy
Asterixis
Fetor hepaticus (sweetish, slightly fecal smell of exhaled breath)
Bleeding
Ascites
Hypoglycemia
Vomiting
Lethargy
Combativeness

Biochemical Parameters
Prolonged PT, PTT
Factors V, VII important in prognosis
Decreased albumin if chronic
Increased bilirubin, ammonia
Decreased fibrinogen, glucose, and albumin if chronic
Follow BUN, creatinine, electrolytes, calcium, phosphorus, magnesium

Abdominal U/S
  Diagnosis
  Assessment of portal vein and flow in case transplantation required
  Follow liver size

Neurological status
  Early stages assess with Trail test

Metabolic screen
  Wilson's disease
  Galactosemia
  Tyrosinemia
  Fructosemia

Viral tests
  Hepatitis A
  Hepatitis B
  Hepatitis C

Transjugular Liver Biopsy
  Contribute to diagnosis and prognosis
  Liver tissue for virology, electron microscopy, antibody staining, histology, enzyme assay
  Venogram and venous pressure
  (Percutaneous biopsy contraindicated because of coagulopathy)

```
EEG: slowing,
triphasic waves
progressive
↓LOC → coma
```

Adenovirus
Enteroviruses
Epstein-Barr virus

Drug screen
Acetaminophen
Cocaine
See Table 13-3 for
drug hepatotoxicity

(See section on drug hepatotoxicity
and tables for further investigations)

Management

Approaches not of proven benefit
Charcoal hemoperfusion
Plasmaphoresis
Hemodialysis
Hemofiltration

Prostaglandin EI
(investigational drug)

Liver transplantation

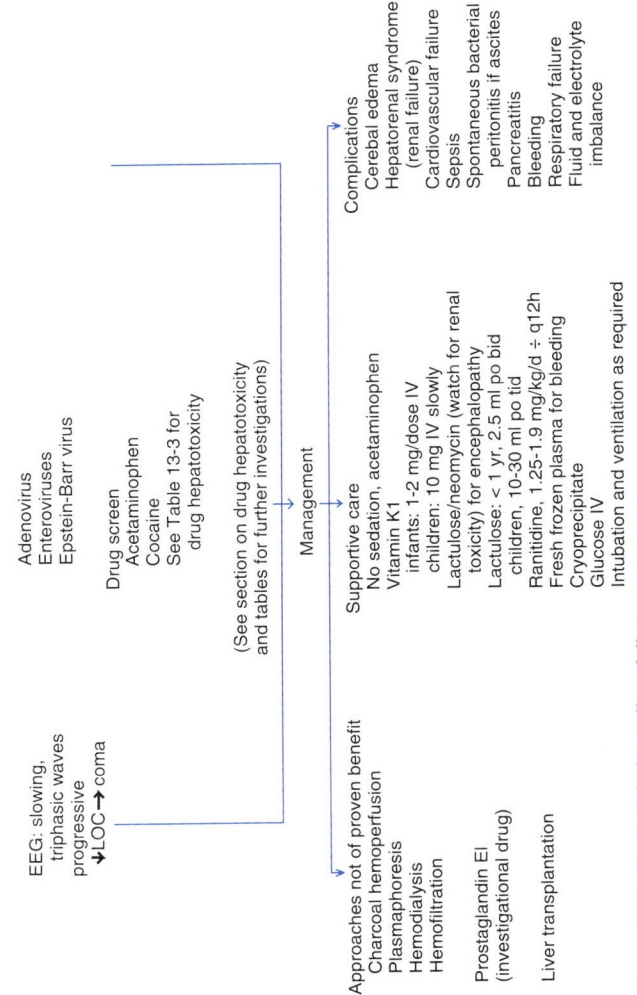

Supportive care
No sedation, acetaminophen
Vitamin K1
  infants: 1-2 mg/dose IV
  children: 10 mg IV slowly
Lactulose/neomycin (watch for renal
  toxicity) for encephalopathy
Lactulose: < 1 yr, 2.5 ml po bid
  children, 10-30 ml po tid
Ranitidine, 1.25-1.9 mg/kg/d ÷ q12h
Fresh frozen plasma for bleeding
Cryoprecipitate
Glucose IV
Intubation and ventilation as required

Complications
Cerebral edema
Hepatorenal syndrome
  (renal failure)
Cardiovascular failure
Sepsis
Spontaneous bacterial
  peritonitis if ascites
Pancreatitis
Bleeding
Respiratory failure
Fluid and electrolyte
  imbalance

Figure 13-2 **Acute fulminant liver failure.**

TABLE 13-2 Clinical Guide to Liver Disorders

Disorder	Investigations	Associated Specific Clinical Features
Infectious		
Toxoplasmosis	Specific IgM antibody, rising IgG titres; detection by CF, IFA, ELISA; isolation of virus from CSF, liver	Chorioretinitis, diffuse intracranial calcifications
Rubella	Isolation of virus from pharyngeal secretions, urine, CSF, liver; IgM specific antibody	Cataracts, hearing loss, patent ductus arteriosus
Cytomegalovirus	Typical inclusion bodies in exfoliated cells in urine, gastric contents, liver; identification of virus in buffy coat and tissue cultures; CF, IFA antibody tests	Chorioretinitis, hearing loss, periventricular intracerebral calcifications
Herpes simplex virus	Isolation of virus from vesicles, cell culture; rising antibody titres	Skin vesicles, signs and symptoms of sepsis
Syphilis	Bone x-rays, darkfield examination, VDRL, FTA-ABS, TPI test	Osteochondritis, periostitis, snuffles, rash
Hepatitis A	IgM anti-HAV virus excreted in stool prior to onset of disease	Usually asymptomatic in infants, young children; fecal–oral transmission; no chronic disease, can present as fulminant liver failure
Hepatitis B	HBsAg, HBeAg, anti-HBc, HBV DNA	Associated immune complex disease (heart, renal, joints), asymptomatic carrier, fulminant liver failure, chronic hepatitis, cirrhosis, hepatocellular carcinoma
Hepatitis C	IgG anti-HCV	Antibody not detectable until 2-3 mo after onset of acute disease, chronic hepatitis, cirrhosis, hepatocellular carcinoma

Hepatitis D ("Delta Ag")	Stain biopsy specimens, polymerase chain reaction for viral RNA, anti-HDV	Requires presence of HBsAg for replication; occurs as acute coinfection, or superimposed on chronic HBsAg carrier; may cause acute fulminant hepatitis; increased risk of chronic liver disease
Coxsackie/echovirus	Isolation from respiratory tract, stool, liver, CSF, blood	Myocarditis, meningoencephalitis, hepatitis, fulminant liver failure
Adenovirus	Isolation from respiratory tract, stool; antibody titers	Pneumonitis, meningoencephalitis, hepatitis, myocarditis
Epstein-Barr virus	Heterophil antibody titer > 1:128 Anti-VCA, Anti-EA	Splenomegaly, lymphadenopathy, usually mild hepatic dysfunction; can be fulminant
Varicella	Isolation from lesions, liver	Disseminated in immunocompromised hosts
Bacterial	Blood, urine, CSF cultures	Liver abscess—fever, weight loss, RUQ tenderness; non-specific liver dysfunction—*E. coli, Klebsiella, Enterobacteriaceae, Staphylococcus, Pseudomonas, Proteus* Neonates: sepsis, meningitis, pneumonitis
Listeria	Isolation of organism from blood culture, CSF, liver	Tender hepatomegaly, granulomatous hepatitis
Tuberculosis	CXR, gastric aspirates	20-30% have hepatitis
Genetic and metabolic		
Trisomy 13, 18	Chromosomes	
α-1-antitrypsin deficiency	Pi typing, α-1-antitrypsin levels	Autosomal co-dominant (chromosome 14) Pi ZZ, Znul, nul deficient; may present at any age, including neonatal hepatitis; 50% develop cirrhosis
Cystic fibrosis	Sweat chloride, increased serum trypsinogen	Autosomal recessive (chromosome 7); neonates; inspissated bile; older children: focal biliary cirrhosis

Continued.

TABLE 13-2 Clinical Guide to Liver Disorders (Cont'd)

Disorder	Investigations	Associated Specific Clinical Features
Genetic and metabolic (cont'd)		
Galactosemia	Non-glucose–reducing substances in urine, decreased galactose-1-phosphate uridyl transferase in RBCs	Autosomal recessive; vomiting, failure to thrive, cataracts; *E. coli* sepsis
Fructosemia	Fructose in urine, decreased or absent hepatic fructose-1-phosphate aldolase B	Autosomal recessive; vomiting, hypoglycemia, FTT; aversion to fructose-containing foods
Tyrosinemia	Positive urinary ferric chloride test, increased urinary succinyl acetone	Autosomal recessive; FTT, hepatocellular failure, renal tubular dysfunction; 100% develop hepatomas
Glycogen storage disease	Liver biopsy for histology and enzyme assay	I—hepatomegaly, hypoglycemia, increased lactic acid, increased uric acid III—hepatomegaly, hypoglycemia, hepatic fibrosis IV—hepatosplenomegaly, cirrhosis, hypotonia VI,IX—hepatomegaly
Gaucher's disease	Gaucher cells in bone marrow; decreased glucosyl ceramide-β-glucosidase in liver, WBC, bone marrow	Hepatosplenomegaly, CNS involvement (neuronopathic) hemolytic anemia, bone pain
Niemann-Pick disease	Decreased sphingomyelinase in WBC, liver; sea-blue histiocytes in liver and BM	Hepatosplenomegaly, progressive dementia, blindness (types A and C); may progress to cirrhosis; may present as neonatal hepatitis
Wolman's disease	Decreased acid esterase in WBC, liver	Vomiting, hepatosplenomegaly, diarrhea, adrenal calcification, steatorrhea, developmental delay, onset in infancy

Cholesterol ester storage disease	Lipoprotein electrophoresis, partial deficiency of acid esterase	Hepatomegaly ± splenomegaly, hyperlipidemia type II, increased triglycerides, onset in late childhood
Zellweger's disease	Increased iron, TIBC, decreased plasmalogens, absence of peroxisomes on liver biopsy	SGA, cataracts, severe hypotonia, microscopic renal cysts, stippled patella, abnormal facies
Perinatal hemochromatosis	Liver biopsy showing end-stage cirrhosis, increased ferritin, hemosiderin-laden macrophages from nasopharynx	Hepatocellular failure, small liver, ascites
Endocrinopathies	See section on *endocrinology*	Hypopituitarism, diabetes insipidus, hypoadrenalism, hypothyroidism, hypoparathyroidism
Wilson's disease	Increased 24-hr urine copper excretion; low serum copper, ceruloplasmin, haptoglobin; ophthalmologic examination for Kayser-Fleischer rings, low ALP with hemolysis; liver biopsy for copper content, specific EM changes	Age of onset > 4 yr; may present as acute or chronic hepatitis, hepatic failure, hemolytic anemia, CNS or psychiatric symptoms
Fatty liver	Liver biopsy, lipoprotein electrophoresis	Obesity; no history of ingestion of alcohol or other toxins; mild aminotransferase elevation
Byler's disease	Liver biopsy	Progressive intrahepatic cholestasis, pruritis, jaundice, malabsorption, hepatomegaly, hepatic fibrosis
Toxic		
Total parenteral nutrition		See p 226
Drugs	In vitro lymphocyte testing	See p 224
Inspissated bile syndrome	Secondary to severe or prolonged hemolysis	Prognosis good
Reye's syndrome	See section on Reye's syndrome	

Continued.

TABLE 13-2 Clinical Guide to Liver Disorders (Cont'd)

Disorder	Investigations	Associated Specific Clinical Features
Vascular		
Congestive heart failure	CXR, ECG, 2-D echo	Hepatomegaly, increased respiratory and heart rate
Budd-Chiari syndrome	Abdominal U/S venography	Oral contraceptive used
Shock	Liver biopsy	Associated with acute tubular necrosis, hypoxic-ischemic encephalopathy; liver dysfunction usually resolves
Veno-occlusive disease	Abdominal U/S venography	Associated with antineoplastic drugs, bush tea
Portal vein	Abdominal U/S and Doppler, venography	Hepatomegaly uncommon; associated with umbilical vein catheters; splenomegaly prominent
Structural		
Alagille's syndrome	Liver biopsy—paucity of bile ducts	Butterfly vertebrae, posterior embryotoxin, peripheral pulmonic stenosis, abnormal facies, jaundice

Non-syndromic bile duct paucity	Liver biopsy—paucity of bile ducts	Jaundice prominent; many causes, including cystic fibrosis, infections
Congenital hepatic fibrosis and caroli's syndrome	Abdominal UIS, ERCP, PTC (percutaneous transhepatic cholangiography) liver biopsy	Hepatosplenomegaly with normal liver function tests, associated renal anomalies
Autoimmune		
Autoimmune Chronic Active Hepatitis	ANA, ESR, liver-kidney microsomal antibody, increased IgG, anti–smooth muscle antibody, antimitochondrial antibody, decreased C4, liver biopsy	Consider diagnosis after 1-2 months liver dysfunction (vs. 6 months in adults), associated with ulcerative colitis, polyserositis, polyarteritis nodosa, Coomb's positive hemolytic anemia, thyroiditis, lupus, arthritis, glomerulonephritis
Primary sclerosing cholangitis	Increased ALP, IgG, ANA, antismooth muscle antibody, ERCP, PTC, liver biopsy	Associated with inflammatory bowel disease, may precede onset of bowel symptoms

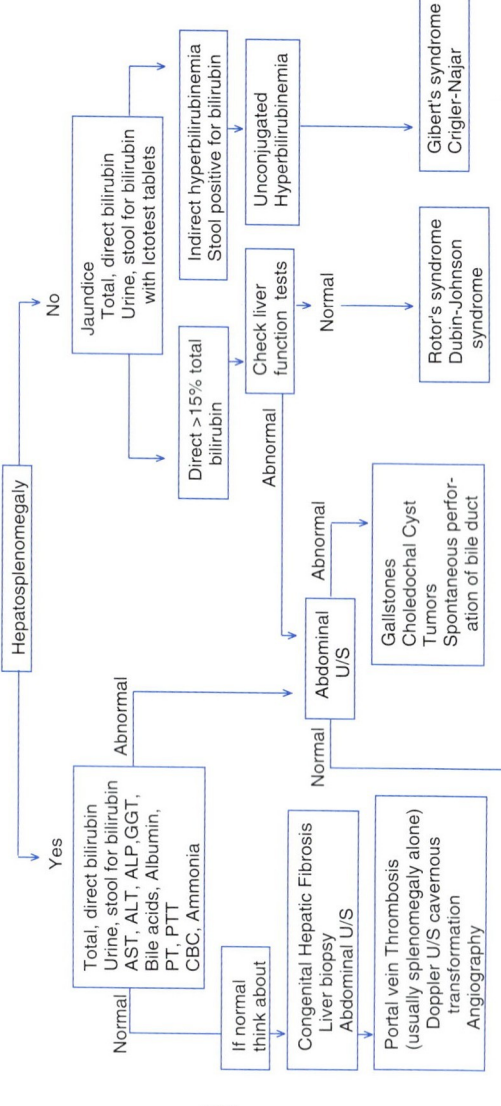

Hepatosplenomegaly

Yes → Total, direct bilirubin, Urine, stool for bilirubin, AST, ALT, ALP, GGT, Bile acids, Albumin, PT, PTT, CBC, Ammonia

- **Normal** → If normal think about:
  - Congenital Hepatic Fibrosis — Liver biopsy, Abdominal U/S
  - Portal vein Thrombosis (usually splenomegaly alone) — Doppler U/S cavernous transformation, Angiography

- **Abnormal** → Abdominal U/S
  - **Normal**
  - **Abnormal** → Gallstones, Choledochal Cyst, Tumors, Spontaneous perforation of bile duct

No → Jaundice: Total, direct bilirubin, Urine, stool for bilirubin with Ictotest tablets

- **Indirect hyperbilirubinemia / Stool positive for bilirubin** → Unconjugated Hyperbilirubinemia → Gibert's syndrome, Crigler-Najar

- **Direct >15% total bilirubin** → Check liver function tests
  - **Normal** → Rotor's syndrome, Dubin-Johnson syndrome
  - **Abnormal** → Abdominal U/S → Gallstones, Choledochal Cyst, Tumors, Spontaneous perforation of bile duct

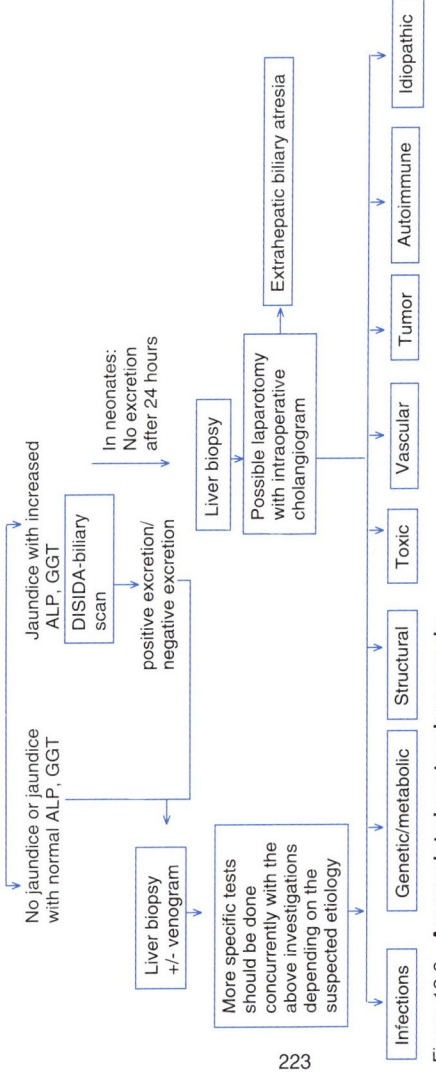

Figure 13-3 **Approach to hepatosplenomegaly.**

TABLE 13-3 Drug Hepatotoxicity

Drug	Type of Liver Injury	Comments
Acetaminophen	Hepatocellular necrosis	Fatality usually due to drug overdose but dose may be in therapeutic range; measure plasma concentrations. Treatment with N-acetylcysteine if given within 24 hours of ingestion. Prognosis is better than other etiologies of fulminant liver failure
Aspirin	Nonspecific focal hepatitis	Association with Reye's syndrome; usually mild-to-moderate dose-dependent rise in serum aminotransferases in patients on high doses of aspirin e.g., rheumatic diseases
Carbamazepine	Granulomatous hepatitis	Rarely can develop hepatic failure; is associated with cholangitis
Cocaine	Hepatocellular necrosis Steatosis	Hepatitis, fulminant hepatic failure, associated myoglobinuria, tachycardia, high fever, rapid increase in aminotransferases; look for cocaine metabolite in urine
Erythromycin	Focal hepatic necrosis Cholestatic reaction	< 6%; onset usually within 1-4 weeks; may be associated eosinophilia; prognosis excellent on withdrawal of drug

Drug	Lesion	Comments
Halothane	Hepatocellular necrosis	Usually requires more than one exposure to halothane; asymptomatic hepatitis to fulminant liver failure; in vitro test for IgG antibodies to halothane-altered liver cell membranes positive in 70%; also reported with methoxyflurane and enflurane
Isoniazid	Hepatocellular necrosis	Mild hepatitis, chronic hepatitis, fulminant liver failure
Methotrexate	Steatosis, fibrosis	May lead to cirrhosis despite normal liver function tests; total dose and duration of treatment important factors; biopsy recommended prior to institution of drug
Phenytoin	Hepatocellular necrosis Granulomatous hepatitis	May be associated rash, fever, lymphadenopathy, absolute eosinophilia; may develop fulminant liver failure; in vitro lymphocyte testing
Rifampin	Hepatocellular necrosis	Hepatitis, impairment of bilirubin uptake by the liver
Sulfonamides	Hepatocellular necrosis	May have associated fever, arthralgia, rash, eosinophilia; chronic active hepatitis, granulomatous hepatitis, fulminant liver failure reported; reaction usually occurs within 2 weeks of starting drug; in vitro lymphocyte testing
Valproic acid	Hepatocellular necrosis Microvesicular steatosis	10% will develop elevation of serum aminotransferases; this is usually asymptomatic and reverses spontaneously; raised ammonia levels may be present; fatal hepatitis usually in children under 10 years, within 6 months of start of therapy, males > females, usually on multianticonvulsant therapy; can also develop Reye's-like syndrome

Total Parenteral Nutrition (TPN) Associated Liver Disease

- Etiology unknown
- Frequency decreases with increasing gestational age
- Other associated factors: sepsis, hypoxia, blood transfusion, intra-abdominal surgery, drugs
- Onset: 10-180 days (onset earlier in premature infants)
- Elevation of AST, GGT, or ALP appears first
- Conjugated hyperbilirubinemia
- Hepatosplenomegaly
- Elevated serum bile acids
- Acute acalculous cholecystitis, biliary sludge, cholelithiasis
- Cholestasis, hepatocellular damage with multinucleated giant cell transformation, mild inflammation
- May progress to fibrosis and cirrhosis
- Hepatocellular carcinoma may complicate

Treatment

- Withdrawal of TPN and start of oral feeds
- Liver function tests usually return to normal within 5 months
- Liver biopsy changes may persist for up to one year
- If TPN continued, progressive liver disease with cirrhosis occurs

Nutrition in Liver Disease

- In general, it is important to maintain nutritional status
- Caloric intake may be supplemented by NG feeds or by TPN to prevent a catabolic state
- Protein intake should be limited but not deleted in the face of hepatic encephalopathy.

Cholestatic Disorders

- Vitamin supplementation (fat soluble vitamins):
  1. Vitamin K_1—dose is variable depending on severity of disease, follow PT
  2. Polyvisol contains vitamin A and D
  3. Vitamin E (Aquasol E)—dose is variable, follow vitamin E levels
  4. Vitamin D—may require supplementations, observe for rickets, follow calcium and phosphorus
- Formula should contain medium chain triglycerides because of fat malabsorption due to decreased intestinal bile salts (e.g., Pregestimil)

FOURTEEN

Infectious Diseases

Immunization

- Premature infants: normal schedule based on postnatal age
- Schedule interruptions: no need to restart from beginning
- Site of injection
  1. Infants: anterolateral thigh
  2. All others: deltoid area
- IM injections: use long needles (e.g., >5/8 inch)
- Acetaminophen 15 mg/kg, at 0 and 4 hr postvaccination and then q4h prn to decrease fever and fussiness
- All routine vaccines can be given safely and effectively at the same time at different sites
- Monitor all children for 15 min postvaccination, and have adrenaline available

CONTRAINDICATIONS

- Febrile illnesses (*not* simple colds)
- Oral egg allergies (anaphylaxis, urticaria): avoid influenza and yellow fever vaccines
- Previous major systemic reaction
- Live vaccines (MMR, OPV, BCG, and yellow fever) contraindicated in
  1. Pregnancy (mother's children still eligible)
  2. Congenital immunodeficiencies (MMR should be given to all HIV patients)
  3. Within 3 mo of chemotherapy or immunosuppressive therapy (vaccinations may not be effective until 3-12 mo post-treatment)

TABLE 14-1A Schedule of Immunizations

Age	Immunization Against		
2 mo	Diphtheria	Pertussis	Tetanus	Poliomyelitis
4 mo	Diphtheria	Pertussis	Tetanus	Poliomyelitis
6 mo	Diphtheria	Pertussis	Tetanus	Poliomyelitis*
12-15 mo‡	Measles	Mumps	Rubella†	
18 mo	Diphtheria	Pertussis	Tetanus	Poliomyelitis
	Haemophilus influenzae type b			
4-6 yr	Diphtheria	Pertussis	Tetanus	Poliomyelitis
14-16 yr	Diphtheria§		Tetanus§	Poliomyelitis*

*This dose may be omitted if live (oral) polio vaccine is being used.
†Rubella vaccine is also indicated for all girls and women of child-bearing age who lack proof of immunity. At all medical visits the opportunity should be taken to check whether such a patient has received rubella vaccine.
‡Canada: MMR vaccine given in a single dose on or after first birthday. United States: Two doses, at 15 mo and at 11–12 yr.
§Diphtheria and tetanus toxoid (Td), a combined adsorbed "adult-type" preparation for use in persons 7 yr of age or more, contains less diphtheria toxoid than preparations given to younger children and is less likely to cause reactions in older persons.

TABLE 14-1B Immunization Schedule for Children Not Immunized in Early Infancy

Timing	Immunization Against		
For children 1 through 6 yr of age			
First visit[#]	Diphtheria	Pertussis	Tetanus	Poliomyelitis
Interval after first visit:			
1 mo	Measles	Mumps	Rubella[†]	
2 mo	Diphtheria	Pertussis	Tetanus	Poliomyelitis
4 mo	Diphtheria	Pertussis	Tetanus	Poliomyelitis[*]
16 mo[¶]	Diphtheria	Pertussis	Tetanus	Poliomyelitis
Preschool—see Note[¶]			
At age:			
18 mo-5 yr	*Haemophilus influenzae* type b		
14-16 yr	Diphtheria[§]		Tetanus[§]	Poliomyelitis[*]

For children 7 yr of age and over

First visit[#]	Diphtheria[§]	Tetanus[§]	Poliomyelitis
Interval after first visit:			
1 mo	Measles	Mumps	Rubella[†]	Poliomyelitis[*]
2 mo	Diphtheria		Tetanus	Poliomyelitis
14 mo	Diphtheria		Tetanus	Poliomyelitis
10 yr	Diphtheria		Tetanus	Poliomyelitis[*]

[*]This dose may be omitted if live (oral) polio vaccine is being used.
[†]Rubella vaccine is also indicated for all girls and women of child-bearing age who lack proof of immunity. At all medical visits the opportunity should be taken to check whether such a patient has received rubella vaccine.
[‡]Canada: MMR vaccine given in a single dose on or after first birthday. United States: Two doses, at 15 mo and at 11–12 yr.
[§]Diphtheria and tetanus toxoid (Td), a combined adsorbed "adult-type" preparation for use in persons 7 yr of age or more, contains less diphtheria toxoid than preparations given to younger children and is less likely to cause reactions in older persons.
[#]Measles, mumps, and rubella vaccines may also be given at the first visit if it is considered likely that a child will not return for further immunization. It has not been shown, however, that full response to all antigens will occur.
[¶]When the last of the above doses are given before the fourth birthday, consideration should be given to administration of an additional dose at time of school entry.

Modified from Canadian Medical Association. CMA policy summary: immunization. Can Med Assoc J 1985; 133:1248B.

Diphtheria, Pertussis, Tetanus, and Poliomyelitis Vaccine

PREPARATIONS

- For use under 7 yr of age: combined DPT-polio (inactivated polio virus, IPV), or DPT and OPV (oral live polio virus) separately. If pertussis vaccine is contraindicated, give DT and IPV separately, or DT and OPV separately.
- For use above 7 yr of age: combined Td-polio (IPV) or Td-OPV

ADMINISTRATION

- A booster dose of Td should be given every 10 yr following primary immunization
- The majority of side effects of DPT-polio are caused by the pertussis vaccine
  1. Minor: 50-75% will have pain, local redness and swelling, fever, or irritability (may be reduced by acetaminophen; see p 228)
  2. Major: persistent crying, 1%; hypotonic hyporesponsive state, 1:1750; seizures, 1:1750
- If a child recovers from culture-proven pertussis, no further doses of the pertussis vaccine are required
- OPV may rarely produce paralytic illness in the recipient (~1 in 8 million doses). Adults are at greater risk.
- Inadequate or unknown status of polio immunity in the household is not a contraindication to immunization of child with OPV. "Household" adults may be advised to update their immunizations with their family doctor (risk to unimmunized "household" contacts, ~1 in 5 million doses).

Infectious Diseases

CONTRAINDICATIONS

Pertussis Vaccine

- Any serious reactions developing within 72 hr following vaccination
  1. Fever >40.5° C
  2. Persistent inconsolable crying (>3 hr)
  3. Collapse episodes (hypotonia, lethargy, pallor)
  4. Convulsions
  5. Acute encephalopathy (within 7 days after vaccination)
- Progressive neurologic disorders (e.g., progressive encephalopathy, uncontrolled epilepsy) but NOT contraindicated in static lesions (e.g., cerebral palsy) or in children with a family history of convulsions or nonprogressive CNS disorders. In a child with a history of seizures there may be an increased risk of a seizure following vaccination.
- Children 7 yr of age or older

Diphtheria and Tetanus Toxoids

- Hypersensitivity or anaphylactic reactions following a previous dose
- Frequent Td doses may produce a local arthus-like reaction

Polio Vaccine

- OPV: pregnancy, immunodeficient children or families with immunodeficient members
- IPV: hypersensitivity reactions in children who are sensitive to streptomycin or neomycin
- All inpatients in a neonatal intensive care setting should receive IPV at scheduled times. If possible, routine polio immunization with OPV should be delayed until after discharge. OPV may be used in specific long-term situations.

Measles, Mumps, and Rubella Vaccine

INDICATIONS

- Measles revaccination if
  1. Measles immunization before 12 mo of age
  2. Previous immunization with killed measles vaccine (before 1970)
  3. Patient has received the present measles vaccine simultaneously with, or within 3 mo after, receiving immune globulin
- Rubella vaccination of susceptible prepubertal and nonpregnant female adolescents

SIDE EFFECTS

- General: fever (day 6 or later), rash, hypersensitivity reactions in children allergic to eggs
- Measles and mumps
  1. Encephalitis (rare)
  2. TB skin test reactivity may be suppressed if administered 1-6 wk following measles vaccination
- Rubella: arthralgia, arthritis

CONTRAINDICATIONS

- Pregnancy: rubella vaccine is contraindicated 3 mo prior to and during pregnancy. However, if vaccine is inadvertently given to a pregnant woman, termination of pregnancy is NOT recommended.
- Hypersensitivity or anaphylactic reactions to eggs or neomycin. Avoid measles and mumps vaccines unless child is first skin tested ± desensitized in hospital setting.
- Administration of immune globulin or blood in preceding 3 mo
- Cell-mediated immune deficiency, malignant disease, and immunosuppression (except HIV infection)

POST-MEASLES EXPOSURE PROPHYLAXIS

- Immune globulin
  1. Infants under 1 yr: Give 0.25 ml/kg IM within 6 days after exposure
  2. Susceptible persons in whom the vaccine is contraindicated (e.g., leukemia): Give 0.5 ml/kg (max 15 ml) IM within 6 days after exposure
- Measles vaccine: might be protective if given to susceptible persons (in whom the vaccine is *not* contraindicated) up to 3 days following exposure.

POST-RUBELLA EXPOSURE PROPHYLAXIS IN PREGNANT WOMEN

- Serology immediately following exposure
  1. If rubella immune, there is no risk of congenital infection; reassure mother
  2. If rubella susceptible, repeat serology in 4 wk. If repeat serology is negative, no infection has occurred. Reassure mother. Arrange for vaccination following delivery. If seroconversion, rubella infection has occurred. Individualized counseling involving patient, geneticist, and obstetrician is recommended.
- If exposure occurs early in pregnancy in a susceptible woman and termination of pregnancy is not an option, immune globulin may be given (0.55 ml/kg; maximum 20 ml) but efficacy is unknown

Prophylaxis for Specific Diseases

HAEMOPHILUS INFLUENZAE TYPE B

Active Immunization (*H. Influenzae* Type B Polysaccharide Vaccine)

- See Table 14-1A and B
- Indications
  1. All children at 18 mo of age
  2. Unimmunized children between 2 and 5 yr of age
  3. Unimmunized high-risk children older than 5 yr (e.g., asplenia, sickle cell disease, or immunosuppression)
- Side effects: local pain and erythema, mild fever (10%)

Post-Exposure Prophylaxis with Rifampin

- In cases of invasive *H. influenzae* type b disease (e.g., meningitis, epiglottitis, arthritis, pneumonia) rifampin is given to
  1. All household contacts and the index case if there is a child (other than index case) less than 4 yr of age at home
  2. Day care center attendees (controversial)
- If two or more cases are detected within 60 days
- In day care homes resembling households with children <2 yr old in which contact is at least 25 hr/wk (same regimen as recommended for household contacts). Not required when all contacts >2 yr old.

NEISSERIA MENINGITIDIS

Active Immunization
- Preparations: quadrivalent (A, C, Y, and W-135)
- Indications
  1. Control of outbreaks (due to serogroups represented in the vaccine) in a closed population
  2. As adjunct to chemoprophylaxis in household contacts during epidemics
  3. Travel to endemic or epidemic areas
  4. May be helpful in children with complement deficiencies or asplenia
- Efficacy: adequate antibody levels are achieved for group A vaccine in children 3 mo or older and with other vaccine groups in children 2 yr or older
- Side effects: local erythema and discomfort (rare), transient fever (2%)
- Postexposure prophylaxis with rifampin
  1. The index case and all household contacts
  2. Day care contacts
  3. Intimate contact, e.g., mouth to mouth resuscitation, intubation or suctioning
  4. Dose: 20 mg/kg/day (maximum, 1200 mg/day) PO ÷ q12h × 2 days
  5. If organism is known to be sensitive to sulfonamides, use sulfisoxazole instead of rifampin
     - <1 yr: 500 mg PO once daily × 2 days
     - 1-12 yr: 500 mg PO q12h × 2 days
     - >12 yr: 1 g PO q12h × 2 days

HEPATITIS A

- Pre-exposure
  1. Travel less than 3 mo: hepatitis A immune globulin 0.02 ml/kg IM once only
  2. Prolonged travel: 0.06 ml/kg IM every 5 mo
- Postexposure: 0.02 ml/kg IM within 2 wk after exposure

HEPATITIS B

Indications

- Pre-exposure
  1. Household and sexual contacts of HBsAg carriers. Treat exposed infants <12 mo old with both hepatitis B Ig and hepatitis B vaccine if the index case involves either parent or a principal caretaker. Vaccinate children >12 mo old only if the index case becomes an HBsAg carrier.
  2. Health care workers frequently exposed to blood or blood products
  3. Residents and staff of institutions for the mentally handicapped
  4. Hemodialysis patients, hemophiliacs, and other recipients of blood products
  5. Sexually active homosexuals
  6. Users of illicit injectable drugs
  7. Heterosexual individuals with multiple partners

Administration

- Three doses of hepatitis B vaccine (suspension of purified surface antigen protein), the second and third doses given 1 and 6 mo, respectively, after the first
- Doses
  1. HEPTAVAX-B
     - <10 yr: 10 μg (0.5 ml) IM
     - ≥10 yr: 20 μg (1.0 ml) IM
  2. RECOMBIVAX-HB
     - <10 yr: 5 μg (0.5 ml) IM
     - ≥10 yr: 10 μg (1.0 ml) IM
- Hemodialysis and immunosuppressed patients: 2 × usual dose for age
- Should be given IM in deltoid (older children and adults) or anterolateral thigh (infants). Suboptimal antibody responses have been seen when vaccine is given in the buttocks.

TABLE 14-2 Post-Exposure Recommendations for Hepatitis B

Type of Exposure	HBIG*	Vaccine†
Perinatal‡	Within 12 hr after birth (repeat at 3 mo if vaccine was not given)	Within 7 days after birth; repeat at 1 and 6 mo
Sexual	Single dose within 14 days after sexual contact (repeat at 3 mo if contact is still HBsAg positive and vaccine was not given)	Recommended for sexual contacts of HBsAg carriers and active homosexual men

Continued.

*Use HBIG unless IG specifically mentioned. Doses of HBIG (or immune globulin [IG]): Perinatal = 0.5 ml IM. Sexual or percutaneous exposure = 0.06 ml/kg IM.
†Give vaccine at a different site than HBIG or IG.
‡Check infant's serology at 7 mo: If HBsAg and anti-HBs are negative, repeat dose of vaccine. If HBsAg is positive: prophylaxis has failed, follow as a carrier. If anti-HBs is positive, vaccination was successful.

TABLE 14-2 Post-Exposure Recommendations for Hepatitis B (Cont'd)

Type of Exposure	HBIG	Vaccine
Percutaneous§		
HBsAg positive blood	Within 24 hr; repeat in 1 mo if vaccine was not given	Initiate vaccine series (or give booster if previously immunized)
Unknown status of blood High-risk source, e.g., acute hepatitis	Within 24 hr. Test source: if positive, repeat in 1 mo if vaccine was not given	Test source: if positive, as above
Intermediate-risk source#	IG within 24 hr. Test source: if positive, give HBIG. Repeat HBIG in 1 mo if vaccine was not given.	Test source: if positive, as above
Low-risk or unknown source	Depends on circumstances. Treatment is optional. If decide to treat, give IG.	Test source: if positive, as above

§If contact has been vaccinated and has a recently documented protective antibody level, no treatment is necessary.
#Blood of immigrants from HBV-endemic areas, residents of custodial institutions, hemodialysis patients, users of illicit drugs, homosexuals.

INFLUENZA

Influenza Vaccine

- Preparations
  1. Vaccine contains polyvalent killed influenza strains (A and B); strains vary by location and year. It is available in two preparations: whole virus and split product (fragments of virus envelope with attached hemagglutinin, used in children <13 yr)
  2. Split product less toxic but less immunogenic
  3. Given annually in autumn; two doses separated by 4 wk
  4. >3 yr: 0.5 ml split product SC or IM
  5. <3 yr: 0.25 ml split product SC or IM
- Indications
  1. Severe chronic disease, e.g., heart disease associated with cardiac failure or pulmonary congestion, chronic pulmonary disease (e.g., cystic fibrosis, severe asthma), chronic renal disease, diabetes mellitus, sickle cell anemia and other hemoglobinopathies, and immunosuppressed children
  2. Long-term ASA therapy (risk of Reye's syndrome in children taking ASA who acquire influenza B)
- Contraindications
  1. Age <6 mo
  2. Hypersensitivity reactions to egg

Amantadine

- Postexposure prophylaxis and treatment for influenza A virus only
- Indications
  1. During outbreaks in custodial institutions
  2. High-risk groups; during influenza A epidemics; when vaccine is contraindicated or expected to evoke inadequate antibody response

- Administration
  1. <9 yr: 4 mg/kg/day (max 100 mg/day) PO ÷ bid
  2. ≥9 yr: 200 mg/day PO ÷ bid
  3. For treatment, start as soon as possible after symptoms begin and continue for 5 days or until asymptomatic × 48 hr
  4. For prophylaxis, give × 10-14 days (may be given throughout an epidemic up to 90 days)
- Precautions
  1. Not recommended for infants <1 yr
  2. Impaired renal function
  3. Active seizure disorder
- Side effects: 5-10% insomnia, lightheadedness, irritability

STREPTOCOCCUS PNEUMONIAE

- Vaccine: purified capsular polysaccharides of 23 serotypes of *S. pneumoniae*
- Indicated in children ≥age 2 yr with
  1. Anatomic or functional asplenia
  2. Sickle cell disease
  3. Nephrotic syndrome
  4. Immunosuppression

Administration

- 0.5 ml IM/SC single dose; if possible, give 2 wk prior to splenectomy or immunosuppression. Revaccination is not recommended at present time (in children who were previously vaccinated at age 2 yr, the need for revaccination is currently being re-evaluated).
- 70-80% of recipients will achieve adequate antibody levels to the antigens in the vaccine (a partial response is seen in Hodgkin's disease or renal transplant patients)

Precautions
- Avoid in pregnancy unless there is a high risk of pneumococcal infection
- This vaccine does not represent all the pneumococcal serotypes; therefore, antimicrobial coverage in certain patients, e.g., asplenic children is still advised
- Side effects: local soreness and erythema, fever, myalgias, anaphylactic reactions (rare)

RABIES

- See Table 14-3 for guide to Post-exposure Prophylaxis.

Administration Following a Bite
- Not previously immunized
  1. HDCV: 1 ml IM—days 0, 3, 7, 14, and 28 (5 doses)
  2. RIG: 20 IU/kg—half IM and half infiltrated around the bite site
  3. Always give HDCV and RIG with different syringes at different sites
- Previously immunized (with HDCV or other type of vaccine with documented positive antibody response), HDCV: 1 ml IM—days 0 and 3 (no RIG)
- Follow-up serology recommended only in immunocompromised patients

Precautions
- Chloroquine interferes with development of active immunity
- Allergies (including anaphylaxis) can occur
- Pregnancy: HDCV and RIG may be given if substantial risk of rabies exists

Side Effects
- HDCV (common): local pain and erythema and swelling, headache, nausea, abdominal pain, myalgias, dizziness, serum-sickness–like reactions following boosters
- RIG: local pain and low-grade fever

TABLE 14-3 Rabies Post-Exposure Prophylaxis Guide*

Animal Species	Condition of Animal at Time of Attack	Treatment of Exposed Person†
Domestic dogs and cats	Healthy and available for 10 days of observation	None, unless animal develops rabies‡
	Rabid or suspected rabid	RIG§ and HDCV
	Unknown (escaped)	Consult public health officials. If treatment is indicated, give RIG§ and HDCV.
Wild Skunk, bat, fox, coyote, raccoon, bobcat, and other carnivores	Regard as rabid unless proven negative by laboratory tests#	RIG§ and HDCV

Other
Livestock, rodents, and lagomorphs (rabbits and hares)

Consider individually. Bites of squirrels, hamsters, guinea pigs, gerbils, chipmunks, rats, mice, other rodents, rabbits, and hares almost never call for antirabies prophylaxis.

---

*These recommendations are only a guide. In applying them, take into account the animal species involved, the circumstances of the bite or other exposure, *the vaccination status of the animal, and presence of rabies* in the region. Local or state public health officials should be consulted if questions arise about the need for rabies prophylaxis.

†*All bites and wounds should immediately be thoroughly cleansed with soap and water.* If antirabies treatment is indicated, both rabies immune globulin (RIG) and human diploid cell rabies vaccine (HDCV) should be given as soon as possible *regardless* of the interval from exposure. Local reactions to vaccines are common and do not contraindicate continuing treatment. Discontinue vaccine if fluorescent-antibody tests of the animal are negative.

‡During the usual holding period of 10 days, begin treatment with RIG and HDCV at first sign of rabies in a dog or cat that has bitten someone. The symptomatic animal should be killed immediately and tested.

§If RIG is not available, use equine antirabies serum (ARS). Do not use more than the recommended dosage.

#The animal should be killed and tested as soon as possible. Holding for observation is not recommended.

From Centers for Disease Control. Rabies prevention: MMWR 1984; 33:393-402.

TETANUS (Table 14-4)

TABLE 14-4 Guide to Tetanus Prophylaxis in Wound Management

Type of Wound	Patient Not Immunized or Partially Immunized (<3 Doses or Unknown)	Patient Completely Immunized Time Since Last Booster* 5-10 Years	>10 Years
Clean, minor (<6 hr, no debris)	Td†; complete the immunization series	None	Td†
All other wounds	Td† TIG‡ 250-500 U IM; complete the immunization series	Td†	Td†

*If patient completely immunized and last booster was within 5 yr, no prophylaxis is necessary.
†For children less than 7 yr, use DPT (DT if pertussis is contraindicated). Attention to wound cleaning and debridement when indicated.
‡Tetanus immune globulin—use separate syringes and deliver at a separate site other than that used for toxoid.
Modified from Giagrasso J, Smith RR. Misuse of tetanus immunoprophylaxis. Ann Emerg Med 1985; 14:573-579.

VARICELLA

- Immunocompromised patients should be tested for varicella antibody titers
- Varicella vaccine: still investigational
- Varicella–zoster immune globulin (VZIG) prepared from plasma of outdated blood with high V-Z antibody titers
- Indications (VZIG)
  1. Immunocompromised susceptible patients exposed to V-Z infection (exposure to household contact, indoor playmate contact >1 hr, or hospital contact—same room or prolonged face-to-face contact)
  2. Neonates whose mothers have developed varicella ≤5 days prior to or within 2 days after delivery
  3. Exposed premature infants <28 wk gestation or ≤1 kg
  4. Exposed premature infants ≥28 wk gestation whose mother lacks a history of chickenpox
- Dose: to be given within 96 hr after exposure (preferably sooner)
  1. <10 kg: 125 U (one vial)
  2. >10 kg: 12.5 U/kg; max 625 U (5 vials)
- Precautions: strict isolation of exposed patient is necessary between days 10 and 21 following exposure. If VZIG was given, isolate until 35 days following exposure.

Diseases and Syndromes

SEPTIC ARTHRITIS

- Neonatal: nosocomial infection; often multifocal; may be subtle, i.e., pain on moving hip to change diaper
- Childhood type often solitary
- *S. pneumoniae, H. influenza* in infants; *Staphylococcus aureus* in older children
- Acute onset of pain; decreased range of motion; hot swollen joint held in flexion

Investigations
- Joint aspiration (hip requires general anaesthetic) for WBC and differential (see p 511), glucose, Gram stain, latex agglutination, culture
- CBC, ESR, blood culture (only 70% positive)
- X-ray exam (may be normal)
- Bone and gallium radionuclide scans may be useful if adjacent osteomyelitis is suspected

Treatment
- *Rapid joint drainage (consult orthopedics) and institution of IV antibiotic treatment are crucial.* Thick pus does not come out through a needle; therefore, surgical drainage required in most cases.
- Continuous passive movement reduces stiffness and speeds healing; avoid weight bearing during the acute illness
- Adequate analgesics for pain control

Antibiotic Therapy
- For empiric therapy, see Table 14-5 (adjust therapy to results of Gram stain and culture)
- Antibiotics should be given IV initially. Once the signs of acute inflammation have resolved, switch to an equivalent dose of antibiotics if the following conditions are met:
  1. Patient can tolerate oral medications and strict compliance is ensured
  2. Serum bactericidal titers (SBT) can be determined; 1-2 hr postlevels should be ≥1:8
  3. Follow-up can be maintained with weekly monitoring of clinical condition, ESR, and SBT. Follow-up x-ray examination should be done if osteomyelitis is suspected.
- Duration (dependent on clinical response)
  1. Antibiotics should be given for a minimum of 2 wk
  2. Shorter courses (1 wk) can be given for gonococcal arthritis
  3. Longer courses (3-4 wk) are advised for *S. aureus* arthritis of hip joint, neonates, immunocompromised patients, gram-negative arthritis or associated osteomyelitis (4-6 wk)
- Intra-articular instillation of antibiotics is unnecessary and frequently causes chemical arthritis

TABLE 14-5 Etiologic Organisms and Empiric Antibiotic Selection for Septic Arthritis*

Age	Potential Organisms	Empiric Antibiotic Therapy
Neonates	Group B strep., S. aureus, coliforms	Cloxacillin + cefotaxime *or* Cloxacillin + ampicillin + aminoglycoside
Infants and children <5 yr	S. aureus, H. influenzae, S. pneumoniae	Cefuroxime *or* Cloxacillin + chloramphenicol
Children >5 yr	S. aureus, S. pneumoniae	Cloxacillin or 1st generation cephalosporin (cefazolin, cephalothin)
Immunocompromised	S. aureus, S. pneumoniae, gram-negative organisms	Cloxacillin + aminoglycoside *or* Cloxacillin + cefotaxime

*In children with hemoglobinopathies, consider *Salmonella* and *H. influenzae* in addition to usual pathogens. In sexually active adolescents consider *N. gonorrhoeae* in addition to usual pathogens.

OSTEOMYELITIS

- Neonate: *S. aureus*, gram-negative bacilli, group B streptococci
- Infants and children: *S. aureus*; less commonly, *S. pneumoniae, H. influenzae*, group A streptococci
- Hemoglobinopathies or other asplenic conditions: consider *Salmonella*
- Puncture wound of foot: *Pseudomonas aeruginosa*
- May be acute, subacute (gradual onset of pain, x-ray changes may resemble osteosarcoma)
- Recurrent, multifocal: bone pain in several sites; x-rays show wide growth plates

Investigations

- WBC, ESR (increased), blood cultures (positive in 70%)
- X-ray: soft tissue swelling, subperiosteal elevation (bone changes not evident for first 10 days)
- Bone scan ± gallium scan. Early stage shows increased uptake; may show decreased uptake in late stages.
- CT scan: useful for vertebral, sacroiliac osteomyelitis
- Needle aspiration or incision and drainage if point tenderness, focal swelling, or an x-ray or nuclear scan suggestive of subperiosteal pus collection

Treatment

- Analgesia, immobilization
- Antibiotic therapy
  1. Neonate: cloxacillin and aminoglycoside, or cloxacillin and cefotaxime
  2. <5 yr: cefuroxime alone or cloxacillin and chloramphenicol in combination
  3. >5 yr: cloxacillin (if allergic to penicillin, can use clindamycin), or first-generation cephalosporin (cefazolin, cephatholin)
  4. Sickle cell disease: add ampicillin or ceftriaxone or cefotaxime

5. Puncture wound of foot: add aminoglycoside or ceftazidime
6. Once organism and sensitivities are identified, switch to appropriate antibiotic
7. Use IV route initially. When switching to oral therapy, observe the same guidelines as outlined in the section on septic arthritis (see p 248).
8. For oral treatment of *S. aureus* osteomyelitis, cephalexin suspension has several advantages over cloxacillin (tastes better, may be given with food, equal cost)

- Duration of antibiotic treatment
  1. Acute osteomyelitis: minimum, 4 wk, until all clinical signs have resolved and ESR is normal
  2. Pseudomonas osteomyelitis secondary to puncture wound of foot: treat for 1-2 wk after surgical debridement
  3. Chronic osteomyelitis requires long-term treatment (minimum, 6 mo)
- Surgical therapy (drainage) if poor response within 72 hr or delayed diagnosis (>4 days), subperiosteal pus, femoral head osteomyelitis with hip joint involvement, or vertebral osteomyelitis with neurologic signs. Puncture wound of foot may require debridement.

BITES

Animal Bites

- Organisms: anaerobes, aerobes including streptococci, *S. aureus, Pasteurella multocida*
- Document the type and health status of the animal as well as the circumstances surrounding delivery of the bite
- Note the location and severity of the wound and any signs of infection

Management

- High-pressure irrigation with copious amounts of sterile saline using a syringe
- Debridement of dead tissues
- Leave unsutured if wound involves the hand or if more than 6-8 hr have elapsed since injury (consult plastic surgeon)
- Prophylactic antibiotics (controversial)—use in facial, hand, or major injuries or when presenting >12 hr after injuries have been sustained
  1. Amoxicillin-clavulanic acid or penicillin × 5 days
  2. Penicillin-allergic patients: tetracycline (if >8 yr) or erythromycin (but 50% of *P. multocida* are resistant)
- Tetanus prophylaxis (see p 246)
- Rabies prophylaxis (see pp 244, 245)
- Instruct parents to return if fever develops, wound becomes infected, or infection is spreading

HUMAN BITES

- Organisms: *S. aureus,* streptococci, anaerobes; more virulent than cat or dog bites
- Document location, severity of wound (involvement of deep structures), and any signs of infection
- Irrigation, debridement as for animal bites
- Leave unsutured
- Elevate extremity
- Tetanus prophylaxis (see p 246)
- Antibiotic prophylaxis
  1. Amoxicillin-clavulanic acid
  2. Penicillin ± cloxacillin
  3. Penicillin-allergic: use clindamycin
- Infection generally requires admission to hospital, early surgical exploration, and debridement. Swab for gram stain, culture; elevate and immobilize affected part. IV antibiotics (penicillin and cloxacillin, clindamycin).
- Joint involvement requires *urgent* referral for surgical exploration and debridement

CELLULITIS

- Nonfacial cellulitis: group A streptococci, *S. aureus;* neonates: group B streptococci
- Buccal cellulitis: as in nonfacial cellulitis plus *H. influenzae*
- If the patient is toxic and the lesion is spreading very quickly and is extremely tender or anesthetic, consider necrotizing fasciitis. Although rare, this requires immediate surgical debridement and IV antibiotics (to cover streptococci, staphylococci, gram-negative organisms, and anaerobes).

Management
- CBC, blood culture
- Needle aspiration of advancing edge for culture
- If etiology unclear:
  1. Nonfacial cellulitis: PO cephalexin or cloxacillin for minor cases; IV cloxacillin or first-generation cephalosporin
  2. Buccal cellulitis: IV cefuroxime, PO cefaclor or amoxicillin-clavulanic acid
- Duration of antibiotics: 7-10 days

PERIORBITAL AND ORBITAL CELLULITIS

- Etiologic organisms: *H. influenzae, S. aureus, S. pneumoniae*
- Often associated with sinusitis or minor skin trauma
- Periorbital cellulitis should be differentiated from orbital cellulitis by absence of proptosis and presence of full ocular movement and normal visual acuity
- CBC, blood culture
- Sinus x-rays
- CT scan if orbital cellulitis is a possibility
- Orbital cellulitis may require urgent surgical drainage in addition to IV antibiotics (in addition to orbital damage, untreated orbital cellulitis can lead to cavernous sinus thrombosis), consult ophthalmology
- Treat with cefuroxime alone, or cloxacillin and chloramphenicol in combination

CERVICAL ADENITIS

- Acute: *S. aureus,* group A streptococci, group B streptococci (neonates); anaerobes, adenovirus, enterovirus less common
- Subacute and chronic (1-3 wk): cat-scratch fever, anaerobes, EBV, CMV, atypical mycobacteria, *Mycobacterium tuberculosis,* toxoplasmosis, histoplasmosis
- Rule out malignancy, drugs (phenytoin, isoniazid), Kawasaki disease, neck anomalies (cystic hygroma, branchial cleft cyst, thyroglossal duct cyst)

Management

- Cultures (skin, throat, ± blood)
- If node is fluctuant, consider incision and drainage (send sample for Gram stain and culture)
- In mild infection, cloxacillin or erythromycin PO × 10 days
- If a dental source is suspected, use penicillin V or clindamycin PO
- Neonatal infections and more severe infections may need IV therapy and surgical drainage
- If no improvement or chronic infection, investigate for mycobacterial (atypical or TB), viral, cat-scratch, or malignant disease

CLOSTRIDIUM DIFFICILE

Investigations

- History of current or recent antibiotic therapy
- Stool for
  1. Anaerobic culture on selective media
  2. Filtration and detection of cytotoxin B
- Sigmoidoscopy – colonoscopy if pseudomembranous colitis suspected

Treatment

- Asymptomatic patients do not require treatment. It is suggested that neutropenic patients be treated even if asymptomatic. Avoid antidiarrheal drugs.
- If symptomatic
  1. Enteric isolation
  2. Discontinue antibiotics if feasible (mildly symptomatic patients may benefit by stopping antibiotics alone)
  3. Metronidazole PO or IV, or vancomycin (metronidazole less expensive and better tolerated)
- Relapses are common (10-20%); may require an additional course of treatment

CONGENITAL INFECTIONS

- Congenital infection may also be caused by: HIV, syphilis, hepatitis B virus (HBV), varicella, and enteroviruses
- Infection occurs in utero (by transplacental transmission) or perinatally (by passage through birth canal)
- Most are asymptomatic at birth, but may still have late sequelae
- CMV most common (0.1-1% of liveborn infants)

TABLE 14-6 Congenital Infections*

CMV	Rubella	Herpes Simplex	Syphilis	Toxoplasmosis
Investigations (see also p 216) CBC, LFTs Culture urine†, throat, gastric contents Serology: IgM‡ X-rays (chest, tibiae with knees) Ophthalmologic examination Audiologic examination CT head	CBC, LFTs Culture urine, throat, stool Serology: IgM‡; IgG§ X-ray (chest, tibiae with knees)# Audiologic examination Ophthalmologic examination	CBC, LFTs EM skin vesicles Culture throat Serology: IgM‡	CBC, LFTs Darkfield examination of nasal discharge VDRL, FTA-ABS X-ray (tibiae with knees)#	CBC, LFTs Serology: IgM‡; IgG§ Ophthalmologic examination CT head
Therapy Consider gancyclovir	No specific therapy	Symptomatic newborn should be treated with acyclovir Treatment of asymptomatic newborn of mother	Penicillin	Complex treatment regimen with sulfadiazine, pyrimethamine, and folinic acid

Isolation	Avoid contact with pregnant women; an infected newborn may excrete the virus for months and even years	Avoid contact with pregnant women; an infected newborn may excrete the virus for months		with active genital herpes is controversial
				None
			Newborns with clinical disease	
Pre- and perinatal prevention	Careful handwashing for nonimmune pregnant women in nurseries and day care centers	Females of child-bearing age should have serology checked; if not immune, should receive vaccination at least 3 mo prior to any planned pregnancy	If mother has genital herpes at or near time of delivery and membranes are intact or ruptured <6 hr, a cesarean section is recommended	Barrier until 24 hr after start of antibiotics
				Pregnant females should have a VDRL; if confirmatory serology is positive, treat
				Avoid ingestion of raw meat
				No contact with cat litter

*Note: Because of overlapping features, a definitive etiologic diagnosis can not be made on clinical grounds alone.
†Urine culture must be taken before 3 wk of age to establish the diagnosis of congenital CMV.
‡Not available at all centers.
§Test *both* infant and mother's serology initially and 12 wk later (see p 637).
#Check for delayed epiphyseal maturation and metaphyseal radiolucent streaks (celery stalking).

HERPES SIMPLEX ENCEPHALITIS

Investigations
- CT scan: focal lesions (usually temporal or frontal; may be normal early in illness)
- Lumbar puncture: CSF usually has normal or increased protein, normal glucose polymorphic or lymphocytic, pleocytosis ($\pm$ increased RBC). If focal signs or signs of increased ICP are present on history or physical exam lumbar puncture should not be done until a CT scan has ruled out space-occupying lesion.
- CSF culture (rarely positive for HSV)
- Blood, CSF serology (rise seen 1 to several weeks later)
- EEG: often focal findings (poor prognostic sign if bilateral)
- Brain biopsy: most definitive way of making diagnosis (used for pathology, EM, IF, viral culture); generally not indicated in normal host, may be indicated if immunocompromised

Treatment
- Supportive care, including treatment of seizures, increased ICP, and monitoring for SIADH
- IV acyclovir for 10 days

HIV INFECTION AND AIDS

- Most children with perinatally acquired HIV infection will become ill in the first 2 yr of life; a small number may remain asymptomatic for several years.

Pediatric Risk Groups for AIDS
- Children who have received blood or blood products (e.g., hemophiliacs) before screening for HIV antibodies (begun in Canada in November 1985, begun April 1985 in U.S.)
- Newborns and infants of a mother with HIV infection; the risk of vertical transmission is approximately 20-50%
- Intravenous drug users
- Sexual contacts of persons with HIV infections; high-risk groups include prostitutes, IV drug users, and homosexual and bisexual men
- Sexually abused

Management
- It is often difficult to distinguish seropositive children <15 mo with true HIV infection from those with only passively acquired maternal antibodies
- Consent with pre- and post-test counseling must be obtained; a pediatric diagnosis may lead to a parental diagnosis

Confirmation of HIV Infection
- Positive serology with confirmatory Western blot
- HIV isolation from blood or tissues (relatively insensitive)
- HIV antigen (serum) or DNA detection tests (polymerase chain reaction)

Other Features Suggestive of HIV Infection
- Hypergammaglobulinemia
- Low T_4 counts
- Low T_4/T_8 ratios
- Lymphopenia
- Anergy
- Thrombocytopenia
- Hemolytic anemia
- CSF pleocytosis, increased protein

TABLE 14-7 CDC Classification System for HIV Infection in Children

Class P-0. Indeterminate infection
Infants <15 mo born to infected mothers but without definitive evidence of HIV infection or AIDS

Class P-1. Asymptomatic infection
Subclass A: Normal immune function
Subclass B: Abnormal immune function—hypergammaglobulinemia, T4 lymphopenia, decreased T4:T8 ratio, or absolute lymphopenia
Subclass C: Immune function not tested

Class P-2. Symptomatic infection
Subclass A: Nonspecific findings (≥2 for ≥2 mo)—fever, failure to thrive, generalized lymphadenopathy, hepatomegaly, splenomegaly, enlarged parotid glands, persistent or recurrent diarrhea
Subclass B: Progressive neurologic disease—loss of developmental milestones or intellectual ability, impaired brain growth, or progressive symmetrical motor deficits
Subclass C: Lymphoid interstitial pneumonitis
Subclass D: Secondary infectious diseases
  Category D-1: Opportunistic infections in the CDC case definition
    Bacterial: mycobacterial infection (noncutaneous, extrapulmonary, disseminated); nocardiosis
    Fungal: candidiasis (esophageal, bronchial, or pulmonary), coccidioidomycosis, disseminated histoplasmosis, extrapulmonary cryptococcosis

TABLE 14-7 CDC Classification System for HIV Infection in Children (Cont'd)

  Parasitic: *Pneumocystis carinii* pneumonia, disseminated toxoplasmosis with onset ≥1 mo of age, chronic cryptosporidiosis or isosporiasis, extraintestinal strongyloidiasis

  Viral: CMV disease (onset ≥1 mo of age), chronic mucocutaneous or disseminated herpes (onset ≥1 mo of age), progressive multifocal leukoencephalopathy

 Category D-2: Unexplained, recurrent, serious bacterial infections (2 or more in a 2-yr period): sepsis, meningitis, pneumonia, abscess of an internal organ, bone and joint infections

 Category D-3: Other infectious diseases including persistent oral candidiasis, recurrent herpes stomatitis (≥2 episodes in 1 yr), multidermatomal or disseminated herpes zoster

Subclass E: Secondary cancers

 Category E-1: Cancers in the AIDS case definition: Kaposi's sarcoma, B-cell non-Hodgkin's lymphoma, or primary lymphoma of brain

 Category E-2: Other malignancies possibly associated with HIV

Subclass F: Other conditions possibly due to HIV infection including hepatitis, cardiopathy, nephropathy, hematologic disorders, dermatologic diseases

---

Adapted from Centers for Disease Control Classification system for human immunodeficiency virus (HIV) infection in children under 13 years of age. MMWR 1987; 36:225-230, 235.

Therapeutic Considerations
- Consult with expert in pediatric HIV infections
- Zidovudine (AZT)
- *P. carinii* pneumonia (PCP) prophylaxis (trimethoprim-sulfamethoxazole)
- IV immune globulin
- All routine vaccinations including MMR are recommended (avoid BCG and OPV)
- Prompt evaluation and treatment of acute infections
- Immune globulin after measles or varicella exposures
- Additional immunizations: influenza (annually); pneumonococcal vaccine
- CMV negative blood transfusions
- Universal blood and body fluid precautions

INFECTIOUS MONONUCLEOSIS

Investigations
- WBC and differential (increased atypical lymphocytes)
- Multiple specific serologic antibody tests available
- Most commonly used: (see p 637 for interpretation)
  1. Heterophile antibodies (Monospot test, Paul Bunnel test)
  2. IgG against viral capsid Ag (VCA)
  3. Anti-EA (early Ag)

Treatment
- Isolation not required
- Symptomatic: bed rest, encourage fluids, warm saline gargles for sore throat, acetaminophen
- Hospitalization and steroids indicated in airway obstruction (start with equivalent of 1-2 mg/kg/day of prednisone; give PO in divided doses and taper over 1-2 wk)

Follow-up
- Usually resolves over 2-3 wk period, although fatigue may persist for weeks
- Contact sports should be avoided if splenomegaly present, due to risk of splenic rupture

BACTERIAL MENINGITIS

- Neonates: group B streptococci, *E. coli, Listeria,* Group D streptococci
- Infants and children <10 yr: *H. influenzae, S. pneumoniae, N. meningitidis*
- Adolescents: *S. pneumoniae, N. meningitidis, H. influenzae* (rare)
- Compromised hosts: in addition to the preceding, *S. aureus,* gram-negative bacilli, *Listeria*

Investigations

- CSF examination (Table 14-8): A lumbar puncture (LP) should be done as soon as the possibility of meningitis is raised (for procedure and precautions, see p 575). If fundoscopic exam not possible in child with closed fontanelle, or if there are focal neurologic signs of increased intracranial pressure, CT should be performed and an LP done only if CT rules out intracranial space-occupying lesion. CSF studies include cell count and differential, Gram stain, culture and sensitivity, protein, glucose, antigen-detection testing (e.g., latex agglutination for encapsulated organisms, e.g., *H. influenzae, N. meningitides, S. pneumoniae,* even if patient has been taking antibiotics); save one tube for additional investigations, e.g., virology, TB.
- CBC, differential, platelet count
- Blood glucose, electrolytes, BUN, creatinine, urine electrolytes
- Blood cultures
- PT, PTT, fibrin split products (if indicated)
- Urine: latex agglutination, specific gravity, electrolytes, and osmolality (if SIADH is suspected)

TABLE 14-8 Interpretation of CSF Findings in Meningitis

	Bacterial	Viral	TB	Partially Treated
Cell count*	Usually >1000	Usually <300	<1000	>1000
Predominant cell	Polymorphs	Early polymorphs, then mononuclear	Lymphocytes	Polymorphs or mononuclear
Gram stain	Usually positive	Negative	Negative (acid-fast stain may be positive)	May be negative
Glucose	Low†	Normal	Low† or normal	Low† or normal
Protein‡	High	Normal or high	Very high	High
Bacterial culture	Usually positive	Negative	Culture for TB may be positive	Often negative

*The WBC count in normal spinal fluid should be at most 5×10^6/L (5/mm^3). Neonates may have higher numbers of WBC, especially if low birth weight. Even though WBC are usually quite high in bacterial meningitis, any count above normal must be viewed suspiciously. RBC to WBC ratios in CSF specimens contaminated with blood must be interpreted with caution; treatment should not be withheld if clinical picture is suggestive of meningitis. Seizures alone do not increase CSF WBC count.
†CSF glucose: <50% of blood glucose.
‡Increased protein seen in meningitis, encephalitis, abscess, leukemia, or intracranial malignancy.

TABLE 14-9 Empiric Antibiotic Selection for Meningitis

Neonate	Ampicillin + aminoglycoside *or* Ampicillin + cefotaxime
Infant 1-2 mo	Ampicillin + cefotaxime
Child 3 mo to 10 yr	Ceftriaxone or cefotaxime *or* Ampicillin + chloramphenicol
>10 yr	Penicillin
Immunocompromised	Cefotaxime (or ceftazidime) + ampicillin
Shunt related	Vancomycin + cefotaxime

Management

- Monitor vital signs, hydration, neurologic status, weight, serum, and urine electrolytes (for SIADH)
- Early management of shock, seizures, raised ICP as necessary
- IV at 60% daily maintenance after ensuring that any dehydration has been corrected; PO intake depending on level of consciousness
- Careful daily assessment: head circumference, skull transillumination (infants), metastatic foci
- Prophylaxis with rifampin for family and index case (see p 236)
- Steroids controversial
- Never delay treatment because an LP cannot be done, or while awaiting CT
- Switch to appropriate antibiotic once organism is identified and sensitivities are known
- Duration
  1. Neonates: 2 wk (3 wk in gram-negative meningitis)
  2. *H. influenzae, S. pneumoniae, N. meningitidis:* 7 days in uncomplicated cases
  3. *S. aureus:* minimum, 3 wk
  4. Gram-negative bacilli: minimum, 3 wk
- Prolonged or recurrent pyrexia (more than 5 days) may be due to
  1. Nosocomial illness, e.g., URI, gastroenteritis
  2. Phlebitis
  3. Secondary focus: arthritis, pneumonia, pleural effusion, pericarditis
  4. Subdural effusions (common; in most cases medical intervention not needed; neurosurgical consultation and aspiration if increasing head circumference, vomiting, seizures, or focal neurologic findings)
  5. Drug fever
  6. Failure of conventional management

Follow-up (All Patients)

- Hearing testing within 1 mo after discharge
- Psychological assessment prior to starting school or before that if developmental delay is suspected
- Neurologic assessment and follow-up if indicated

MUMPS

Confirmation of Diagnosis
- Saliva, urine, CSF (if indicated) for viral isolation
- Mumps serology (p 638)

Treatment
- Respiratory isolation (may be contagious as long as 7 days prior to parotid swelling and 9 days after onset)
- Symptomatic treatment only (acetaminophen for pain; cold or warm packs to areas of swelling)

SELECTED PARASITIC INFECTIONS

TABLE 14-10 Selected Parasitic Diseases

Disease	Treatment*
I. Intestinal nematodes	
Ascariasis	Pyrantel pamoate or mebendazole
Hookworm (*Ancylostoma duodenale, Necator americanus*)	Mebendazole or pyrantel pamoate
Pinworm (*Enterobius*)	Pyrantel pamoate or mebendazole
II. Protozoa	
Amebiasis	
Asymptomatic intestinal disease	Iodoquinol
Symptomatic intestinal or invasive disease	Metronidazole and iodoquinol
Giardiasis	Metronidazole or quinacrine PO × 7 days or furazolidone PO × 10 days
Malaria	
1. Vivax, ovale and malariae	Chloroquine
	Oral or NG (bitter taste)
	If very ill or vomiting, use the parenteral route (IM, SC)
	If dehydrated, rehydrate with 20 ml/kg bolus of IV normal saline prior to injection
	Monitor BP closely
	Switch to oral dose when tolerated

	To achieve radical cure (prevention of relapses) for vivax and ovale†
2. Chloroquine-sensitive falciparum malaria‡ (if unsure of sensitivity, consider resistant— see ‡)	Following chloroquine Rx, give primaquine PO × 14 days (test for G6PD deficiency prior to Rx) Chloroquine (as above)

3. Chloroquine-resistant falciparum malaria‡	Oral Route
	  Quinine sulphate§ for 3-9 days plus either clindamycin for 7 days
	    or
	  Single-dose pyrimethamine-sulfadoxine
	Parenteral route
	  Unable to tolerate oral Rx
	  Parasitemia >5%
	  IV quinidine-load with quinidine sulfate
	    Give in 2 mg/ml of saline with dextrose
	    Cardiac monitor and frequent BP readings
	    Monitor serum glucose q2-4h at bedside
	    Switch to PO quinine as soon as feasible
	    If patient still severely ill after 72 hr of Rx, decrease dose by 1/3 because of expected impaired hepatic clearance
	  Plus either
	  Pyrimethamine-sulfadoxine or clindamycin (see 3A)

*See formulary for dosages and methods of administration.
†Not necessary for congenital or transfusion-related malaria.
‡Potentially rapidly fatal or severe. Suggest urgent infectious disease referral.
§Duration of quinine or quinidine duration variable: African-acquired—3-5 days; Southeast Asian acquired—5-9 days.
See also: Lynk A, Gold R. A review of 40 children with imported malaria. Pediatr Infect Dis J 1989; 8:745-750.

PERTUSSIS

- WBC and differential (lymphocytosis)
- Nasopharyngeal swab or aspirate (Auger suction) for culture
- Admit if severe illness or apnea
- Supportive care: clear airway secretions; O_2 for cyanotic episodes
- Antibiotics
  1. Erythromycin estolate may prevent paroxysmal stage if started in catarrhal stage and may shorten period of communicability
  2. Treat secondary bacterial infections

Prevention

- Chemoprophylaxis
  1. Indications: household or close contacts if <1 yr regardless of immunization status, or <7 yr and not fully immunized. Some authorities believe that all contacts should receive chemoprophylaxis
  2. Erythromycin estolate (dose as for infection); alternatively, trimethoprim-sulfamethoxazole
- Active immunization of contacts. Give DPT if <7 yr and either
  1. Unimmunized or immunizations are not up to date
  2. Partially immunized and third dose was ≥6 mo ago or
  3. No DPT in last 3 yr

STREPTOCOCCAL PHARYNGITIS

- Diagnosis: throat culture or latex agglutination test for rapid detection of group A streptococcal antigen in pharyngeal secretions
- Rationale of therapy: prevents suppurative complications (e.g., peritonsillar abscess), prevents rheumatic fever, and alleviates symptoms. Role in prevention of nephritis uncertain
- Antibiotics
  1. Penicillin V PO × 10 days or benzathine penicillin G as a single IM dose
  2. Penicillin-allergic patients: erythromycin estolate × 10 days
- Follow-up cultures not necessary unless patient or member of family has rheumatic fever; then culture, and if positive, re-treat
- Carriers are not treated unless a family member has rheumatic fever
- Clindamycin alone × 10 days, or rifampin × 5 days together with penicillin × 10 days, is more effective than oral penicillin therapy alone in eradicating carrier state

SEPTIC SHOCK

Management

- For monitoring and the acute management of shock and its complications, see p 547
- Use of steroids controversial
- Obtain necessary specimens (blood, urine, appropriate swabs, ± CSF) for microscopy, Gram stain, cultures, latex agglutination
- Remove intravascular catheters; send tip for culture
- Radiologic (e.g., CXR, ECHO, CT scan) or nuclear scan studies if indicated
- Prompt institution of antibiotics

TABLE 14-11 Empiric Antibiotic Selection for Septic Shock or Severe Illness

Neonate	Ampicillin + aminoglycoside ± cloxacillin if risk for *S. aureus* *or* Ampicillin + cefotaxime
Infant, 1-2 mo	Ampicillin + cefotaxime ± cloxacillin if risk of *S. aureus*
Child, 3 mo-10 yr	Cefuroxime (ceftriaxone or cefotaxime if risk of meningitis)
>10 yr	Cefuroxime
Immunocompromised	Extended-spectrum penicillin (e.g., ticarcillin) + aminoglycoside *or* Vancomycin + ceftazidime
Line or shunt related	Vancomycin + ceftazidime
Intra-abdominal	Clindamycin *or* metronidazole + ampicillin + aminoglycoside
Urinary tract	Ampicillin + aminoglycoside
Respiratory tract	Cefuroxime ± erythromycin If aspiration suspected: clindamycin + aminoglycoside

SINUSITIS

- Acute: *S. pneumoniae, H. influenzae, Branhamella catarrhalis*
- Chronic: *Bacteroides,* anaerobic and aerobic streptococci, *S. aureus, H. influenzae,* fungus

Management
- Sinus x-ray: (diagnostic specificity in children not proven)
- Antimicrobials
  1. Acute: amoxicillin, trimethoprim-sulfamethoxazole, amoxicillin-clavulanic acid or cefaclor $\times$ 10 days
  2. If severe and periorbital cellulitis see p 253
  3. If persistent, may require ENT referral (sinus lavage, drainage)
- Antihistamines and decongestants: clinical efficacy not proven and also may reduce local resistance
- Complications: brain abscess, parameningeal infection, cavernous sinus thrombosis

TABLE 14-12 Characteristics of Cephalosporins

1st Generation*	2nd Generation†	3rd Generation‡
Excellent gram-positive coverage (*S. aureus*, group A strep, *S. pneumoniae*)	Good gram-positive coverage (*S. aureus*, group A strep, *S. pneumoniae*)	Ceftriaxone, good gram-positive coverage; all others poor
Poor enterococcus	Poor enterococcus	Poor enterococcus
Poor gram-negative coverage	Active vs *H. influenzae*	Good gram-positive coverage
Sometimes used in UTIs	Spotty vs gram-negative enterics	Ceftazidime, good *P. aeruginosa* coverage; all others poor
No CSF penetration	± CSF penetration	Good CSF penetration

*Cefazolin, cephalexin.
†Cefuroxime, cefaclor.
‡Cefotaxime, ceftriaxone, ceftazidime, cefixime.

TUBERCULOSIS

Investigations
- History of exposure
- Skin testing
  1. Mantoux/PPD 5TU 0.1 ml intradermally
  2. Positive if ≥10 mm of induration at 48-72 hr (5-10 mm may be significant in household contacts or individuals previously immunized with BCG)
  3. Radiologic evidence: CXR (AP and lateral)
  4. Stains for acid-fast bacilli and TB cultures: sputum, gastric aspirate, urine, CSF (if indicated)
  5. Histologic study and TB culture when indicated: lymph nodes, liver, pleura, bone marrow

General Treatment
- Isolation not required for primary TB in children; isolate only if cavitary or endobronchial disease is present
- Inform public health department
- Supportive care
- Give pyridoxine when INH is used in patients with meat- and milk-poor diets, malnutrition, CNS disease, pregnancy

Pulmonary TB

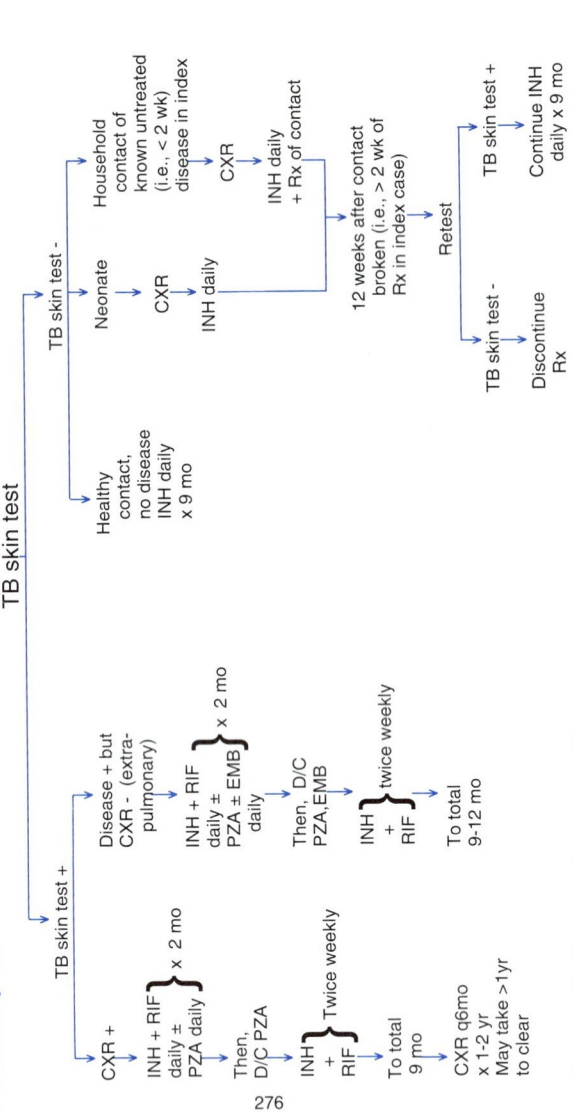

TB skin test +

CXR +
→ INH + RIF daily ± PZA daily } × 2 mo
→ Then, D/C PZA
→ INH + RIF } Twice weekly
→ To total 9 mo
→ CXR q6mo × 1–2 yr. May take >1yr to clear

Disease + but CXR − (extra-pulmonary)
→ INH + RIF daily ± PZA ± EMB daily } × 2 mo
→ Then, D/C PZA, EMB
→ INH + RIF } twice weekly
→ To total 9–12 mo

TB skin test −

Healthy contact, no disease INH daily × 9 mo

Neonate → CXR → INH daily

Household contact of known untreated (i.e., < 2 wk) disease in index → CXR → INH daily + Rx of contact

→ 12 weeks after contact broken (i.e., > 2 wk of Rx in index case) → Retest
- TB skin test + → Continue INH daily × 9 mo
- TB skin test − → Discontinue Rx

Figure 14-1 **For legend, see opposite page.**

Extrapulmonary TB

- Meningitis
  1. INH and rifampin × 12 mo
  2. Streptomycin or pyrazinamide for first 4-8 wk
  3. Prednisone × 4-6 wk (if there is evidence of decreasing level of consciousness, increased ICP, or focal signs); start with 1-2 mg/kg/day and taper after 1-2 wk
- Adenitis: INH and rifampin
- Indications for steroids:
  1. Meningitis
  2. Problematic hilar adenopathy (airway, atelectasis)
  3. Pericardial effusion
  4. Tension pleural effusion

Figure 14-1 **Management of tuberculosis. TB should be managed in consultation with infectious diseases specialist. INH = isoniazid: no need to monitor LFTs unless clinical indication; RIF = rifampin; PZA = pyrizinamide: used if resistance suspected; EMB = ethambutol: bacteriostatic only—main use is to prevent emergence of resistant organism.**
N.B.: Additional drugs available for resistance (streptomycin, ethionamide).
Follow up x-ray, cultures, public health officials.

VARICELLA (CHICKEN POX)

- Incubation period: 10-21 days (35 days if patient has received VZIG)
- Contagious 48 hr prior to appearance of rash until lesions are dried and scabbed, approximately 6 days after onset (immunosuppressed patients may be contagious for longer periods)

Management
- Isolation (strict)
- Symptomatic therapy: baking soda baths, calamine, topical antipruritic, systemic antihistamines if severe itching
- IV acyclovir in immunosuppressed patients
- VZIG prophylaxis for specific contacts (see p 247)

VIRAL HEPATITIS

Investigations
- CBC, bilirubin (total, direct), AST (SGOT), ALT (SGPT), PT, PTT
- Viral studies (see pp 216-217)

Treatment
- Supportive; no diet or exercise restriction necessary
- Steroids not indicated
- Hospitalize if high temperature, dehydration, renal impairment, severe jaundice, prolongation of PT (abnormal synthetic function of liver), impaired neurologic function, or social considerations
- Fulminant liver failure; see pp 214-215
- Hepatitis A and B postexposure prophylaxis of patient and household contacts; see pp 237-240

Follow-up

- Advise patient or parents to return in case of increased jaundice, impaired neurologic function, recurrence of vomiting, or bleeding—i.e., signs of fulminant hepatitis
- Monthly follow-up necessary until clinical resolution to exclude chronic disease
- Acute hepatitis may be possible presentation of either chronic active hepatitis, nonviral hepatitis (toxic, drugs) or Wilson's disease (see Chapter 13)

Infections in the Immunocompromised Host

- Early consultation with infectious diseases specialist is advisable.
- All isolated organisms in immunocompromised patients should be considered as potential pathogens
- Fever represents infection until proved otherwise (e.g., versus tumor lysis, transfusion or drug reactions)
- Start empiric therapy early against the most common, serious pathogens; from the beginning, consider clinical endpoints for changing or discontinuing treatment.

TABLE 14-13 Common Risk Groups and Associated Infectious Disease Syndromes

Risk Group	Infectious Disease Syndrome
Post-chemotherapy neutropenia	Polymicrobial sepsis Fungi (late)
Immunosuppressive therapy (Malignancies, post-transplant, collagen vascular disease, renal disease)	Polymicrobial sepsis CMV, varicella *Pneumocystis* pneumonia
Splenic dysfunction	Overwhelming encapsulated *(Pneumococcus)* bacterial sepsis
Hypogammaglobulinemia	Sinopulmonary bacterial
Low-birth-weight premature infants with CVLs plus broad-spectrum antibiotics	Fungi

AGGRAVATING FACTORS

- Indwelling catheters (IV, Foley; remove or replace when possible); other foreign bodies (e.g., shunts)
- Malnutrition
- Skin and mucosal breakdown
- Prolonged broad-spectrum antibiotics (increased fungal risk)
- Prolonged hospitalization (resistant organisms, nosocomial infections)
- Graft-vs-host disease (increased CMV risk)

INVESTIGATIONS FOR ALL PATIENTS

- Complete physical examination with special attention to fundi, oropharynx, chest, catheter sites, skin, and perianal area
- Central line and peripheral blood cultures (bacteria and fungi)
- Urine cultures (bacteria and fungi)
- Drainage cultures
- CXR
- LFTs, creatinine

INVESTIGATIONS FOR SELECTED PATIENTS

- Bronchoalveolar lavage (BAL) if pulmonary focus suspected (cultures for bacteria, CMV and respiratory viruses, fungi and mycobacteria; stains for fungi, bacteria, mycobacteria, and *Pneumocystis*)
- Esophagoscopy (bacterial, CMV, HSV, and fungal cultures)
- CSF culture, Gram stain cell count, chemistry, latex agglutination
- Buffy coat and urine cultures for CMV
- Ophthalmology consult (CMV, fungal retinitis)
- Abdominal and renal U/S (abscesses, fungal balls)
- Vesicular scrapings for EM and cultures (varicella, herpes simplex)

PRINCIPLES OF MANAGEMENT OF FEVER AND NEUTROPENIA

- Sepsis may be polymicrobial, so maintain broad antibiotic coverage while neutropenic even if specific bacteria are cultured
- Inflammatory signs such as abscesses or CXR findings may be absent until neutrophils increase
- Fungal infections are more common with severe (<100/mm^3) or prolonged (>7 days) neutropenia. They are difficult to detect and may be present despite negative cultures, abdominal or renal U/S and eye exams.
- At the onset of fever, start a broad-spectrum penicillin (e.g., ticarcillin) and an aminoglycoside (e.g., gentamicin) or ceftazidime
- If the patient is ill, if fever persists for >72 hr, or if IV catheter sepsis is suspected, add vancomycin
- If deterioration occurs after 72 hr of therapy, or if fever and neutropenia persist for >7 days, add amphotericin B (arrange abdominal and renal U/S and ophthalmology consult)
- If fever lasts <7 days but neutropenia persists without a focus, continue broad-spectrum antibiotics until:
  1. Neutrophils >500/mm^3 or
  2. Total of 14 days of antibiotics, then monitor expectantly (30% relapse with fever and neutropenia)
- With significant oral mucositis or gingivitis, peritoneal signs or perianal inflammation, add metronidazole to tobramycin and ticarcillin combination
- If esophagitis is suspected, add amphotericin B and consider reactivation of herpes viruses; arrange for esophagoscopy (usually deferred until no longer neutropenic)
- In patients with pneumonitis who deteriorate despite 72 hr of initial antibiotics, add amphotericin B, TMP-SMX (high-dose) and erythromycin. These patients generally require bronchoalveolar lavage.

Childhood Exanthems

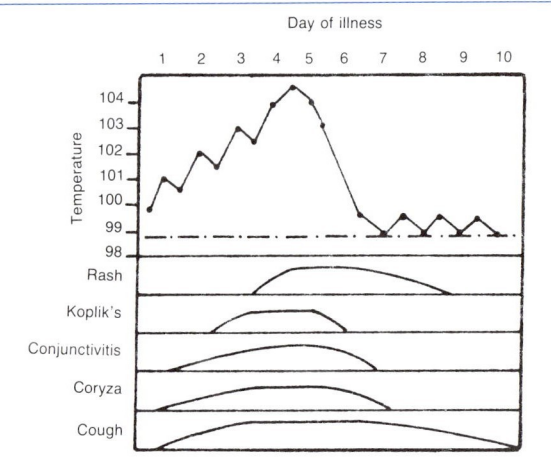

1. Measles

Rash
- Erythematous
- Maculopapular
- Starts at hairline, behind ears and upper neck
- Spreads to face and neck and then extends to trunk and extremities
- Fades in order of appearance
- Desquamates (except palms, soles)

Incubation period
- 8–13 days

Period of communicability
- 1–2 days before symptoms to 4 days after rash appears

Therapy
- See p 235 for post-exposure prophylaxis

Isolation
- Respiratory

Figure 14-2 **Common childhood exanthems.** (Diagrams from Krugman S, Katz S, Gershon AA, Wilfert C. Infectious diseases of children, 8th ed. St Louis: CV Mosby, 1985:456.)

Continued.

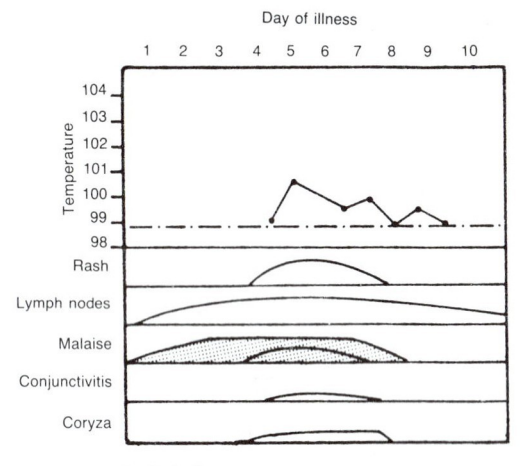

2. Rubella

Rash
- Pink
- Maculopapular
- Lesions on extremities may be discrete
- Starts on face, neck→trunk, extremities (spreads more quickly than measles)

Incubation period
- 14–21 days

Period of communicability
- 7 days pre-rash to 7 days after rash appears

Therapy
- None

Isolation
- Respiratory

Figure 14-2, continued.

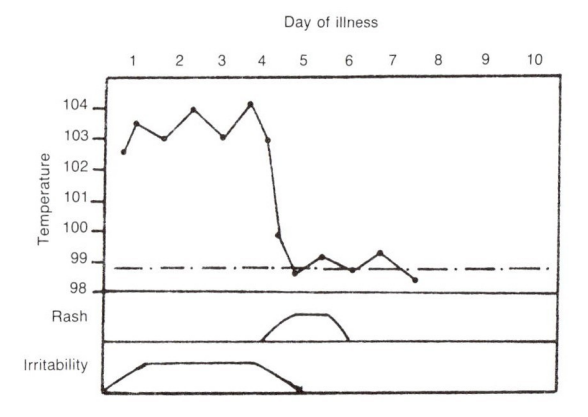

3. Roseola infantum

Rash
- Macular-maculopapular
- Neck-arms-trunk ± face
- Onset of rash accompanies disappearance of fever

Incubation period
- 5–15 days

Period of communicability
- Unknown

Therapy
- None

Isolation
- None

Figure 14-2, continued.

Continued.

4. Erythema infectiosum (a parvovirus infection)

Rash
- Red flushed face, slapped-cheek appearance
- Maculopapular rash over trunk and extremities with lacelike appearance

Incubation period
- 4–14 days

Period of communicability
- Unknown

Therapy
- None

Isolation
- Respiratory (for 7 days following onset of illness)

Figure 14-2, continued.

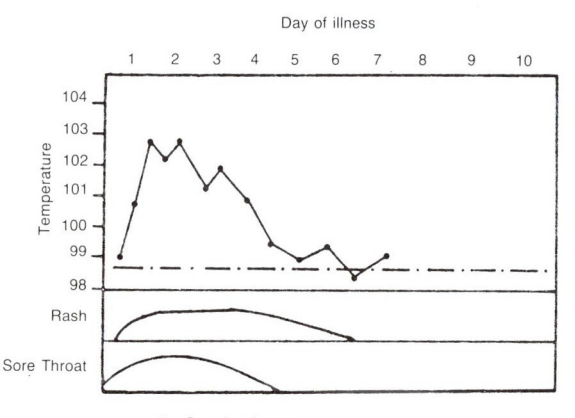

5. Scarlet fever

Rash
- Erythematous
- Blanches on pressure
- Starts in axillae, groin, and neck → generalized
- Circumoral pallor
- Desquamates (palms, soles involved)

Incubation period
- Occurs 2–5 days following streptococcal pharyngitis or impetigo

Period of communicability
- Maximum during the acute infection

Therapy
- Penicillin or erythromycin × 10 days

Isolation
- Barrier until on antibiotics for 24 hr

Figure 14-2, continued.

FIFTEEN

Metabolic Disease

Recognition and Management of Inherited Metabolic Disease (Tables 15-1 to 15-3)

- Inherited metabolic disease generally manifests clinically as:
  1. A neurologic syndrome
  2. A hepatic syndrome
  3. Acute metabolic acidosis

IN THE NEWBORN

- Metabolic disease should be excluded in any newborn who becomes acutely ill after a period of normal behavior and feeding
- Illness attributed to inborn errors of metabolism usually progresses rapidly; delay in recognition and initiation of appropriate management may lead to permanent neurologic impairment
- Acute metabolic disease in the newborn is generally "small molecule" in origin—i.e., involving carbohydrate and amino acid metabolism

IN INFANCY AND CHILDHOOD

- Any of the inherited metabolic diseases presenting acutely in the newborn period may present later in infancy or childhood as acute illness

- Conditions presenting at this age may be milder variants of conditions presenting in the newborn and are often precipitated by intercurrent illness or infection
- The manifestations of inherited metabolic disease may be superimposed on a chronic history of failure to thrive or developmental delay of varying severity. Metabolic diseases that cause a slowly progressive encephalopathy generally affect the biosynthesis and degradation of macromolecules—i.e., storage diseases such as the lysosomal hydrolase deficiencies.

INITIAL LABORATORY INVESTIGATIONS

Test	Comments
Electrolytes, ABG	Rule out congenital adrenal hyperplasia; calculate anion gap
CBC, differential, platelets, blood smear	Neutropenia and/or thrombocytopenia may be seen with organic acidemia; leukocyte inclusions may be suggestive of a storage disease (may be reported as "atypical lymphocytes")
Routine urinalysis, Clinitest	Ketonuria should always be considered as abnormal in the newborn; absent urine-reducing substances does not rule out galactosemia. Determine feeding status.
Blood glucose	
Blood ammonia	Pulmonary hemorrhage or primary respiratory alkalosis may be the first clue of hyperammonemia

Continued.

Test	Comments
Plasma calcium, magnesium	
Liver function tests including PT, PTT	
Galactosemia screen (from RBCs) *prior to transfusion*	Classical galactosemia in infants may be associated with *E. coli* sepsis
Uric acid	
Amino acid screen (serum and urine)	
Urine organic acid	If necessary, sample may be frozen at $-20°$ C if analysis is delayed
CSF glycine	May be elevated in presence of normal urine and plasma screens in nonketotic hyperglycinemia; primarily in newborns with therapy-resistant seizures
Urine mucopolysaccharide spot test and oligosaccharide screen; x-rays hands, chest, spine; peripheral smear, bone marrow	As an initial evaluation of a storage disease

GUIDELINES FOR EARLY MANAGEMENT

- Discontinue dietary or parenteral intake of protein and fat
- Give IV 10% dextrose and 0.2% NaCl ± KCl at 1.5 times maintenance fluids to promote diuresis and excretion of water-soluble toxic metabolites. Avoid fluid overload in children with acute encephalopathy.
- Treat shock, hypoglycemia, metabolic acidosis, electrolyte imbalances, infections, and coagulopathies by conventional methods. Plasma bicarbonate, <10 mmol/L, should be cautiously half-corrected to treat metabolic acidosis.
- Consider treating potential vitamin-responsive enzymopathies with pharmacologic doses of the relevant vitamin
  1. Thiamine HCl—100 mg IV
  2. Biotin—20 mg IV
  3. Vitamin B_{12}—1 mg IV
  4. Riboflavin—20 mg IV or PO daily
  5. Pyridoxine (Vitamin B_6)—100–200 mg IV for intractable seizures
- Consider administering detoxifying agents in the case of suspected UCED or organic acidopathy: arginine, sodium benzoate, sodium phenylacetate
- Consider peritoneal dialysis for worsening or resistant metabolic acidosis, or hemodialysis for severe hyperammonemia associated with UCED

TABLE 15-1 Clinical Presentation of Inherited Metabolic Disease—The Newborn

Primary Manifestation	Characteristics	Metabolic Differential Diagnosis
Neurologic syndrome		
Acute encephalopathy	Lethargy, coma, feeding problems, vomiting, hypotonia, seizures, hyperventilation, ↑ICP	Amino acid disorder (MSUD); organic acidemia (MMA, PA); UCED; THAN; fatty acid oxidation defect (MCAD)
Intractable seizures	Early onset, complex in type and often resistant to control with conventional anticonvulsants	Nonketotic hyperglycinemia; pyridoxine dependency; Menkes syndrome; peroxisomal disorder (Zellweger syndrome)
Hepatic syndrome		
Severe hepatocellular dysfunction	Recurrent hypoglycemia (± ketosis) with a combination of hepatomegaly, seizures, vomiting, jaundice, bleeding diathesis, renal tubular defects, aminoaciduria and hyperammonemia (although levels are lower than seen in UCED, THAN or an organic acidemia)	Galactosemia; HFI; hereditary tyrosinemia; defects in fatty acid oxidation; defects in glycogenolysis (GSD I, III)

Acute metabolic acidosis		Generally nonspecific findings; most consistent feature is *failure to thrive*; anorexia and vomiting often intractable and out of proportion to the severity of any intercurrent illness; associated with dehydration, ketoacidosis, tachypnea	
	Normochloremic	↓HCO$_3^-$, normal Cl$^-$; anion gap >20 (normal = 12-15 mmol/L) = [Na] − ([Cl] + [HCO$_3$])	Amino acid disorder (MSUD); organic acidemia (MMA, PA); congenital lactic acidosis; disorders of gluconeogenesis (PDH deficiency,* PC deficiency,* GSD I)
	Hyperchloremic	↓HCO$_3^-$, ↑Cl$^-$; normal anion gap (characterizes proximal renal tubular acidosis)	Cystinosis; galactosemia; HFI; hereditary tyrosinemia

MSUD = maple syrup urine disease; MMA = methylmalonic acidemia; PA = propionic acidemia; UCED = urea cycle enzyme defect; THAN = transient hyperammonemia of the newborn; MCAD = medium chain acyl-CoA dehydrogenase deficiency; HFI = hereditary fructose intolerance; GSD = glycogen storage disease; PDH = pyruvate dehydrogenase; PC = pyruvate carboxylase.

TABLE 15-2 Clinical Presentation of Inherited Metabolic Disease Infants and Children

Primary Manifestation	Characteristics	Metabolic Differential Diagnosis
Neurologic syndrome Developmental arrest or regression ± seizures	May be associated with chronic failure to thrive Often associated with specific neurologic deficits—i.e., ataxia or deficits of special senses (vision, hearing) May evolve insidiously over a protracted time	Mucopolysaccharidosis Sphingolipidosis and disorders of lipid metabolism Tay-Sachs Niemann-Pick Krabbe disease Metachromatic leukodystrophy Mucolipidosis Neuronal ceroid lipofuscinosis Peroxisomal disorders Mitochondrial disorders Disorders of amino acid, organic acid, and carbohydrate metabolisms UCED
Ataxia	Can be associated with evidence of encephalopathy	Lipidosis Peroxisomal disorders—Refsum's disease Mitochondrial disorders Amino acid disorders—MSUD UCED

Peripheral neuropathy		Abetalipoproteinemia
		Krabbe disease
		Metachromatic leukodystrophy
		Acute intermittent porphyria
		Refsum's disease
		Adrenoleukodystrophy
Psychiatric symptoms	Often associated with neurologic findings	Acute intermittent porphyria
		Fabry's disease
		Wilson's disease
		Metachromatic leukodystrophy
		Adrenoleukodystrophy
		Hartnup disease
		Homocystinuria
Hypotonia	Cerebral, cortical	Sphingolipidosis, mucopolysaccharidosis, mucolipidosis
	Nerve fibers	See "Peripheral neuropathy" above
	Muscle	GSD II
Hypertonia	Early spasticity	Krabbe Disease
		Neuronopathic Gaucher's disease
	Late spasticity	Tay-Sachs Disease
		Niemann-Pick
		GM_1 gangliosidosis

Continued.

TABLE 15-2 Clinical Presentation of Inherited Metabolic Disease (Cont'd)

Primary Manifestation	Characteristics	Metabolic Differential Diagnosis
Hepatic syndrome Hepatomegaly	Liver dysfunction in childhood associated with metabolic disease usually presents with hepatomegaly as prominent feature Generally, liver enlargement is slow and progressive as a result of fatty infiltration, accumulation of glycogen, complex lipids, or expanded number or size of one or more cell types Cirrhosis: generally secondary to diffuse chronic liver injury with loss of normal structure and function	**Hepatomegaly with associated hypoglycemia** Disorders of carbohydrate metabolism: GSD I, III, HFI, galactosemia, fatty acid oxidation defects Disorders of amino acid metabolism: (only a few manifest hepatomegaly) cystinosis (late onset hepatomegaly), lysinuric protein intolerance, hereditary tyrosinemia **Hepatomegaly with psychomotor retardation** Disorders of lipid metabolism: GM$_1$ gangliosidosis, Gaucher's disease I/III, Niemann-Pick disease (A, C, D), Wolman's disease, cholesterol-ester storage disease, fucosidosis, mannosidosis **plus distinctive somatic features**

		Wilson's Disease (Kayser-Fleischer rings)
		Mucopolysaccharidosis
		Zellweger syndrome (Cerebrohepatorenal syndrome)
		Other metabolic causes of hepatomegaly
		Abetalipoproteinemia
		Hyperlipoproteinemia (I, V)
		Porphyria
		UCED
		Alpha-1-antitrypsin deficiency
		Tyrosinemia
		Wilson's disease
		Galactosemia
		HFI
		GSD III, IV
		Alpha-1-antitrypsin deficiency
Maladaptation to starvation	Principal adaptations are glycogenolysis, gluconeogenesis, and increased fat utilization	GSD I
		Fructose 1,6,diphosphatase deficiency
	Hereditary defects tend to present later in infancy with fasting hypoglycemia and metabolic acidosis	Pyruvate carboxylase deficiency
		Phosphoenolpyruvate carboxykinase
		Disorders of fatty acid oxidation (MCAD)
		Systemic carnitine deficiency

MCAD = medium chain acyl-CoA dehydrogenase deficiency; UCED = Urea cycle enzyme defect; MSUD = Maple syrup urine disease; GSD = Glycogen storage disease; HFI = Hereditary fructose disease.

TABLE 15-3 Clinical Presentation of Inherited Metabolic Disease—Other Recognizable Features

Feature	Description	Condition
Odor	Burnt sugar	MSUD
	Sweaty feet	Isovaleric aciduria, glutaric aciduria, type II
	Musty	PKU
	Cabbage-like	Tyrosinemia
	Ammonia-like	MMA, PA, UCED
Skin	Hypopigmentation	Albinism
	Hyperpigmentation	Gaucher disease, Niemann-Pick, adrenoleukodystrophy
	Rash/eczema	PKU, Hartnup disease, biotinidase deficiency, porphyria
	Icthyosis	Steroid sulfatase deficiency, multiple sulfatase deficiency, neutral lipid storage disease, Refsum's disease
	Xanthomas	Hyperlipoproteinemias I-III
Hair	Alopecia	Homocystinuria, Menkes syndrome
	Hirsutism	Hunter's syndrome, Hurler's syndrome, Scheie's disease, porphyria
	Abnormal architecture	Homocystinuria, Menkes syndrome, argininosuccinic aciduria
	Fair coloring	Albinism, PKU, homocystinuria, histidinemia, isovaleric acidemia, cystinosis, Menkes syndrome

Eyes

Cornea	Clouding	Mucopolysaccharidosis (Hurler's, Scheie's, Maroteaux-Lamy, (NB.: Not Hunter's)
	Crystals	Cystinosis
Lens	Cataracts	Galactosemia, mannosidosis, Refsum's disease, Wilson's disease
	Dislocation	Homocystinuria, hyperlysinemia (persistent), sulfite-oxidase deficiency
Retina	Macular cherry red spot	GM_1, GM_2 gangliosidosis, mucolipidosis I, neuraminidase deficiency (sialidosis), Niemann-Pick, metachromatic leukodystrophy
	Pigment retinopathy	Albinism, cystinosis, Refsum's disease, neuronal ceroid lipofuscinosis, Hunter's, Hurler's, mitochondrial disorders
	Optic atrophy	GM_2 gangliosidosis, Krabbe disease, Leigh's syndrome, metachromatic leukodystrophy

MMA = methylmalonic acidemia; PA = propionic acidemia; UCED = urea cycle enzyme deficiency; PKU = Phenylketonuria; MSUD = Maple syrup urine disease.

SIXTEEN

Neonatology

Abbreviations

CAH	congenital adrenal hyperplasia
CHF	congestive heart failure
CPAP	continuous positive airway pressure
ETT	endotracheal tube
IDM	infant of diabetic mother
IPPV	intermittent positive pressure ventilation
IVH	intraventricular hemorrhage
LGA	large for gestational age
NEC	necrotizing enterocolitis
NPT	nasopharyngeal tube
PDA	patent ductus arteriosus
PFC	persistent fetal circulation
PPHN	persistent pulmonary hypertension of the newborn
PROM	premature rupture of membranes
RDS	respiratory distress syndrome
SEH	subependymal hemorrhage
SGA	small for gestational age
TAPVR	total anomalous pulmonary venous return
TGA	transposition of the great arteries
UAC	umbilical artery catheter
UVC	umbilical venous catheter
VSD	ventricular septal defect

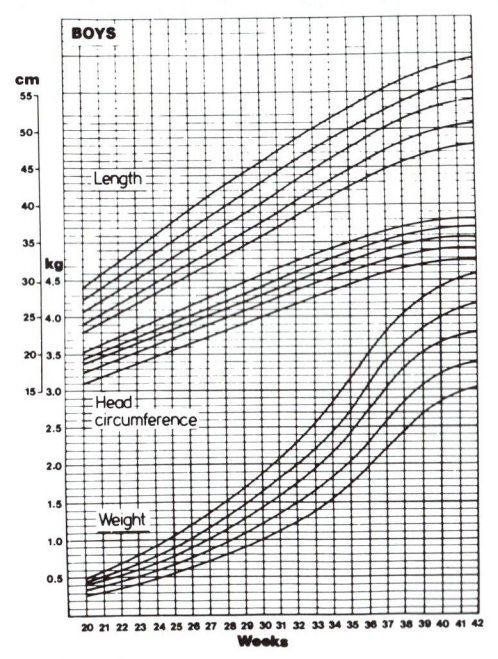

Figures 16-1 and 16-2 **Growth parameters: boys (means ± 1 and 2 SDs) and girls (means ± 1 and 2 SDs).** (From Keen DV, Pearse RG. Weight, length, and head circumference curves for boys and girls of between 20 and 42 weeks gestation. Arch Dis Child 1985; 60:44.)

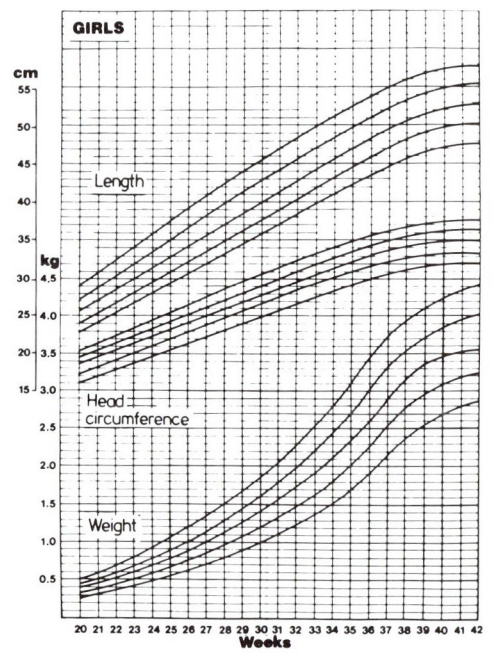

Figure 16-2 **For legend, see opposite page.**

GESTATIONAL AGE ASSESSMENT (Ballard)

NAME _____   DATE TIME OF BIRTH _____   BIRTH WEIGHT _____
HOSPITAL NO _____   DATE TIME OF EXAM _____   LENGTH _____
                               AGE WHEN EXAMINED _____   HEAD CIRC. _____
RACE _____   SEX _____   EXAMINER _____
APGAR SCORE: 1 MINUTE _____ 5 MINUTES _____

NEUROMUSCULAR MATURITY

NEUROMUSCULAR MATURITY SIGN	0	1	2	3	4	5	RECORD SCORE HERE
POSTURE							
SQUARE WINDOW (WRIST)	90°	60°	45°	30°	0°		
ARM RECOIL	180°		100°–180°	90°–100°	<90°		
POPLITEAL ANGLE	180°	160°	130°	110°	90°	<90°	
SCARF SIGN							
HEEL TO EAR							

TOTAL NEUROMUSCULAR MATURITY SCORE

SCORE
Neuromuscular _____
Physical _____
Total _____

Figure 16-3 **Modified Dubowitz assessment. Sample of a form used to estimate gestational age by evaluation of various aspects of maturity.** (Reproduced with permission of the Mead Johnson Nutritional Group, Evansville, IN 47721). N.B.: Accuracy is ± 1 wk at more than 32 wk; unreliable at less than 32 wk. Neurologic component in compromised infants is unreliable.

PHYSICAL MATURITY

PHYSICAL MATURITY SIGN	0	1	2	3	4	5	RECORD SCORE HERE
SKIN	gelatinous, red, transparent	smooth, pink, visible veins	superficial peeling and/or rash, few veins	cracking, pale area, rare veins	parchment, deep cracking, no vessels	leathery, cracked, wrinkled	
LANUGO	none	abundant	thinning	bald areas	mostly bald		
PLANTAR CREASES	no crease	faint red marks	anterior transverse crease only	creases anterior 2/3	creases cover entire sole		
BREAST	barely perceptible	flat areola, no bud	stippled areola, 1-2mm bud	raised areola, 3-4mm bud	full areola, 5-10mm bud		
EAR	pinna flat, stays folded	slightly curved pinna, soft with slow recoil	well-curved pinna, soft but ready recoil	formed & firm with instant recoil	thick cartilage, ear stiff		
GENITALS (Male)	scrotum empty, no rugae		testes descending, few rugae	testes down, good rugae	testes pendulous, deep rugae		
GENITALS (Female)	prominent clitoris & labia minora	majora & minora equally prominent	majora large, minora small	clitoris & minora completely covered			

TOTAL PHYSICAL MATURITY SCORE

Reference:
Ballard JL, Novak KK, Driver M. A simplified score for assessment of fetal maturation of newly born infants. J Pediatr 95:769-774, 1979. Reprinted by permission of Dr. Ballard and Journal of Pediatrics.

MATURITY RATING

TOTAL MATURITY SCORE	GESTATIONAL AGE (WEEKS)
5	26
10	28
15	30
20	32
25	34
30	36
35	38
40	40
45	42
50	44

GESTATIONAL AGE (weeks)
By dates _____
By ultrasound _____
By score _____

Figure 16-3, continued.

TABLE 16-1 Parkin Assessment of Gestational Age

Soft tissue assessment
Skin texture
Tested by picking up a fold of abdominal skin between finger and thumb, and by inspection
- 0: Very thin, with gelatinous feel
- 1: Thin and smooth
- 2: Smooth and of medium thickness; irritation rash and superficial peeling may be present
- 3: Slight thickening and stiff feeling with superficial cracking and peeling; especially evident in hands and feet
- 4: Thick and parchment-like with superficial or deep cracking

Skin color
Estimated by inspection when baby is quiet
- 0: Dark red
- 1: Uniformly pink
- 2: Pale pink, although the color may vary in different parts of the body; some parts may be very pale
- 3: Pale—nowhere really pink except on the ears, lips, palms, and soles

Breast size
Measured by picking up breast tissue between finger and thumb
- 0: No breast tissue palpable
- 1: Breast tissue palpable on one or both sides, neither being more than 0.5 cm in diameter
- 2: Breast tissue palpable on both sides, one or both being 0.5-1.0 cm in diameter
- 3: Breast tissue palpable on both sides, one or both being more than 1.0 cm in diameter

TABLE 16-1 Parkin Assessment of Gestational Age (Cont'd)

Ear firmness

Tested by palpation and folding of upper pinna

- 0: Pinna feels soft and is easily folded into bizarre positions without springing back into position spontaneously
- 1: Pinna feels soft along the edge and is easily folded, but returns in places
- 2: Cartilage can be felt to the edge of the pinna, although it is thin in places and the pinna springs back readily after being folded
- 3: Pinna firm with definite cartilage extending peripherally; springs back immediately into position after being folded

Score	Gestational age (in weeks)
1	27
2	30
3	33
4	34½
5	36
6	37
7	38½
8	39½
9	40
10	41
11-12	>41

From Parkin M, Hey E, Clowes YS. Rapid assessment of gestational age at birth. Arch Dis Child 1976; 51:529.

TABLE 16-2 **APGAR Score**[*]

APGAR	Sign	0	1	2
Appearance	Color	Blue, pale	Body pink; extremities blue	Completely pink
Pulse	Heart rate	Absent	<100 beats/min	>100 beats/min
Grimace	Reflex irritability	No response	Grimace	Cry
Activity	Muscle tone	Limp, flaccid	Some flexion of extremities	Active, well flexed
Respiration	Respiratory effort	Absent	Gasping; slow, irregular	Regular, good lusty cry

[*]N.B.: An APGAR score should be done at 1 and 5 min, and thereafter at 5-min intervals until a score of 7 is achieved. Modified from Ostheimer GW. Resuscitation of the newborn infants. Clin Perinatol 1982; 9(1):183.

Delivery of the High-Risk Neonate

- Equipment in case room
  1. Laryngoscope
  2. Endotracheal tubes (sizes 2.5, 3.0, 3.5, 4.0)
  3. Magill forceps
  4. Radiant heater *on,* clean warm towels
  5. O_2 bagging equipment with masks (sizes 0, 1, 2)
  6. Suction *on*
  7. Umbilical catheterization tray (catheter sizes 3.5, 5.0 F)
  8. Emergency drugs
     - Na bicarbonate, 4.2% concentration (0.5 mEq/ml)
     - Dextrose (10%, 25%)
     - 5% albumin
     - Naloxone
     - Epinephrine 1:10,000
- Normal sequence of response to resuscitation: increased heart rate → reflex activity → color improves → apnea resolves → tone and responsiveness improve
- Threshold for intubating premature infants (<32 wk) is low
- Special problems in initial management (Fig. 16-4 and Table 16-3)
  1. SGA infant: hypothermia, hypoglycemia, hyperviscosity syndrome (secondary to polycythemia)
  2. LGA infant: birth trauma, asphyxia, hypoglycemia, hyperbilirubinemia

Neonate delivered

Transfer to radiant warmer
Dry thoroughly
Gently suction to avoid vagal stimulation
Immediatly resuscitate for bradycardia, APGAR <6-7

Mild asphyxia

HR >100 min
RR slow, irregular
Color: blue extremities
APGAR 6-7

↓

Gentle tactile stimulation
± gentle nasopharyngeal suction

↓

Minimal or no improvement

↓

100% O_2 by mask with tight seal (CPAP)

↓

Color improves and cry vigorous

Moderate asphyxia

HR <100, >50
RR slow, irregular
Color: blue
APGAR 3-5

↓

Gentle suction, tactile stimulation, 100% O_2 by mask

↓

Minimal or no improvement

↓

Bag and mask IPPV 40-60/min
100% O_2

→

Severe asphyxia

HR <50
RR, apneic
Color: blue, pale
APGAR < 3

↓

Nasal/oropharyngeal suction + immediate oral intubation
100% O_2
IPPV 40-60/min
Peak pressures 30-40 mm Hg initially thereafter, decrease to minimum pressure required to move chest

→ FiO_2 →
Wrap, observe

Peak pressures of 30-40 mm Hg may be required to move chest initially; thereafter decrease to minumum pressure required to move chest

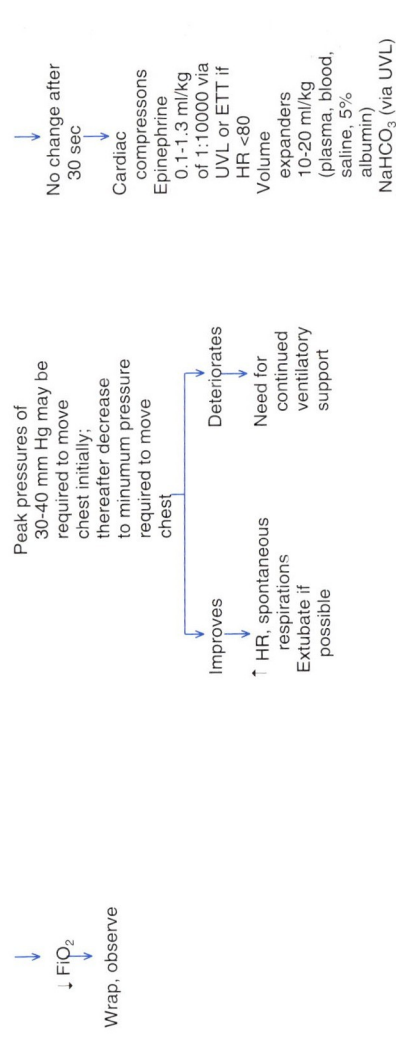

Improves → ↑ HR, spontaneous respirations
Extubate if possible

Deteriorates → Need for continued ventilatory support

→ No change after 30 sec →
Cardiac compressons
Epinephrine 0.1-1.3 ml/kg of 1:10000 via UVL or ETT if HR <80
Volume expanders 10-20 ml/kg (plasma, blood, saline, 5% albumin)
$NaHCO_3$ (via UVL) 1-3 ml/kg of 4.2% (2-6 ml/kg) for prolonged resuscitation with metabolic acidosis

Figure 16-4 **Guide to assessment and management of neonate at delivery.**

TABLE 16-3 Thick ("Pea Soup") Meconium-Stained Liquor Noted During Delivery*

Nasal suction by obstetrician when "crowning" occurs is recommended

Radiation heater; supine. *Do not stimulate.*

Intubate

Suction trachea by using ETT as suction catheter, apply wall section to ETT directly

Reintubate and suction until clear

Dry thoroughly; place dry blanket under infant; do not wrap.

O_2 by mask, keeping tight seal, to improve color if necessary (may need some IPPV)

Aspiration of stomach early to avoid further aspiration of swallowed meconium

---

*Thinly stained liquor in a *well* baby requires gentle nasopharyngeal suction only.

Modified from Merritt TA. Respiratory distress. In: Ziai M, Clarke TA, Merritt TGA, eds. Assessment of the newborn. Boston: Little, Brown, 1984:167-168.

Sedation and Paralysis

- Sedation can generally be accomplished with morphine in boluses, or by continuous infusion, if necessary
- Paralysis: pancuronium bromide, 0.1 mg/kg q2-4 hr PRN
- Morphine should be used routinely when paralyzing

Neonatal Seizures

- "Jitteriness" can be differentiated from seizures by restraint or change in position: will stop former, not latter. Causes include birth asphyxia; CNS anomalies; SGA; hyperviscosity (usually secondary to polycythemia); decreased glucose, Ca, or Mg levels.

Seizure Control
- ABCs
- Phenobarbital is first choice; apnea, hypotension may occur
- Lorazepam, diazepam
- Phenytoin
- Paraldehyde PR or IV
- *Treat underlying cause*

Investigations
- Always check glucose, Ca, Mg, electrolytes, arterial blood gases
- CBC, differential
- Septic work-up (blood, CSF, urine cultures, CXR examination); work-up of congenital infection as indicated (see p 255)
- Head U/S, CT scan
- Neurologic function, EEG, evoked potentials
- Metabolic screen, NH_4, liver function tests, as indicated
- Consider *drug withdrawal*

TABLE 16-4 Etiology of Neonatal Seizures and Approximate Time of Onset

	0-3 Days	4-7 Days	After 10 Days
Brain Injury*	+		
Complicated hypocalcemia	+		
Benign hypocalcemia		+	
Hypoglycemia	+		
Pyridoxine dependency	+	+	+
Infection (congenital, meningitis, sepsis)	+	+	+
Malformation	±	+	+
Metabolic defects†	+	+	+
Subdural injury			+
Drug withdrawal	+	+	+
IVH/SEH	+		

*Most common cause (includes asphyxia, trauma).
†Urea cycle disorders, e.g., MSUD, PKU (see Chapter 15, Metabolic Disease).
Modified from Weiner HL, et al., eds. Pediatric neurology. 2nd ed. Baltimore: Williams & Wilkins, 1982:50.

Fluids and Electrolytes

- High surface area to weight ratio
- Immature renal function
- Immature skin; higher losses in premature infants
- Insensible fluid losses: (approximate values)
  1. <1500 g: 30-60 ml/kg/24 hr
  2. 1500-2500 g: 15-35 ml/kg/24 hr
  3. >2500 g: 10-15 ml/kg/24 hr
- Urine output: 50-100 ml/kg/day
- Weight is the most useful parameter of fluid status monitoring
- High urinary Na losses (up to 10-12 mmol/kg/day in premature infants)
- 3% NaCl = 0.5 mmol/ml = 0.5 mEq/ml; KCl = 2 mmol/ml = 2 mEq/ml; 10% Ca gluconate = 0.2 mmol/ml = 0.4 mEq/ml

TABLE 16-5 Guidelines for Fluid and Electrolyte Therapy—Prediuretic Phase*

BW	Water†	Na‡	K	Ca	Glucose§
(g)	(ml/day)	(mmol/kg/day)			(%)
<750	125-150	nil	nil	—	5
750-1000	75-125	nil	nil	—	5-10
1000-1500	60-80	nil	nil	—	10
>1500	50-60	nil	nil	—	10

*Prediuretic phase (days 1-2, urine output <1-2 ml/kg/h).
†Add 30% for radiant heater, add 10% for phototherapy, subtract 10% for heat shield and/or cellophane wrap.
‡In infants <750 g with a tendency to early hypernatremia, saline may be hazardous even in arterial line.
§Change up or down may be needed, according to blood glucose concentration.
From Perlman M, Kirpalani H. Residents handbook of neonatology. Philadelphia: B.C. Decker, 1992.

TABLE 16-6 Guidelines for Fluid and Electrolyte Therapy—Postdiuretic Phase*

BW	Water†	Na‡	K§	Ca	Glucose
(g)	(ml/day)	(mmol/kg/day)			(mg/kg/min)
<750	150-200	3-4	1-2	1-2	4-8
750-1000	120-160	3	1-2	1-2	4-8
1000-1500	80-150	3	1-2	1-2	4-8
>1500	70-130	2-3	1-2	1-2	4-8

*"Obligatory" diuretic phase (water and Na balance negative by definition, 1-5 days age) and
"Postdiuretic" phase (water and Na balance stabilize and then should become positive after >2-4 days age).

†Adjust water intake according to environmental conditions as indicated in Table 16-5.

‡*Add Na to IV fluid when* —
  Diuretic phase established (urine output >1-2 ml/kg/h for >6-8h) Serum Na is <140mmol/L and not rising.
  Much larger doses may be required in the post-diuretic phase in infants <750g in whom urine losses of Na may be excessive. *This must be determined by measurement of urine Na concentration and urine output before large IV doses of sodium are given, owing to the tendency of these infants to become hypernatremic from excessive IWL.*

§*Add K to IV fluid when* —
  Diuretic phase established
  Serum K is <5.5mmol/L and not rising

From Perlman M, Kirpalani H. Residents handbook of neonatology. Philadelphia: B.C. Decker, 1992.

HYPONATREMIA

- Na <130 mmol/L

Excess Na Loss

- Renal tubular immaturity, hypoxic injury
- Diuretics
- GI losses
- Salt-losing 21-hydroxylase deficiency
- "Late hyponatremia of prematurity" (>1 wk) may be caused by inadequate intake in addition to above causes

Treatment

- Calculate deficit $(Na_{desired} - Na_{actual}) \times 0.6 \times wt\ (kg)$
- Replace over 24-48 hr in addition to providing maintenance and an estimate of ongoing losses
- Calculated deficit is often an underestimate in infants weighing <1500 g
- Monitor serum Na q6-12h

Water Retention

- Iatrogenic overload (excess dextrose solutions)
- SIADH
- CHF

Treatment

- Fluid restriction (½-⅔ maintenance)
- If symptomatic: 3% NaCl to correct to 125 mmol/L ± diuretics
- Monitor serum Na q6-12h

HYPERNATREMIA

- Na >150 mmol/L

Excess H_2O Loss

- Dehydration from increased insensible losses (especially from radiant warmer)
- GI losses
- Osmotic diuresis (rare)

Excess Na Administration

- Normal saline
- NaHCO$_3$

Treatment (Dehydration Most Common)

- Assume fluid deficit 10-15% (100-150 ml/kg) and correct by replacing deficit over 24-48 hr to avoid too rapid a decrease in Na
- If patient hypotensive, resuscitate with 10-15 ml/kg colloid or crystalloid, subtracting volume given from total deficit to be replaced
- If the initial Na >160, use normal saline to replace deficit, use 5% dextrose and 0.45 saline (D$_5$/0.45 NS) or 3.33 dextrose and 0.33 saline (⅔-⅓) as maintenance fluid (to provide usual requirements of 3 mmol/kg/day)
- If initial Na <160, use D$_5$/0.45 NS for deficit; continue as above
- For infants <1.5 kg, deficits may be 20-25% of body weight. Initially, use 5% dextrose with or without 0.2 saline for replacement of deficit; monitor and adjust further based on Na, wt, urine output, urine Na.

HYPOKALEMIA

- Most commonly iatrogenic—e.g., inadequate intake, excessive urinary losses from diuretic therapy, or respiratory alkalosis

HYPERKALEMIA

- K >7 mmol/L
- Excess input (IV)
- Cellular leak (damage, necrosis, resorbed blood)
- Renal failure
- Adrenal insufficiency (CAH, hemorrhage, infarct; associated with decreased Na)

Management

- Ensure that blood sample not hemolyzed
- Obtain ECG; monitor continuously
- Serum K $\geq$8 mmol/L without ECG changes, $\geq$7 mmol/L with ECG changes

Alkalinize with $NaCO_3$, 1.5-2 mmol/kg/15 min, + 1 kayexalate g/kg PR

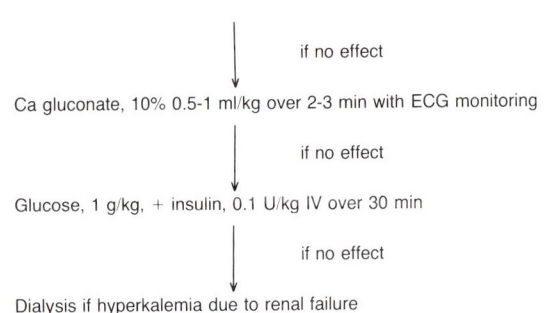

↓ if no effect

Ca gluconate, 10% 0.5-1 ml/kg over 2-3 min with ECG monitoring

↓ if no effect

Glucose, 1 g/kg, + insulin, 0.1 U/kg IV over 30 min

↓ if no effect

Dialysis if hyperkalemia due to renal failure

Acid-Base Status

RESPIRATORY ACIDOSIS

- Corrected by ventilation, *not* $NaHCO_3$

RESPIRATORY ALKALOSIS

- Generally in ventilated infants

METABOLIC ACIDOSIS

- HCO_3^- <20 mmol/L
- Sepsis (consider septic work-up)
- Hypoxia
- Shock
- PDA with CHF
- HCO_3^- losses (renal tubular acidosis)
- Metabolic (amino acidemia, organic acidemia, congenital lactic acidosis)
- Excess protein load
- SEH, IVH

Management
- Treat underlying cause
- $NaHCO_3$ (4.2%) for pH <7.2 and base excess >10
- Base deficit: [$HCO_{3\ desired}$ − $HCO_{3\ actual}$] × wt (kg) × 0.6
- Correct half of calculated deficit initially, usually over 1-4 hr. Do not infuse in Ca-containing solutions
- 2 mmol/kg of $NaHCO_3$ increases pH by 0.1 unit.

METABOLIC ALKALOSIS

- Usually secondary to excessive $NaHCO_3$ therapy
- May be seen with hypokalemia, PO_4 excess, hypochloremia, and postexchange transfusion

HYPERGLYCEMIA

- Glucose >10 mmol/L ± glycosuria
- Iatrogenic (TPN, dextrose solutions)
- Stress: *sepsis must be excluded*

Management
- Monitor urine, blood glucose, Chemstrip
- Decrease glucose infusion in stages of 2.5% Dextrose
- Monitor weight, fluid balance
- Insulin therapy rarely required

HYPOGLYCEMIA

- Full term: glucose <2.2 mmol/L
- Preterm: glucose <1.65-2.5 mmol/L
- Clinical: lethargy, apnea, cyanosis, tremor, tachypnea, seizures
- Decreased carbohydrate stores (SGA, postmature, premature, RDS, maternal hypertension
- Endocrine: excess insulin, often LGA, IDM, erythroblastosis fetalis, Beckwith-Wiedemann syndrome, islet cell dysplasias, suppression of hypothalamopituitary adrenal axis
- Metabolic disease
- Miscellaneous mechanisms (not fully understood): shock, asphyxia, sepsis, hypothermia, polycythemia, rapid wean of IV glucose

Management

- Identify and monitor infants at risk q3-4h prefeed; every second or third feed after 48-72 hr
- PO feeds optimal
- IV glucose if above inadequate
  1. Asymptomatic: IV glucose, 5-8 mg/kg/min (3-5 ml/kg/hr of 10% dextrose); may increase infusion as necessary
  2. Symptomatic: IV glucose bolus, 1 ml/kg of 25% dextrose followed by infusion of 10-12 mg/kg/min
  3. If unsuccessful, consider glucagon, 0.5-1 mg/24 hr infusion; dose may be increased to 2 mg/24 hr
  4. Prednisone, diazoxide for refractory cases (consult with endocrinologist)

HYPOCALCEMIA

- Full term: Ca <1.9 mmol/L
- Preterm: Ca <1.75 mmol/L (due to lower albumin)
- Ionized Ca <0.75 mmol/L
- Monitor Mg

Management

- Identify high-risk infants (premature, SGA, sepsis, cardiovascular compromise)
- Treat high-risk infants with maintenance Ca as continuous infusion for 48-72 hr starting at 6 hr: 0.6-1 mmol/kg/day or 25-45 mg/kg/day elemental Ca
- Acute symptomatic hypocalcemia: irritability, jitteriness, cyanosis, stridor, increased reflexes, prolonged QT interval, seizures (may be multifocal or migratory with alert periods between spells)
- Dilute 10% Ca gluconate solution to 2% and give 0.05-0.1 mmol/kg infusion over 10 min with ECG monitoring (bradycardia, asystole can occur), followed by maintenance infusion as above
- Asymptomatic infants: variable, may treat when Ca <1.8 mmol/L with PO supplementation or IV infusion as for high-risk infants
- *Observe IV sites closely for extravasation*
- Vitamin D PO for high-risk infants: 400-800 IU/day

Neonatal Respiratory Distress (Fig. 16-5 and Tables 16-7 and 16-8)

- Goal of therapy is to maintain $P{CO_2}$ <50 mm Hg; $P{O_2}$ 50-70 mm Hg; and pH >7.25
- All term neonates with respiratory distress should be treated with antibiotics (penicillin or ampicillin and aminoglycoside) until sepsis ruled out
- Criteria for ventilation
  1. Marked hypoxia, rising $P{CO_2}$
  2. Shock with poor perfusion and hypotension, regardless of arterial blood gases
  3. Frequent apnea (see below)

TABLE 16-7 **Differential Diagnosis of Respiratory Distress in Newborn Period**

Pulmonary Disorders

Common	Less Common
Respiratory distress syndrome Transient tachypnea (TTN) Meconium aspiration Pneumonia Pneumothorax	Pulmonary hypoplasia Upper airway obstruction Ribcage anomalies Space-occupying lesions (e.g., diaphragmatic hernia) Pulmonary hemorrhage Immature lung syndrome

Extrapulmonary Disorders

Vascular	Metabolic	Neuromuscular
Persistent pulmonary hypertension of the newborn Congenital heart disease Hypovolemia-anemia Polycythemia	Acidosis Hypoglycemia Hypothermia	Cerebral hypertension Cerebral hemorrhage Muscle or NMJ disorders Spinal cord problems Phrenic nerve palsy Drugs (morphine, phenobarbitol)

Modified from Klaus MH, Fanaroff AA, eds. Care of the high risk neonate. Philadelphia: W.B. Saunders, 1986:179.

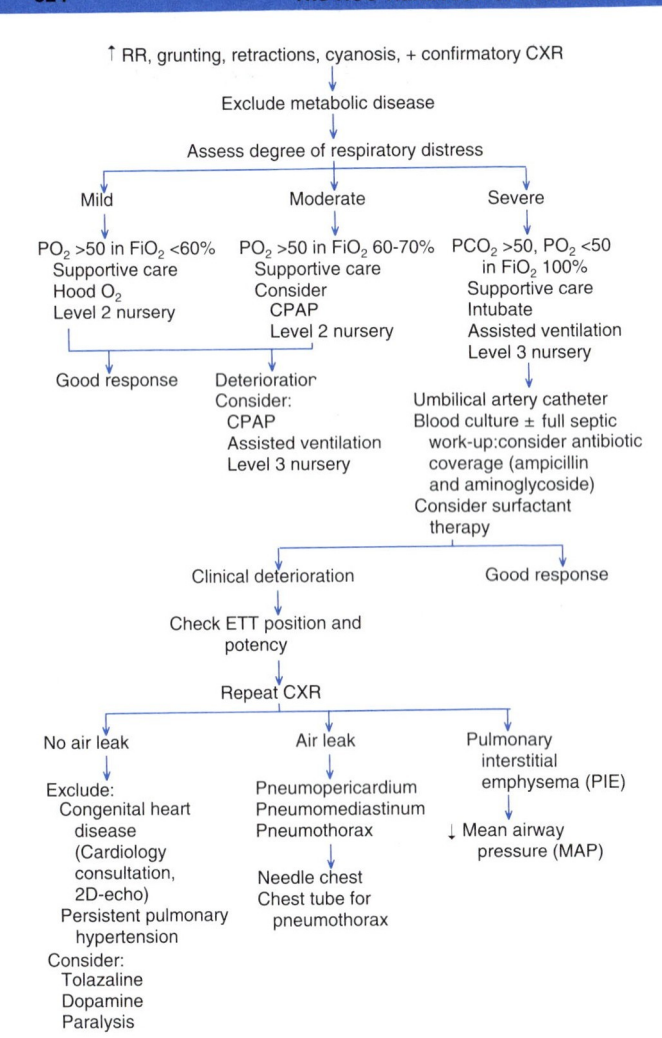

```
↑ RR, grunting, retractions, cyanosis, + confirmatory CXR
                            ↓
              Exclude metabolic disease
                            ↓
         Assess degree of respiratory distress
          ↓              ↓               ↓
        Mild          Moderate         Severe
```

- **Mild**: PO_2 >50 in FiO_2 <60%; Supportive care; Hood O_2; Level 2 nursery
- **Moderate**: PO_2 >50 in FiO_2 60-70%; Supportive care; Consider CPAP; Level 2 nursery
- **Severe**: PCO_2 >50, PO_2 <50 in FiO_2 100%; Supportive care; Intubate; Assisted ventilation; Level 3 nursery

Mild → Good response

Moderate → Deterioration, Consider: CPAP, Assisted ventilation, Level 3 nursery

Severe → Umbilical artery catheter; Blood culture ± full septic work-up: consider antibiotic coverage (ampicillin and aminoglycoside); Consider surfactant therapy

→ Clinical deterioration | Good response

Clinical deterioration → Check ETT position and potency → Repeat CXR

- **No air leak**: Exclude: Congenital heart disease (Cardiology consultation, 2D-echo), Persistent pulmonary hypertension. Consider: Tolazaline, Dopamine, Paralysis
- **Air leak**: Pneumopericardium, Pneumomediastinum, Pneumothorax → Needle chest, Chest tube for pneumothorax
- **Pulmonary interstitial emphysema (PIE)**: ↓ Mean airway pressure (MAP)

Figure 16-5 **Initial management of respiratory distress syndrome.** (Modified from Berman S, ed. Pediatric decision making. Toronto: B.C. Decker, 1985:219)

TABLE 16-8 Management of Nonresponse to IPPV

Cause of Nonresponse	Diagnostic Features	Action
ETT not in correct location	Observe chest movement Auscultate for asymmetric air entry CXR to confirm	Reposition if ETT in right mainstem bronchus Reintubate and reassess
Tension pneumothorax	Displaced apex beat ± hemodynamic compromise Decreased or unequal air entry CXR or transilluminate to confirm	Urgent drain with butterfly needle until stable then insert chest tube
Massive meconium aspiration	History of fetal distress and "pea-soup" liquor staining Characteristic CXR ↑ Risk of PFC ↑ Risk of pneumothorax	Suction trachea and oropharynx using ETT Intubate and ventilate, if indicated
Diaphragmatic hernia	Scaphoid abdomen noted at birth ± respiratory distress Bowel sounds heard over chest CXR diagnostic ↑ Risk of PPHN	Pass N/G tube and connect to low-gomco Intubate IPPV and transfer to tertiary center Sedate and paralyze
Hypoplastic lungs	History of oligohydramnios ± PROM ± Potter's facies Characteristic CXR	Urgent intubation Ventilatory support Require high peak pressures
Sepsis neonatorum ± congenital pneumonia	History of PROM or maternal fever CXR suspicious, but may look like RDS Cultures may be positive	Antibiotics Ventilatory support ± Volume expanders ± Inotropes

Apnea

- Cessation of respiration of >15-20 sec duration, with fall in heart rate to <100/min or cyanosis. After 30-45 sec of apnea, pallor and hyptonia will occur. Apnea may be central, obstructive, or mixed.
- Do not attribute apnea automatically to prematurity, especially in infants of gestational age >30 wk
- Always exclude underlying cause

TABLE 16-9 Management of Apnea

Immediate resuscitation
Surface stimulation
Gentle nasopharyngeal suction
Ventilation with inflating bag and mask
Intubation and IPPV

	Cause	Action
1. Infection	Neonatal sepsis Meningitis Necrotizing enterocolitis (NEC)	Full septic work-up including LP Antibiotics
2. Thermal instability	Hypo/hyperthermia	Assess body and isolette temperature
3. Metabolic disorders	Hypoglycemia Hypocalcemia Hypo/hypernatremia Hyperammonemia	Dextrostix ± blood glucose Serum Ca, ECG Electrolytes, BUN; fluid balance, weight Serum NH_4, amino acids, organic acids, liver function tests

Continued.

TABLE 16-9 Management of Apnea (Cont'd)

	Cause	Action
4. CNS problems	Asphyxia Intracranial hemorrhage Cerebral malformation Seizures	Observation EEG, Head U/S Head U/S ± CT scan Consider anticonvulsants
5. Decreased O_2 delivery	Hypoxemia Worsening RDS ± complication Anemia/shock Left to right shunt (PDA) Pneumothorax	Check ETT CXR CBC, electrolytes, BUN, ABG ECG, 2D-ECHO Needle + chest tube
6. Upper airway obstruction	Choanal atresia Macroglossia Reflux	Attempt passage of N/G tube Oropharyngeal airway CXR for aspiration
7. Drugs	Maternal pre- or postnatal exposure	Drug/toxic screen depending on history and clinical findings

Continuing management to prevent recurrences, and monitoring
Continuous TCPO$_2$ monitoring. Adjust FiO$_2$ accordingly
Minimize handling of small infants
± "Rocking mattress" stimulation
Consider altering feeding pattern—i.e., slow continuous orogastric, or IV
Drug therapy:
  1. Caffeine citrate; lower incidence of side effects with caffeine vs. theophylline
  2. Aminophylline or theophylline are alternatives
Recurrent attacks: Consider short-term assisted ventilation:
  1. NPT or nasal prong CPAP
  2. ETT CPAP
  3. IPPV (often need only slow rate—i.e., ~6-10/min)

Modified from Forfar JL, Arneil GC. Textbook of paediatrics. 2nd ed. New York: Churchill Livingstone, 1978:156.

Cyanosis of the Newborn

HYPEROXIC CHALLENGE

- To exclude cardiac disease, place in 100% FiO_2 with $TcPO_2$ monitor in situ until P_{O_2} >150
- Normal hyperoxic challenge: P_{O_2} will rise to >500 mm Hg. With normal physiologic shunting, P_{O_2} may be 450-500 mm Hg.
- Pulmonary disease: P_{O_2} will usually rise to >100 mm Hg
- If P_{O_2} remains <100-150 mm Hg, highly suggestive of right to left shunting

DIFFERENTIAL

- Pink arms and blue legs: coarctation + PDA, PPHN, hypoplastic left heart + PDA
- Blue arms + pink legs: TGA + aortic arch interruption + PDA
- If cyanosis with P_{O_2} >50 and decreased O_2 saturation, consider methemoglobinemia

Acyanotic

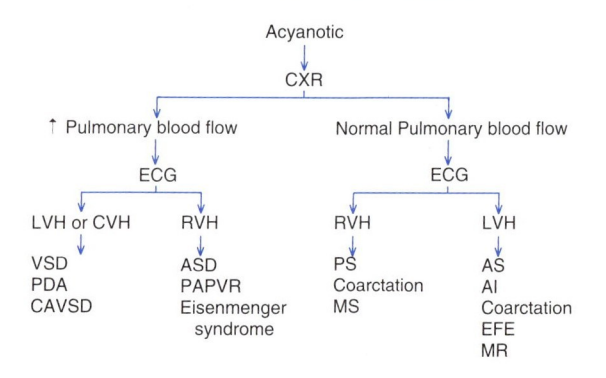

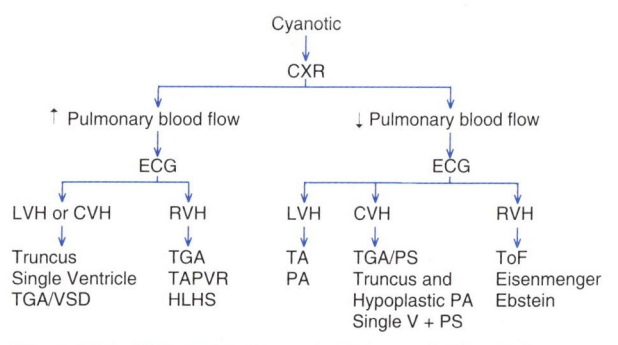

CXR
├── ↑ Pulmonary blood flow
│   └── ECG
│   ├── LVH or CVH
│   │   ├── VSD
│   │   ├── PDA
│   │   └── CAVSD
│   └── RVH
│   ├── ASD
│   ├── PAPVR
│   └── Eisenmenger syndrome
└── Normal Pulmonary blood flow
    └── ECG
        ├── RVH
        │   ├── PS
        │   ├── Coarctation
        │   └── MS
        └── LVH
            ├── AS
            ├── AI
            ├── Coarctation
            ├── EFE
            └── MR

Cyanotic

CXR
├── ↑ Pulmonary blood flow
│   └── ECG
│   ├── LVH or CVH
│   │   ├── Truncus
│   │   ├── Single Ventricle
│   │   └── TGA/VSD
│   └── RVH
│   ├── TGA
│   ├── TAPVR
│   └── HLHS
└── ↓ Pulmonary blood flow
    └── ECG
        ├── LVH
        │   ├── TA
        │   └── PA
        ├── CVH
        │   ├── TGA/PS
        │   ├── Truncus and Hypoplastic PA
        │   └── Single V + PS
        └── RVH
            ├── ToF
            ├── Eisenmenger
            └── Ebstein

Figure 16-6 **Differential diagnosis of congenital heart disease. LVH** = left ventricular hypertrophy; **CVH** = combined ventricular hypertrophy; **RVH** = right ventricular hypertrophy; **CAVSD** = combined atrioventricular septal defect; **PAPVR** = partial anomalous pulmonary venous return; **AS** = aortic stenosis; **AI** = aortic insufficiency; **PS** = pulmonary stenosis; **MS** = mitral stenosis; **MR** = mitral regurgitation; **EFE** = endomyocardial fibroelastosis. **TGA** = transposition of great vessels; **HLHS** = hypoplastic left heart; **ToF** = tetrology of Fallot; **TA** = tricuspid atresia. **PA** = pulmonary atresia; **TAPVR** = total anomalous pulmonary venous return; **PDA** = patent ductus arteriosus; **VSD** = ventricular septal defect.

Dysrhythmias

- Supraventricular tachycardia: may be cause of intrauterine CHF or hydrops
- Bradycardia: may be secondary to complete heart block (rule out maternal systemic lupus erythematosus)
- See pp 41-49 for management

Patent Ductus Arteriosus (PDA)

- Common association with RDS in premature infants; 80% of infants <1000 g, 20% of all premature infants
- Clinical signs: characteristic harsh systolic murmur continuing into diastole, active precordium, bounding pulses, wide pulse pressure, worsening respiratory status, CHF
- Signs may be absent ("silent ductus")
- When available, 2D-ECHO to confirm diagnosis

Management

- Fluid restriction: ⅔ maintenance
- Indomethacin: 0.2 mg/kg for first dose, followed by 0.1 mg/kg for up to total of 3 doses at 12-hr intervals. Second course can be repeated 48 hr later in the absence of side effects.
- Adverse effects of indomethacin: platelet dysfunction, decreased renal artery flow leading to decreased GFR and urine output, fluid retention ± hyponatremia, increased creatinine, bowel perforation (rare)
- 80% success rate after first dose with 25% reopening; 18% reclose without further therapy
- Contraindications to indomethacin
  1. Increased creatinine (>100-120 μmol/L)
  2. Increased urea (>7 mmol/L)
  3. Oliguria <0.5-1 ml/kg/hr
  4. Necrotizing enterocolitis
  5. Thrombocytopenia, <80,000
  6. Hyperbilirubinemia
  7. IVH

Duct-Dependent Cardiac Lesions

- Interruption of aortic arch, coarctation or severe aortic isthmus narrowing, severe tetralogy of Fallot, pulmonary atresia, tricuspid atresia, transposition of the great arteries, Ebstein's anomaly, hypoplastic left heart syndrome
- To maintain duct patency
  1. Prostaglandin E_1, 0.05-0.1 μg/kg/min; monitor P_{O_2} or O_2 saturation; maintain P_{O_2} >30 mm Hg
  2. Side effects: apnea, hyperthermia, jitteriness, flushing, lethargy, diarrhea
- *Be prepared to intubate in case of apnea*

Cardiac Failure

TABLE 16-10 Cardiac Failure in the Neonatal Period*

A. Birth
   - Arrhythmias
   - Anemias
   - A-V fistula
   - Perinatal asphyxia

B. Day 1
   As in *A* plus:
   - Hypoplastic left heart syndrome
   - Metabolic abnormalities
   - Tricuspid atresia/Ebstein's
   - Critical pulmonary stenosis

C. Weeks 1-2
   As in *B* plus:
   - Arrhythmias
   - Coarctation
   - TGA with VSD
   - TAPVR (obstructed)
   - Myocarditis
   - Endocardial fibroelastosis
   - Pompe's disease
   - PDA in premature infant

D. Weeks 2-4
   As in *C* plus:
   - TAPVR (unobstructed)
   - Truncus arteriosus
   - A-V canal

*For management, see p 30; for abbreviations see p 301.

Persistent Pulmonary Hypertension of the Newborn (PPHN)

- Right-to-left shunt occurs through foramen ovale and/or PDA; associated with pulmonary arteriolar spasm or thickening (primary)
- May be 1° or 2°
- Most are term or post-term infants
- Secondary causes include
  1. Transient tachypnea of the newborn
  2. Meconium aspiration syndrome
  3. Hyaline membrane disease
  4. Group B streptococcal pneumonia
  5. Pulmonary hypoplasia ± diaphragmatic hernia
  6. Severe asphyxia
  7. Polycythemia
- Clinical: marked cyanosis, acidosis, and RV heave

Investigations

- Hyperoxic challenge
- CXR: oligemic lung fields, or consistent with underlying disease; cardiomegaly; may look normal
- ECG: RV strain

Treatment

- Sedation ± paralysis usually required
- Hyperventilate to achieve respiratory alkalosis (CO_2 in 25-30 mm Hg range with pH, 7.45-7.55); causes pulmonary arteriolar vasodilatation and decreases pulmonary vascular resistance
- Inotropes: dopamine, dobutamine to increase systemic resistance and decrease right to left shunting
- Tolazaline: 1-2 mg/kg IV bolus then 0.5-2 mg/kg/hr. Patients should be on continuous inotrope infusion to counteract fall in systemic BP; may need colloid/crystalloid support.

Jaundice

<24 Hr of Age

- Hemolytic (Rh or ABO incompatibility) anemia until proven otherwise
- Sepsis or congenital infection should be considered

24-72 Hr

- Mostly "physiologic" N.B.: Premature infants have later onset (day 6 or 7) and longer duration (up to day 14) of physiologic jaundice
- Hemolytic anemia (unrelated to major blood group incompatibility): G6PD deficiency, pyruvate kinase deficiency, spherocytosis, Duffy or Kell incompatibility
- Polycythemia (SGA, late clamping of the cord, maternal-fetal and fetofetal transfusions)
- Sepsis or congenital infection
- Bruising, hemorrhage, or swallowed blood

>72-96 Hr

- "Physiologic" ± breast milk jaundice most common
- Infection: sepsis (including UTI) or hepatitis (congenital infection)
- GI obstruction (increased enterohepatic circulation)

>1 Wk (Prolonged Neonatal Jaundice)

- Hypothyroidism (may not have typical features)
- Galactosemia
- Breast milk (benign) (see p 391 for management)
- Prolonged physiologic (e.g., preterm)
- Crigler-Najjar syndrome, Gilbert's disease
- Obstructive jaundice (e.g., "neonatal hepatitis," biliary atresia, inspissated bile syndrome, choledochal cyst, alpha-1-antitrypsin deficiency)

TABLE 16-11 Nonphysiologic Jaundice (Jaundice Requiring Investigation or Treatment)

Clinically apparent jaundice in first 24 hr of life
Increase in total serum bilirubin concentration of >85 mmol/L per day
Total serum bilirubin concentration >220 mmol/L within the first 4 days of life in term infants
Direct serum bilirubin concentration higher than 34 mmol/L
Visible jaundice lasting >1 wk in term infants or 2 wk in premature infants

Modified from Foetus and Newborn Committee, Canadian Paediatric Society. Use of phototherapy for neonatal hyperbilirubinemia. Can Med Assoc J 1986; 134:1237-1245.

INVESTIGATIONS

Jaundice Occurring <1 Wk of Age

- Family history of jaundice, maternal history, blood group and Rh status, previous pregnancies, transfusions, Rhogam
- Physical exam: hepatosplenomegaly, enclosed hemorrhage
- Laboratory: infant's blood group, direct Coomb's test (negative test does not rule out hemolytic anemia), total bilirubin or microbilirubin, CBC, hematocrit ± reticulocyte count, blood smear
- Septic work-up as indicated

Prolonged Jaundice (>1 Wk of Age)

- Above features and investigations plus thyroid function tests, galactosemia screen (including urine for non–glucose-reducing substances), total and direct bilirubin, liver function tests

PHOTOTHERAPY

- Should be first line of therapy depending on rate of rise and independent of etiology
- More effective when combined with oral feeds
- More effective in controlling bilirubin in high-risk situations if initiated at low levels, than in abruptly reducing established high levels
- Blue light most effective, but affects ongoing assessment of infant by altering observer perception
- May use either continuous or intermittent (6 hr on, 6 hr off) with similar efficacy
- "Double" phototherapy indicated when bilirubin levels approach within 35 mmol/L of exchange level (but may be initiated earlier)
- Insensible fluid loss may increase by up to 35%, necessitating increased fluid intake, especially in very low birth-weight (VLBW) infants
- Serum bilirubin levels should be followed every 6 hr, or more often depending on level and cause
- Delaying initiation of phototherapy until bilirubin levels are >200 mmol/L by 24 hr after birth may significantly reduce the number of infants receiving phototherapy for ABO incompatibility without increasing the need for exchange transfusions (assuming no other high-risk factor present—e.g., preterm)
- Exclude treatable causes of jaundice (e.g., sepsis, metabolic); many initially respond to phototherapy, thus delaying primary treatment
- Phototherapy treatment can be used prophylactically in high-risk infants—e.g., markedly bruised premature infants (controversial), and as an adjunct, but not replacement for, exchange transfusion
- Contraindicated in the presence of conjugated hyperbilirubinemia ("bronzed" baby)
- Complications and adverse effects include hypernatremic dehydration, hyperthermia, masking of potentially serious underlying cause (e.g., sepsis), possible retinal damage if eyes uncovered, transient rashes, loose stools
- Watch for "delayed" anemia in hemolytic disease of the newborn—often overlooked during initial management of hyperbilirubinemia

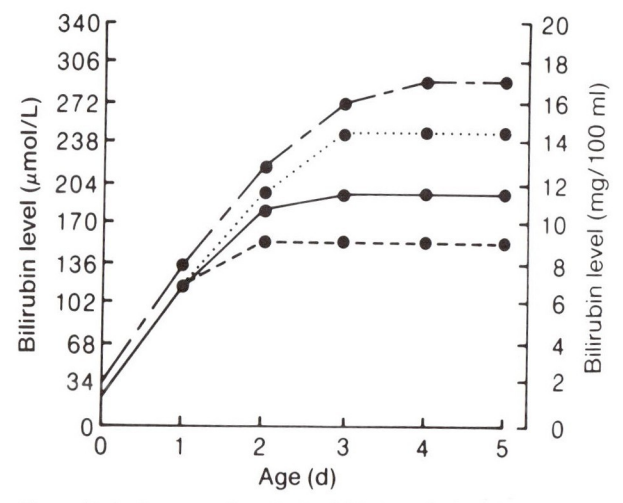

Figure 16-7 **Suggested guide for initiation of phototherapy in neonatal hyperbilirubinemia. Curves represent serum unconjugated bilirubin level at which phototherapy should be considered. ●— - —● = birth weight >2,500 g; ●·····● = 2,001-2,500 g; ● – ● = 1,500-2,000 g; ●---● = <1,500 g.** (From Foetus and Newborn Committee, Canadian Paediatric Society. Use of phototherapy for neonatal hyperbilirubinemia. Can Med Assoc J 1986; 134:1238. Reprinted by permission of the publisher.)

TABLE 16-12 Suggested Values of Serum Unconjugated Bilirubin at Which Phototherapy Should Be Considered for Neonatal Hyperbilirubinemia*

Birth weight, g	Bilirubin level, μmol/L (mg/100 ml)	
	Uncomplicated course	Complicated course†
<1250	136 (8)	85 (5)
1250-1499	170 (10)	136 (8)
1500-1999	205 (12)	170 (10)
2000-2499	220 (13)	205 (12)
≥2500	255 (15)	220 (13)

*Includes asphyxia neonatorum, prolonged hypoxemia, severe acidosis, hypotermia (rectal temperature less than 35°C), septicemic meningitis, deterioration of or insult to the central nervous system and birth weight less than 1000 g.
Modified from Foetus and Newborn Committee, Canadian Pediatric Society. Use of phototherapy for neonatal hyperbilirubinemia. Can Med Assoc J 1986;134:137.

EXCHANGE TRANSFUSION

- Always performed in level 3 nursery setting
- Indications in hemolytic disease of newborn
  1. Cord hemoglobin <120 g/L or cord bilirubin >85 mmol/L
  2. Postnatal rate of rise of unconjugated bilirubin >17 mmol/L/hr in Rh incompatibility
  3. Serum unconjugated bilirubin >340 mmol/L in first 48-72 hr of life (controversial)
  4. Rapid progression of anemia despite satisfactory control of jaundice
  5. Hydrops fetalis may require immediate exchange transfusion with packed cells to correct anemia
- Postexchange (30-60 min); anticipate "rebound" rise in bilirubin due to redistribution (of bilirubin)
- Much controversy exists about safe or critical levels of unconjugated bilirubin. Threshold for intervention in the "sick," low birth weight (LBW), or VLBW infant should be low.
- Complications
  1. Embolization of air bubbles, or small thrombi
  2. Hypocalcemia, hypoglycemia, acidosis, hyperkalemia
  3. Hypothermia, hyperthermia
  4. Sepsis
  5. Volume overload, cardiac arrhythmias

TABLE 16-13 Exchange Transfusion Guidelines*

Birth Weight (kg)	Serum Bilirubin Concentration, μmol/L (mg/100ml) Post-natal age <96 hours	Post-natal age >96 hours
>2.5	340-425 (20-25)	375-460 (22-27)
1.5-2.5	225-340 (15-20)	290-375 (17-22)
1.0-1.5	240-305 (14-18)	220-255 (13-15)
<1.0	205-240 (12-14)	220-255 (13-15)

*Authors' criteria for exchange transfusion in mmol/L and mg/dl, according to birth weight and postnatal age. The levels for these various interventions should be individualized if additional risk factors are present (see rationales and correction factors in text).

Authorities differ on the question of whether these criteria should refer to "indirect" bilirubin or total bilirubin. "Indirect" bilirubin should be used in patients with high "direct" bilirubin concentrations, i.e., >17 mmol/L (>1 mg/dL).

From Perlman M, Kirpalani H. Residents handbook of neonatology. Philadelphia: B.C. Decker, 1992.

Nutrition

TPN

- See p 397. Principles for starting and maintaining TPN are similar to those in older children. For lower glucose needs or intolerance, 5% or 7.5% glucose solutions (P 7.5) are available. Monitoring and complications are similar to those in older children.

TABLE 16-14 Approximate Daily Nutritional Requirements of Term and Preterm Infants

	Term	Preterm*
Energy (kcal/kg)	100	110-165
Protein (g/kg)	2.2-1.3	2.9-4.0
Carbohydrate (g/kg)	10	8-16
Fat (g/kg)	3.3	4.0-9.0
Na (mmol/kg)	1.2-0.8	1.3-3.0
Cl (mmol/kg)	1.2-0.8	2.1-3.3
K (mmol/kg)	1.2-0.8	2.0-5.0
Ca (mmol/kg)	1.0-1.1	2.2-4.5
P (mmol/kg)	0.7	2.1-3.8
Vitamin A (ug/kg)		120-195
Vitamin D (IU/day)	400 (10)	800-2000 (20-50)
Vitamin E (mg/100 kcal)		0.6
Vitamin K	0.5-1.0 mg at birth	

*Requirements should be computed according to BW until BW is regained, after which actual weight is used. The "requirements" are based on *enteral* nutrition.

From Perlman M, Kirpalani H. Residents handbook of neonatology. Philadelphia: B.C. Decker, 1992.

Infection

- High-risk infants include <37 weeks gestational age, prolonged membrane rupture (>24 hr) maternal fever, instrumental vaginal delivery, indwelling catheters, maternal UTI, use of broad-spectrum antibiotics
- Wide spectrum of clinical presentation; must consider in any infant with the following:
  1. Respiratory distress
  2. Apnea
  3. Increasing O_2 and ventilation requirements
  4. Feed intolerance
  5. Abdominal distension or ileus
  6. Temperature instability
  7. Seizures, lethargy
  8. Metabolic: hyperglycemia, hypoglycemia, acidosis, hyperbilirubinemia
  9. Obvious focus: skin, bones, joints, omphalitis

Investigations

- "Surface" and ETT cultures may be of little value
- Blood cultures
- Urinalysis, microscopy, urine culture: suprapubic aspiration is preferred method, see p 575; catheter sample acceptable
- CSF Gram stain; protein, glucose determinations; culture (LP not performed if cardiorespiratory instability)
- CXR (nonspecific for infection)
- Urine, CSF for antigen detection (latex agglutination); may be useful in infant in whom antibiotics already initiated

Antibiotic Therapy

- Common organisms include Group B streptococci, coliforms, *Listeria,* and coagulase-negative staphylococci, (in infants >7 days who have had intravenous catheters)
- Consider *S. aureus* in skin, bone, and joint disease; *Shigella* or *Salmonella* in gastroenteritis
- Superinfection with *Candida* must be considered in all infants with prolonged or recurrent illness, indwelling shunt or intravenous catheter, or congenital heart disease (bacterial endocarditis)
- *Ureaplasma urealyticum* increasingly implicated in respiratory infection
- Initial coverage depends on clinical presentation:
  1. Ampicillin + aminoglycoside
  or
  2. Ampicillin + cefotaxime
  ±
  3. Cloxacillin if *Staphylococcus* is a consideration
- Vancomycin used in prolonged or recurrent illness, especially if indwelling shunt or catheter
- *Pseudomonas* requires coverage with ceftazidime or ticarcillin
- NEC (see p 523)
- For *Candida* sepsis, amphotericin B (see p 699)

Drug Withdrawal

- Opiates, cocaine, alcohol most common. Usually incomplete history. Must have high index of suspicion for multiple drug use.
- CNS: high-pitched cry, sleeplessness, hyperactive Moro reflex, tremors, increased muscle tone, myoclonus, seizures, areas of skin excoriation 2° to excess activity
- GI: excessive sucking, poor feeding, regurgitation and vomiting, loose and watery stools, prolonged postnatal weight loss
- Autonomic: fever, tachypnea, apnea, nasal stuffiness, mottling, fever, sneezing, yawning

- Time of onset: usually within 72 hr after birth; may appear up to age 2 wk. Will vary depending on drug, timing of use before delivery, labor, presence of other illness
- Duration ranges from 6 days-8 wk; may last up to several months
- Neonatal abstinence scoring sheets used to monitor symptoms and response to pharmacotherapy. Scores are dynamic (every 2-4 hr), based on CNS, GI, vasomotor, respiratory, and metabolic disturbances.

Treatment

- Phenobarbital (loading dose followed by titrated maintenance dose based on abstinence scores and/or clinical picture; usually 20 mg/kg load followed by 6-12 mg/kg/day
- Paregoric 0.8-2 ml/kg/day, titrated as above; morphine an alternative
- Treatment generally 3-5 days, then gradually taper
- Must follow for long-term effects of pre- and perinatal drug exposure, general increase in caloric requirements, risk of HIV infection, neurodevelopmental delay, child abuse

Figure 16-8 **Neutral thermal environment for premature infants. The charts indicate the neutral thermal environment and are used as guidelines to set incubator temperature. The charts relate to infants of 26-35 wk gestation. No data are available for infants <26 wk. For naked infants >35 wk and >1 wk postnatal age in the incubator, the neutral thermal environment is 32.0° C. Axillary temperature of 36.7 to 37.2° C is accepted as normal. If incubator temperature required to maintain this axillary temperature differs from that indicated in the guidelines, consider the possibility of (a) artefact, e.g., error in measurements of either incubator or axillary temperature, or lack of humidity, or (b) disturbed homeostasis for age, e.g., illness.** (Modified from Sauer PJJ, Dane HJ, Visser HKA. New standards for neutral thermal environment of healthy very low birthweight infants in week one of life. Arch Dis Child 1984; 59:19.)

TEMPERATURE CONTROL IN PREMATURE INFANTS

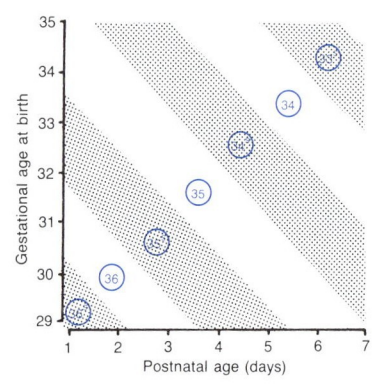

Neutral thermal environment during the first postnatal week for infants of 26–35 wk gestation.

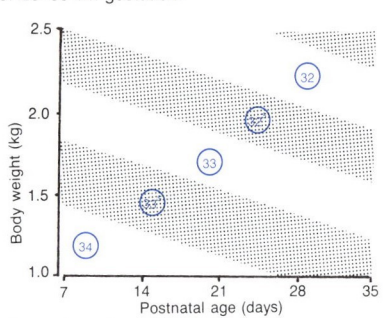

Neutral thermal environment for infants 26–35 wk gestation between 1–5 postnatal wk.

Figure 16-8 **For legend, see opposite page.**

SEVENTEEN

Nephrology

Acute Renal Failure

- Sudden decrease in renal function with disturbed water and electrolyte balance, and retention of nitrogenous wastes
- Differentiate type of ARF (see Fig. 17-1)

Management

- Prerenal: rehydration (saline, Ringer's lactate, albumin, plasma, blood)
- Renal: insensible losses (400 ml/m^2/day or 20 ml/kg/day) + urine output + ongoing losses (GI, hemorrhage). (↑ temperature: ↑ insensible losses sign by 12% per 1°C)
- Monitor: weight daily or twice daily, electrolytes, acid-base status, urine output, vital signs, ± CVP)
- *Infection is major cause of death in ARF.*

Management of Complications

- Acidosis (see p 98); hypertension (see p 359)
- Hyperphosphatemia: dietary restriction, phosphate binders, dialysis
- Hyperkalemia
  1. Stat ECG: peaked T waves, wide QRS, increased PR interval, decreased P and R waves, ST segment depression, prolonged QT interval
  2. Treatment: Na$^+$ − K$^+$ exchange resin—e.g., kayexalate, 1 g/kg PO (action within 12 hr) or PR (action within 30 min; may repeat q1-2h)
- If K$^+$ > 7 mmol/L:
  1. NaHCO$_3$ 1-3 mmol/kg (shifts K$^+$ intracellularly); risk of hypocalcemic tetany with decreased pH
  2. Dextrose 0.5 g/kg/hr (10% dextrose at 5 ml/kg/hr) until blood glucose reaches 14 mmol/L (shifts K$^+$ intracellularly)

```
Acute renal failure
            │
            ▼
Rule out obstructive causes (U/S most useful)
            │
            ▼
Determine type of ARF
(Prerenal or renal)
            │
      ┌─────┴─────────────────┐
      ▼                       ▼
  Laboratory           Theraputic challenge
      │                       │
      │          20 ml/kg IV crystalloid/colloid over 1-2 hr x 2 maximum
      │                (preferably with CVP monitor)
      │                       │
      │              ┌────────┴────────┐
      │              ▼                 ▼
      │         >2 ml/kg hr urine   Oliguria:
      │                             Neonates: <0.5 ml/kg/hr urine
      │         Prerenal            <Older: 2 ml/kg/hr
      │                                 │
      │                                 ▼
      │                             Furosemide
      │                             2 mg/kg IV
      │                             q4h x 2
      │                                 ±
      │                             Mannitol
      │                             0.5-1 g/kg/IV
      │                                 │
      │                        ┌────────┴────────┐
      │                        ▼                 ▼
      │                   Oliguria persists   Diuresis
      │                        │                 │
      │                        ▼                 ▼
      │                   Renal (intrinsic)  Prerenal oliguria
      │                   disease                or
      │                                      Oliguric ATN
      │                                      converted to
      │                                      nonoliguric ATN
      ▼
```

	Prerenal	Renal (intrinsic)
*Urine specific gravity	<1.020	<1.015
*Urine Na+ (mmol/L)	<10	>25
Urine/plasma osmolality	>1.3	<1.1
Sediment	Hyaline fine granular casts	Cellular casts

*Not useful if diuretics have been used. NB false ↑ SG with proteinuria, glycosuria, mannitol, and radio-opaque dyes.

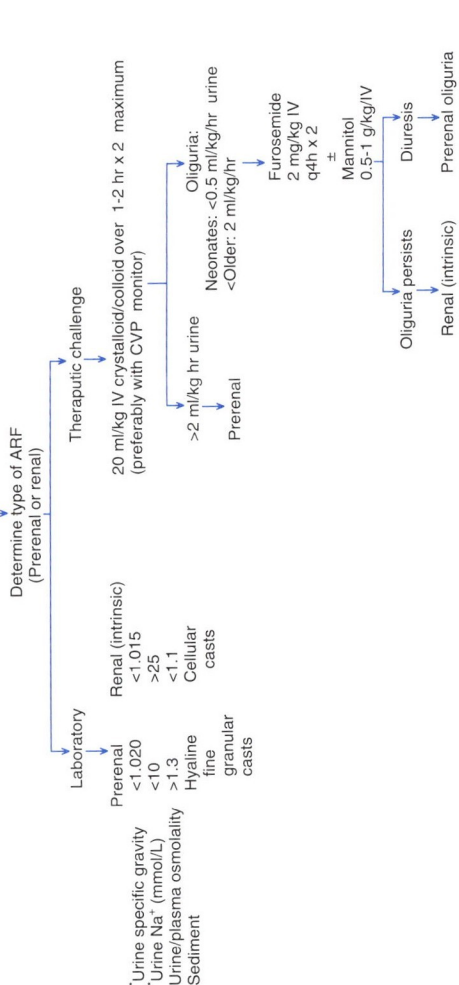

Figure 17-1 **Approach to acute renal failure.**

- If ECG changes
  1. 10% calcium gluconate 0.5 ml/kg IV over 3-5 min (do not mix with bicarbonate)
  2. Insulin plus concurrent glucose infusion: 1 U Regular insulin per 5 g of infused glucose
- Indications for dialysis
  1. Uncontrollable fluid overload (hypertension or pulmonary edema)
  2. Uncontrolled hyperkalemia
  3. Severe metabolic acidosis
  4. Progressive uremia
  5. Dialyzable nephrotoxin
  6. Hyperammonemia
  7. Facilitation of TPN (re: volume)

Urinary Tract Infection (UTI)

- Definition: more than two clean voided urine specimens with $\geq 10^5$ colonies/ml of single organism *or* 10^3 colonies/ml in a catheter specimen *or* any concentration in a suprapubic specimen
- Bacteriology: *Escherichia coli* in 85% of females, *Proteus* species in males; also, *Streptococcus faecalis, Klebsiella, Pseudomonas, Staphylococcus epidermidis*
- Differential diagnosis of pyuria: bacterial UTI, fever, dehydration, mycoplasma, appendicitis
- Investigations
  1. Screening tests, e.g., nitrate dipsticks
  2. Urine for microscopy (cell count, bacteria, casts)
  3. Urine culture and sensitivity
  4. In systemic illness, CBC, blood culture, renal function tests
- Management
  1. Push fluids
  2. Antibiotics: trimethoprim-sulphamethoxazole (TMP-SMX) PO; amoxicillin or pivampicillin, or nitrofurantoin for uncomplicated cases, × 7-10 days. Ampicillin plus aminoglycoside parenterally for systemic illness × 10-14 days.

- Follow-up
  1. Cultures
     - Repeat cultures at 48 hr (should be sterile), then 3 days after cessation of therapy
     - Follow with monthly cultures × 3 (for normal anatomy), then only if symptomatic or febrile illness
  2. Radiologic evaluation
     - U/S all ages
     - Vesicoureterogram (VCUG) in all boys, and in girls <6 yr with first UTI. Should be done after UTI treated. IVP only for further anatomic detail or if obstruction suspected.
  3. Chemoprophylaxis (TMP-SMX, amoxicillin, pivampicillin)
     - All grades reflux
     - >3 UTIs/yr
     - For children <1 mo, TMP-SMX is relatively contraindicated due to sulfa component and potential for hyperbilirubinemia. May use trimethoprim alone, 2 mg/kg/day (single or divided doses) or amoxicillin/pivampicillin. For children >1 mo: TMP-SMX and nitrofurantoin are best choices.
     - Amoxicillin and pivampicillin are inadequate for prophylaxis; cephalexin may be used in specific clinical situations.
  4. Reflux (Fig. 17-2)
     - May be 1° or 2° to obstructive uropathy (posterior urethral valves), mechanical abnormality (bladder wall, duplicated collecting system), functional abnormality (neurogenic bladder)
     - Grades I and II 1° reflux: antibiotic prophylaxis until free of reflux × 1-2 yr (85% will resolve). Follow with VCUG q6mo.
     - Grades III and IV 1° reflux, and all 2° reflux: refer to urologist; may require surgery

5. Nuclear scans
   DMSA (Dimercaptosuccinic acid)
   - Assess renal shape (scarring)
   - History of pyelonephritis
   - Increasing frequency of lower tract infections
   - Increasing reflux on VCUG

   DTPA (Diethylenetriaminepentacetic acid)
   - Assesses renal urine flow and function

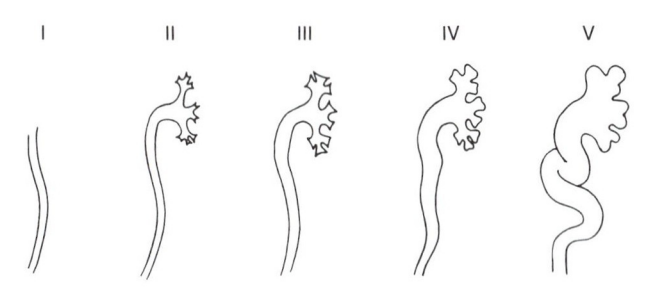

Figure 17-2 **Grades of vesicoureteral reflux (International Classification).**

Chronic Renal Failure

- Monitor biochemistry, hematology, growth
- Psychologic and educational support
- Diet
  1. Increase calories (NG or G-tube supplementation *early*)
  2. Multivitamins
  3. Decrease total protein, generally when creatinine >50 mmol/L in infant and >100 mmol/L in older child. Will depend on previous nutrient intake. To allow for growth, should not be less than recommended daily intake.
  4. Decrease Na^+: restricted Na^+ diet = 2-5 g/day; should not go below 1-3 mmol/kg/day to allow for growth (1 mmol = 23 mg). Will depend on current intake, i.e., often "no added salt" sufficient (vs. actual restriction).
  5. Decrease K and PO_4
  6. Oral PO_4 binder: calcium carbonate (acts as Ca supplement as well), *not* aluminium (except acute short-term)
  7. Ca, vitamin D supplements. Alphacalcidol = 1 α-(OH)-vitamin D_3. Dosage = 0.01 µg/kg/day. Advantage: available in liquid, allows for smaller infant doses. Rocaltrol = Calcitriol = 1,25 $(OH)_2$ Vitamin D_3. Dose = 0.01 µg/kg/day (more potent).
- Fluid and electrolytes
  1. Restrict fluid if edema, elevated BP, CHF
  2. Diuretics, antihypertensives, kayexelate, bicarbonate as needed
- Anemia: Erythropoietin is effective in preventing and correcting anemia of CRF; decreases need for repeated transfusions. Complications include hypertension, flu-like illness, seizures, cerebrovascular accidents, ↑ K^+, clotting of vascular access. Fe therapy may be required to prevent Fe deficiency. Dosage = 50 U/kg IV or SC 3 times per week; thereafter, titrate dose.
- Renal osteodystrophy (RODS): delayed bone age, subperiosteal resorption on radial aspect of phalanges, rachitic changes. Dietary management: Ca supplementation, PO_4 binding.

Glomerulonephritis

- May be characterized by:
  1. Nephritic syndrome: oliguria (<300 ml/m^2/day), hematuria, edema, elevated BP
  2. Nephrotic syndrome
  3. Mixture of nephritic and nephrotic
- Etiology see Table 17-1
- Glomerulonephritis can occur after Group A streptococcal throat or skin infection; rheumatic fever occurs after throat infection only

TABLE 17-1 Causes of Glomerulonephritis

↓ C_3	Normal C_3
Poststreptococcal GN	IgA nephropathy (Berger's)
Membranoproliferative GN	Hereditary nephritis (Alport's)
Systemic lupus erythematosus	Rapidly progressive GN
Bacterial endocarditis	Henoch-Schönlein purpura
Shunt nephritis	Goodpasture's syndrome and anti-GBM disease (membranoproliferative GN type 1)

Management

- Family history of high frequency deafness, hematuria
- Urinalysis, including microscopy
- Total hemolytic complement and C_3
- Electrolytes, BUN, creatinine, acid-base status
- CBC, smear, ESR
- Throat swab, antistreptolysin-O titre (ASOT), antihyaluronidase titre
- ± Protein electrophoresis, cholesterol, and triglycerides
- ± CXR (cardiomegaly, pulmonary edema, effusion)
- ± Renal biopsy
- Treatment
  1. Fluids: restrict for oliguria or circulatory overload to insensible losses (400 ml/kg/day) + urine output
  2. Diet: decreased Na^+ if increased BP, decreased K^+, normal protein
  3. Positive throat swab requires antibiotic therapy
  4. Manage ARF and secondary complication (see p 348)
  5. Hospitalization indicated for decreased renal function, elevated BP ± diagnostic evaluation

Hemolytic Uremic Syndrome

Investigations

- CBC and smear: decreased Hb anisocytosis; fragmented, helmet-shaped, and burr cells; increased reticulocytes; platelets normal early, then decreased
- Urinalysis: hematuria; proteinuria; RBCs and granular casts on microscopy
- Stool cultures (e.g., *Shigella,* verotoxin-producing *E. coli.* N.B.: Must ask for these cultures specifically on laboratory requisition).
- Manage ARF (see p 348). Supportive management of anemia, thrombocytopenia.
- Antibiotics not indicated, even with positive stool cultures

Proteinuria

- Definition: >150 mg/24 hr, or >140 mg/m^2 in small children
- Intermittent proteinuria
  1. Functional: strenuous exercise, fever, extreme cold
  2. Orthostatic: related to upright position; may be seen in resolving pyelonephritis or glomerulonephritis
  3. Transient, idiopathic
- Persistent proteinuria is usually abnormal

Management

- Exclude transient proteinuria
- Exclude orthostatic proteinuria
  1. Urine sample should be tested *immediately* on rising, and again after walking or standing for 2 hr or more. (Repeat twice).
  2. Two 12-hr urine collections (12 hr while ambulant, 12 hr while recumbent)
- History
  1. Family history of renal disease, deafness
  2. Medications, e.g., gold, penicillamine, probenecid, amphotericin
  3. Other symptoms related to urinary tract or other systemic diseases
- Physical signs: height, weight, BP
- Complete urinalysis (including specific gravity, microscopy), culture
- Renal function
  1. 24-hr urine collection for protein, and creatinine clearance
  2. BUN, creatinine, electrolytes
- Further work-up if associated features dictate (e.g., U/S, protein electrophoresis, C_3, serum lipids)
- Renal biopsy may be indicated (see below)

Nephrotic Syndrome

- Characteristics
  1. Proteinuria (>50 mg/kg/day or >40 mg/m^2/hr)
  2. Hypoproteinemia (often <25 g/L albumin)
  3. Edema
  4. Hyperlipidemia
- Etiology: may be 1° (renal) or 2° (systemic disease). Minimal change commonest (70%), focal glomerulosclerosis next most common.
- Initial investigations as per proteinuria
- Indications for renal biopsy
  1. Age <1 yr
  2. Marked nephritic syndrome components (↑ BP, renal failure, gross hematuria) of unknown etiology
  3. Low C_3
  4. No response *once on steroid therapy* for 4-8 wk
- Complications:
  1. Diminished resistance to infection (*Pneumococcus, H. influenza,* coliforms), especially peritonitis
  2. Hypovolemia with postural hypotension, circulatory collapse, renal failure (in minority of patients with minimal change lesion)
  3. Protein depletion
  4. Increased coagulability of blood, leading to thrombosis (especially of renal vein)
  5. Complications of therapy (diuretics, steroids, cytotoxics)

Management

- Diet: decreased Na$^+$; no protein restriction unless in renal failure
- Exclude and treat bacterial infection, e.g., peritonitis
- Edema
  1. If edema severe, restrict fluid intake
  2. For respiratory distress, impending skin breakdown, marked ascites, pulmonary edema, or effusions: infuse 1 g/kg of salt-poor 25% albumin IV over ~ 1-2 hr, followed by IV furosemide, 1-2 mg/kg

3. Avoid overly aggressive efforts at diuresis, as this may produce intravascular depletion and further aggravate oliguria and hypercoagulable state
- Remission induction
  1. Prednisone, 2 mg/kg/day (60 mg/m^2/day) in 3-4 doses (maximum, 80 mg/day)
  2. Treat until urine trace positive or negative for 5-7 days, or for a total of 28 days
  3. If no remission in 28 days, consider referral to nephrologist and biopsy. If biopsy consistent with steroid-responsive (minimal-change pathology) type, resume therapy for another 28 days *or,* alternatively, consider addition of cyclophosphamide. If compatible with steroid-resistant (i.e., after 8-wk steroid therapy) type, treat with appropriate therapy, if available or applicable.
- Maintenance therapy
  1. Prednisone, 1.5-2.0 mg/kg/day (45-60 mg/m^2/day)—maximum dose, 80 mg/day; single daily dose on alternate days for 28 days, then taper by 10 mg q2-4wk to 30 mg, then ↓ by 5 mg q2-4wk until discontinued
  2. Monitor first morning void for albumin at home
- Relapse (~ ⅔ of patients)
  1. 2+ or heavier proteinuria for 7 consecutive days
  2. Treat as above to induce remission; then alternate-day treatment
  3. Cytotoxic drugs (e.g., chlorambucil, cyclophosphamide) are used for steroid-dependent or steroid-resistant cases or frequent relapsers, but because of serious potential side effects, this should be done in consultation with a nephrologist
  4. Steroid-resistant cases should be considered for renal biopsy
  5. Alternatives for steroid-resistant and immunosuppressive-resistant cases or high-steroid requirements with frequent breakthroughs: ASA + dipyrimadole, levamisole (immunostimulant)

Hypertension

- Secondary hypertension most common <13 yr
- Consider diagnosis of essential or primary in adolescent
- Refer to Figures 17-3 and 17-4 for percentiles of blood pressure values by age

Text continued on p 364.

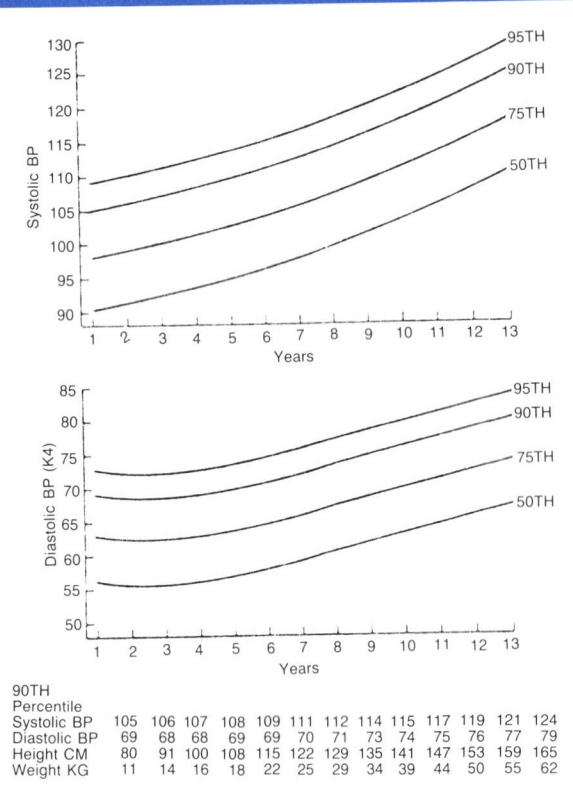

90TH Percentile													
Systolic BP	105	106	107	108	109	111	112	114	115	117	119	121	124
Diastolic BP	69	68	68	69	69	70	71	73	74	75	76	77	79
Height CM	80	91	100	108	115	122	129	135	141	147	153	159	165
Weight KG	11	14	16	18	22	25	29	34	39	44	50	55	62

A. Boys: 1–13 yr of age

Figure 17-3 **Percentiles of blood pressure measurement in boys and girls.** (From Report of the Second Task Force on Blood Pressure Control in Children—1987. Reproduced with permission from Pediatrics 1987; 79:5-6.)

Nephrology

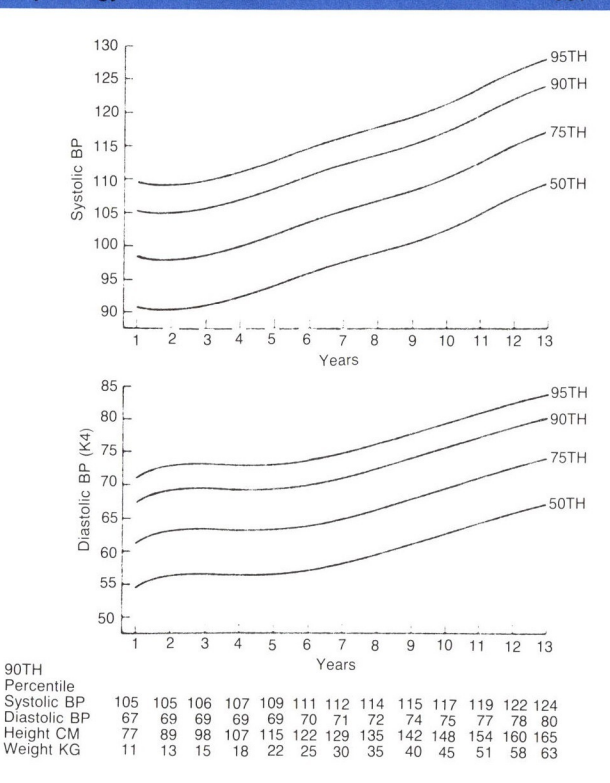

90TH Percentile													
Systolic BP	105	105	106	107	109	111	112	114	115	117	119	122	124
Diastolic BP	67	69	69	69	69	70	71	72	74	75	77	78	80
Height CM	77	89	98	107	115	122	129	135	142	148	154	160	165
Weight KG	11	13	15	18	22	25	30	35	40	45	51	58	63

B. Girls: 1–13 yr of age

Figure 17-3, continued.

Continued.

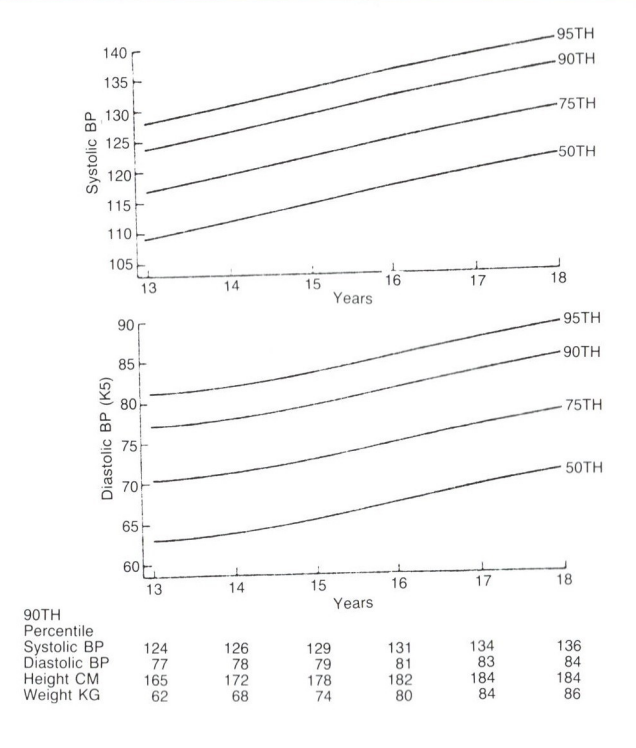

90TH Percentile						
Systolic BP	124	126	129	131	134	136
Diastolic BP	77	78	79	81	83	84
Height CM	165	172	178	182	184	184
Weight KG	62	68	74	80	84	86

C. Boys: 13–18 yr of age

Figure 17-3, continued.

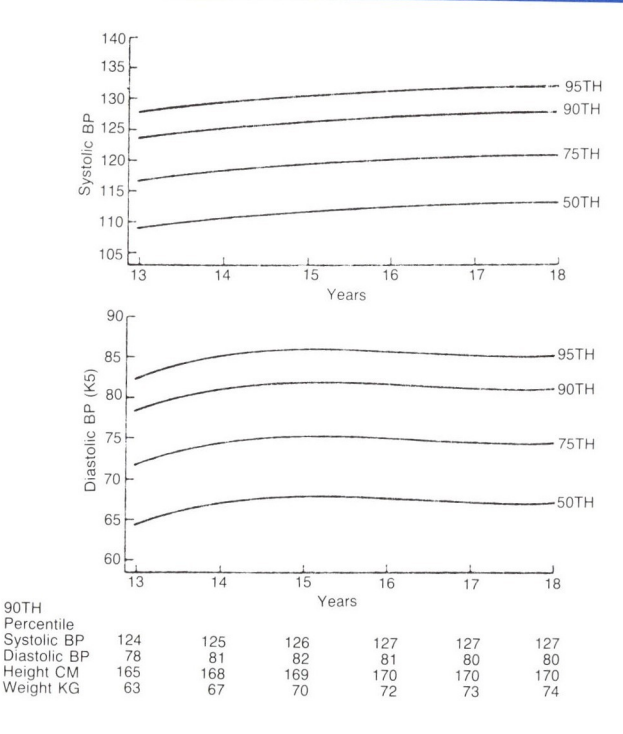

90TH Percentile						
Systolic BP	124	125	126	127	127	127
Diastolic BP	78	81	82	81	80	80
Height CM	165	168	169	170	170	170
Weight KG	63	67	70	72	73	74

D. Girls: 13–18 yr of age

Figure 17-3, continued.

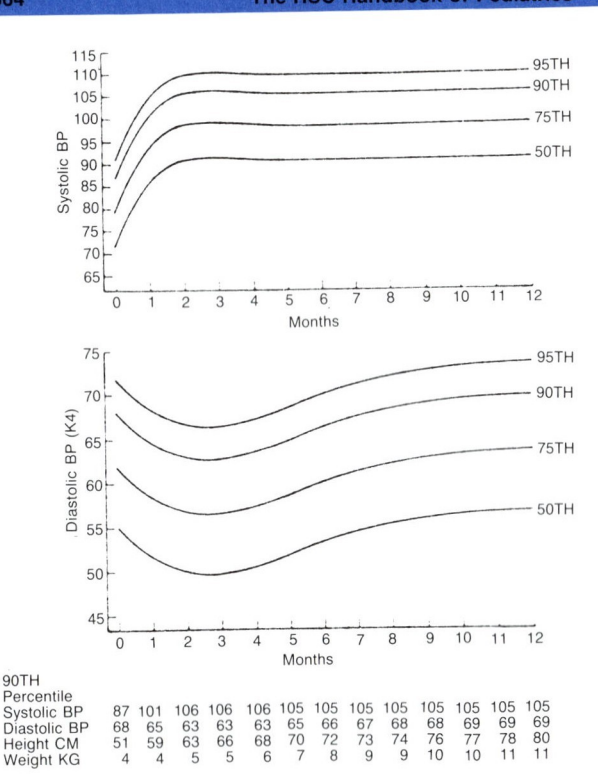

90TH Percentile													
Systolic BP	87	101	106	106	106	105	105	105	105	105	105	105	105
Diastolic BP	68	65	63	63	63	65	66	67	68	68	69	69	69
Height CM	51	59	63	66	68	70	72	73	74	76	77	78	80
Weight KG	4	4	5	5	6	7	8	9	9	10	10	11	11

A. Boys

Figure 17-4 **Percentiles of blood pressure in infants awake (birth to 12 months of age).** (From Report of the Second Task Force on Blood Pressure Control in children—1987. Reproduced with permission from Pediatrics 1987; 79:5-6.)

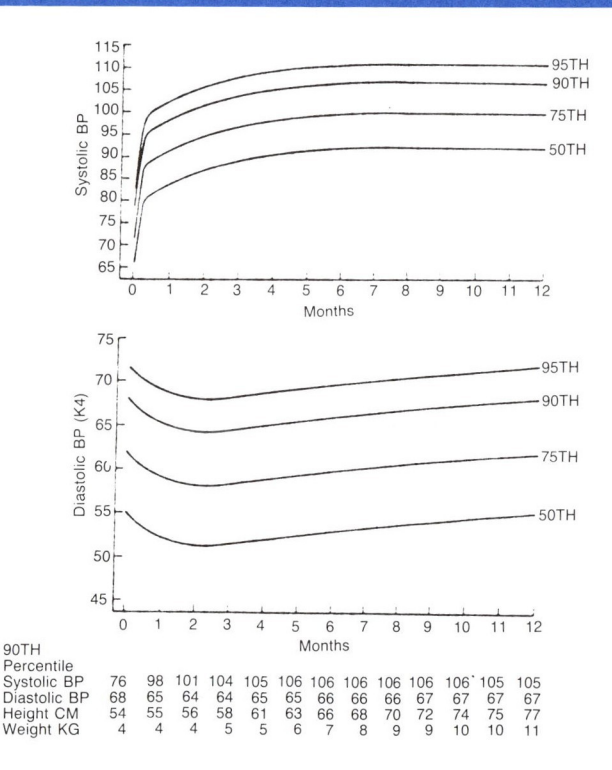

90TH Percentile													
Systolic BP	76	98	101	104	105	106	106	106	106	106	106	105	105
Diastolic BP	68	65	64	64	65	65	66	66	66	67	67	67	67
Height CM	54	55	56	58	61	63	66	68	70	72	74	75	77
Weight KG	4	4	4	5	5	6	7	8	9	9	10	10	11

B. Girls

Figure 17-4, continued.

Investigations

- Confirmation of BP by frequent measurements with an appropriately sized cuff (two-thirds of arm, and bladder to encircle arm completely). If cuff is too small, BP reading is falsely high; if cuff is too large, falsely low.
- Renal
  1. Urinalysis, microscopy, and urine specific gravity
  2. Urine culture
  3. Plasma electrolytes, BUN, creatinine, blood acid-base status, uric acid
  4. Creatinine clearance
  5. U/S of abdomen (anatomy of GU system)
  6. IVP, renal scan
  7. Renins (peripheral ± renal vein)
  8. ± Arteriogram
- Cardiac: CXR, ECG, 2 DEcho
- Endocrine
  1. 24-hr urine for vanillymandelic acid (VMA) and catecholamines
  2. Cortisol, aldosterone, renin (plasma), 17-OH progesterone
  3. Thyroid function tests

Treatment

- General
  1. Low Na^+/no added salt diet. Will depend on current intake. Generally, 2-5 g/day; not <1-3 mmol/kg/day (1 mmol = 23 mg).
  2. Weight reduction and control
  3. Physical activity (dynamic or aerobic exercise)
  4. Avoid smoking
- Indications for drug therapy (Table 17-2)
  1. Symptomatic
  2. Target organ damage
  3. BP persistently >95th percentile
- Acute hypertension: clinical features include encephalopathy (including seizures), LV failure, accelerated increase in BP. Treat with nifedipine PO or hydralazine IV as first-line. Continuous infusion (labetalol, nitroprusside) should be done in ICU setting (Table 17-3).

TABLE 17-2 Management of Hypertension*

Diuretics
  Hydrochlorothiazide
  Spironolactone: use with caution in CRF because of ↑ K^+; may be given in combination with above as novospirozine, Aldactazide
  Furosemide

β-blockers
  Propranolol: avoid in asthmatics, diabetics, Raynaud's, CHF
  Metoprolol: headache, bronchospasm, fatigue, dizziness
  Nadolol: advantage of once daily use (precautions as per propranolol)

Vasodilators
  Hydralazine
  Minoxidil: hirsutism, Na^+ and fluid retention
  Prazosin: α-blockade as well (may induce positive ANA)

Sympathetic inhibitor and peripheral norepinephrine depletion
  α-Methyldopa: Coomb's positive hemolytic anemia, ↑ liver enzymes

Calcium-channel blockers
  Nifedipine: peripheral edema, dizziness, headache, nausea, and vomiting
  Long- and short-acting formulations available.

Angiotensin-converting enzyme inhibitor
  Captopril
  Enalapril: dosage not yet established in pediatric age group; advantage—once daily use (side effects as per captopril)

---

*Notes:
  1. All vasodilators are associated with fluid retention; therefore, it is often necessary to combine with diuretics.
  2. Drug therapy often starts with diuretics, then sympatholytics (e.g., β-blockers, α-methyl-dopa) and vasodilators are added systematically. This approach, however, may be modified according to etiology (e.g., captopril in patients with "renal" hypertension may be introduced earlier in certain situations).
  3. Nifedipine is first choice for breakthrough or exacerbation of chronic hypertension.

TABLE 17-3 Drug Therapy for Acute Hypertension

Drug and Dosage	Duration	Side Effects
Vasodilators*		
Diazoxide: 1-2 mg/kg/dose IV bolus (over 30 sec) q5-15 min until BP controlled (onset within minutes → arteriolar dilatation)	Up to 24 hr (mean, ~ 5 hr)	Acute hypotension, ↑ glucose, tachycardia, Na^+ and fluid retention, headache
Nitroprusside, 0.5-8.0 µg/kg/min IV, titrated to response (immediate onset → arteriolar and venous dilatation)	During infusion only	Hypotension, tachycardia, headache, nausea, chest pain; ↑ *risk of cyanide poisoning if used >48 hr*
Hydralazine, 0.2-0.5 mg/kg IV (max., 25 mg IV) (arteriolar dilatation—onset within 30 min)	4-12 hr	Hypotension, tachycardia, fluid retention, vomiting, lupus-like syndrome

Sympathetic blocking agents*

Labetalol, 1-3 mg/kg IV (α and β blocker — onset within minutes). Useful as infusion. — Up to 24 hr — GI upset, headache, dizziness

Phentolamine, 0.1-0.2 mg/kg IV (α-blocker used in pheochromocytoma → immediate onset) — 30-60 min — Tachycardia, ↓ BP, nausea, vomiting, abdominal pain

Others

Captopril, 0.3-2 mg/kg per dose PO (angiotensin-converting enzyme inhibitor onset within 15 min) — 8-12 hr — Neutropenia; proteinuria; reversible renal failure in renovascular disease; rash

Nifedipine, 0.25-0.5 mg/kg bite and swallow: maximum, 20 mg (calcium channel blocker — onset within 20-30 min) — 6 hr — Dizziness and facial flushing

Clonidine, 2-6 μg/kg IV† (central α adrenergic stimulation — onset within 30 min) — 8 hr — Sedation, dry mouth, rebound ↑ BP

*May require ICU setting.
†Not available in Canada.

Hematuria

- Definition: 5-10 RBCs/hpf in spun sample
- History: previous episodes, intercurrent illness, recent pharyngitis, drugs, trauma, family history of stones
- Physical examination: BP, plot growth, hearing, renal mass or cysts

Investigations

- CBC, platelets
- Urinalysis, microscopy, culture
- If casts, throat swab for culture
- BUN, creatinine
- U/S
- ± 12- or 24-hr urine collection protein, calcium, creatinine clearance
- ± PT, PTT
- ± TB test
- ± Work-up collagen vascular disease
- Indications for biopsy: strong suspicion of glomerulonephritis, recurrent hematuria (microscopic or gross) × 1 yr, hypertension, coexistent nephrotic features, collagen vascular disease

Enuresis

- All enuretics should have the following basic screening evaluations:
  1. Urinalysis (protein, glucose, specific gravity), microscopy ± urine culture
  2. Height and weight plotted on standard growth charts
- Nocturnal enuresis
  1. Demystify, and educate child about etiology and prognosis
  2. Positive reinforcement techniques and no punitive action by caregivers
  3. Explore psychosocial issues

4. Enuresis alarms
   - Consider in motivated and willing child, usually after 8 yr
   - Cures attained slowly, but success rate is higher than with other modes of therapy alone
5. Drugs
   - DDAVP administered by nasal spray: moderate success rate
   - Imipramine: potentially lethal drug; use with caution for limited period after other modalities have failed; high relapse rate (40-60%)
6. Behavior modification
- Diurnal enuresis
  1. Most are secondary to functional immaturity but consider underlying pathology such as UTI, diabetes mellitus, spinal dysraphism or lesions, renal anomalies
  2. In addition to basic screening tests, consider urodynamics, lumbosacral x-rays, VCUG, renal U/S as indicated
  3. Explore psychosocial issues
  4. For decreased bladder capacity, consider bladder exercises and oxybutynin

Peritonitis in Chronic Ambulatory Peritoneal Dialysis (CAPD)

- Etiologic agents: *S. epidermidis, S. aureus, S. viridans,* gram-negative organisms—e.g., *E. coli, Pseudomonas* species
- Clinical diagnosis: cloudy effluent, abdominal pain, fever
- Laboratory diagnosis: dialysate WBC > 100/mm^3 with >50% PMNs ± positive Gram stain; positive culture

Treatment

- Using 1.5% dianeal, three exchanges (in and out) with heparin (500 U/L) added
- To the fourth bag add the following: Cefazolin 500 mg/L, Tobramycin 1.7 mg/kg/bag, Heparin 500 U/L
- To subsequent bags add the following: Cefazolin 250 mg/L, Tobramycin 8 mg/L, Heparin 500 U/L; if bag is still cloudy, continue heparin until bag clears
- Adjust antibiotics according to sensitivities
- *S. aureus* peritonitis
  1. Cloxacillin: loading dose 1 gm/L, then maintenance 100 mg/L
  2. Rifampin 10-20 mg/kg/day divided bid PO
- Continue therapy for minimum of 2 wk for proven cases; resistant cases may need longer therapy

Renal Function Tests

GLOMERULAR FILTRATION RATE (GFR)

- Creatinine clearance
  1. Creatinine clearance can vary, especially with severe disease
  2. Some secretion of creatinine does occur, especially with reduced renal function
  3. Consumption of red meat can increase serum creatinine
  4. <1L urine volume in 24 hr gives falsely low reading in older children
- Calculation based on urine collection, corrected for surface area

$$C_{cr} = \frac{U \times V}{P \times t} \times \frac{1.73}{SA}$$

where: U = urine concentration of creatinine
V = total urine volume in ml
t = duration of collection of urine
P = serum concentration of creatinine
SA = surface area in m^2

- To check adequacy of urine collection
  1. Adult females and children produce 135-175 μmol (15-20 mg) creatinine/kg/day
  2. Adult males produce 175-220 μmol (20-25 mg) creatinine/kg/day
- Renal scan using [99m]Technetium-labeled DTPA
- Rough estimation of GFR

$$\text{GFR} = \frac{k \times L}{[\text{creatinine}] \text{ mg/dl}} = \text{ml/min}/1.73 \text{ m}^2$$

where: L = height in cm
  k = 0.33 low birthweight infants
  0.45 term AGA infants
  0.55 children, adolescent girls
  0.70 adolescent boys

[creatinine] μmol/1 × 0.0113 = mg/dl
(Normal GFR, ~ 120-140ml/min/1.73 m^2)

Urinalysis

- Clinistix—specific for glucose (uses glucose oxidase)
- Clinitest tablets—positive with glucose, fructose, galactose, lactose, ascorbic acid, homogentisic acid, pentose, tyrosine, chloramphenicol, chloral hydrate, sulfonamides, salicylate metabolites. Method: add 2 drops urine to 10 drops water, then add tablet.
- Hematuria: Dipstix positive with hemoglobinuria and myoglobinuria
- Nitrites: screening test for UTIs; only positive with gram-negative organisms
- DNPH: (dinitrophenylhydrazine) test positive (presence of keto acids) in maple syrup urine disease, phenylketonuria, ketotic hyperglycinemia, lactic acidosis, methylmalonic-aciduria, etc.
- Cyanide nitroprusside test: screen for cystinuria and homocystinuria
- Unspun urine: test for WBCs and bacteria
- Spun urine (centrifuge at 2000 rpm for 2 min): test for formed elements—e.g., casts (look at peripheries of cover slip)

EIGHTEEN

Neurology

Seizures (Tables 18-1 to 18-3)

TABLE 18-1 Classification of Seizures

ILAE* Classification	Other Terminology
I. Partial seizures	
A. Simple partial seizures	
1. With motor signs	Jacksonian seizures or focal motor seizures
2. With somatosensory or special sensory symptoms (visual, auditory, olfactory, gustatory, vertiginous)	Sensory seizures
3. With autonomic symptoms or signs	Abdominal epilepsy or epileptic equivalent
B. Complex partial seizures	Psychomotor or temporal lobe seizures
II. Generalized seizures	
A. Absence seizures	
1. Typical	Petit mal
2. Atypical	Petit mal variant or complex petit mal
B. Myoclonic seizures	
C. Atonic seizures	Akinetic seizures or drop attacks
D. Tonic-clonic seizures	Grand mal, major motor seizures, generalized convulsive seizures

*International League Against Epilepsy

TABLE 18-2 Differentiation: Seizure, Syncope, Breath Holding

Symptom	Seizure (Generalized Type)	Syncope	Breath Holding "Blue"	Breath Holding "White"
Precipitating event	Usually none but occasionally in response to hyperventilation or flickering lights	Usually present	Frustration, anger	Pain, surprise
Loss of consciousness	May be prolonged	Brief	May occur	May occur
Onset	Aura may occur and is often stereotyped	Light-headed, queasy, blurred vision	Frustration, crying	Pain, injury
Appearance	Rubor, cyanosis, sweating	Pale, clammy, cold	Cyanosis, holds breath in inspiration	Same as syncope

Continued.

TABLE 18-2 Differentiation: Seizure, Syncope, Breath Holding (Cont'd)

Symptom	Seizure (Generalized Type)	Syncope	Breath Holding "Blue"	Breath Holding "White"
Motor activity	Prominent, prolonged, jerking	Minimal: occasional eyelid flutter or isolated jerk can occur	Occasional clonic movements; can terminate (rarely) in generalized tonic-clonic seizure	Same as syncope
Postictal	Drowsy: may sleep	Wakes up	Rapid return to normal	Rapid return to normal
EEG (between episodes)	Usually abnormal	Normal	Normal	Normal
Age	Not specific	Older child, adolescent	6 mo-4 yr	1-4 yr
Treatment	Conventional anticonvulsants, if recurrent	Semiprone position	None	None

TABLE 18-3 Long-term Seizure Management

Seizure Type	First Choice*	Alternates
Generalized tonic-clonic	Carbamazepine	Phenytoin[†] Phenobarbital[‡] Valproate Primidone
Partial complex, simple partial	Carbamazepine	Phenytoin Phenobarbital Valproate Primidone
Absence	Valproate[§]	Clonazepam Ethosuximide
Myoclonic	Valproate	Nitrazepam Clonazepam Clobazam
Atonic	Valproate	Nitrazepam Clonazepam Primidone
Infantile spasms	Nitrazepam or ACTH	Clonazepam Primidone

*General guidelines only; will depend on clinical situation.
†Avoid in young children <6 yr when possible, because of cosmetic side effects
‡Phenobarbital is drug of first choice in most generalized seizures in children <age 2.
§Avoid use with multiple anti-epileptic drugs and in children <2 yr

STATUS EPILEPTICUS

- Definition: a single generalized (tonic-clonic, myoclonic, tonic, or absence) or focal (clonic or jacksonian) seizure lasting 30 min or longer; this includes any series of seizures without intervening return of consciousness with a duration of greater than 30 minutes.

Management

- Secure airway; oxygenation, assisted ventilation if necessary
- Establish intravenous line with 5% dextrose and normal saline, at ⅔ maintenance
- Diazepam 0.3 mg/kg IV, to be given at 2 mg/min. Repeat every 10 min if needed for maximum of three doses. If IV access is not available, give same preparation PR at dose of 0.5 mg/kg once only. Maximal dose for children ≤5 yr is 5 mg; for those >5 yr, 10 mg. (Alternatively, use lorazepam, 0.05 mg/kg IV, to maximum of 4 mg. Infuse no faster than 2 mg/min. Maximum, two doses.) To administer PR diazepam or lorazepam, draw up desired dose in 1 ml or 3 ml syringe; dilute with normal saline. When syringe is withdrawn, squeeze buttocks firmly together for 1-2 min.
- Blood for glucose (Dextrostix can be done at the bedside) plus electrolytes, BUN, CBC, calcium, magnesium, toxic screen, anticonvulsant levels. Urine for toxic and metabolic screen as indicated.
- Low blood glucose (<2.2 mmol/L), give 25% dextrose 2 ml/kg
- Monitor respirations; O_2 saturation or blood gases; ECG must be prepared to manage airway and ventilation if apnea occurs.

- Begin maintenance anticonvulsant therapy with phenytoin 20 mg/kg IV (maximum 1 g) at 50 mg/min; slow infusion rate if hypotension or bradycardia occur. Administer staged doses of 10 mg/kg IV; to maximum of 30 mg/kg.
- *If seizure continues* after 25-30 min: phenobarbital 20 mg/kg IV at 60 mg/min; staged doses of 10-15 mg/kg; may go up to 40 mg/kg. (maximum IV loading dose 600 mg). Risk of apnea increased when barbituates given in conjunction with benzodiazepines. In children <2 yr, may use phenobarbital as drug of first choice.
- *If seizure continues:* may give 1-2 doses of paraldehyde, PR 0.2-0.4 ml/kg/dose (undiluted). Dilute in syringe with equal volume of vegetable or olive oil. Rectal administration as for diazepam and lorazpam. Maximum 10 g/dose
- *If seizure continues,* patient will require intubation and thiopentone infusion in ICU setting with continuous EEG monitoring
- Investigations: evaluation depends on history and physical findings
  1. Urgent CT head scan (or MRI) if history suggestive of focal lesion (trauma, bleed, space-occupying lesion), or presence of persistent focal neurologic signs, or evidence of raised ICP.
  2. Lumbar puncture if there is a history consistent with meningitis, meningismus or fever, and no evidence of raised intracranial pressure
  3. EEG when available
  4. Further metabolic investigations (see Chapter 15, Metabolic Disease)

FEBRILE SEIZURES

- Most febrile seizures have stopped before the child reaches hospital; treat a continuing seizure as for status epilepticus.
- Acetaminophen PR or PO if temp > 38.5° C
- Judicious search for infectious focus with antibiotic treatment as appropriate
- Investigations depend on history and physical findings: Consider CBC, blood culture, electrolytes, glucose, calcium, magnesium, urine culture
- If clinical situation warrants, lumbar puncture if no evidence of raised intracranial pressure. A high index of suspicion for meningitis is needed in children <1 yr and in children with recurring or prolonged febrile seizures in the previous 24 hr.
- Hospitalization may not be necessary if the following criteria are met
    1. Brief (<15 min) febrile seizure with full recovery
    2. The cause of the fever is identified, and appropriate outpatient treatment is initiated
    3. Follow-up arranged
- Parent education
    1. Febrile seizures are common, occurring in 4% of children under 5 yr of age
    2. ⅔ of these children will have only one seizure
    3. Recurrent febrile seizures are more likely if there is a family history of febrile seizures or if the first febrile seizure occurs at <1 yr of age
    4. Subsequent nonfebrile seizures likely in approximately 5%; the major risk factors and features of "atypical febrile seizures" are
        - Complicated febrile seizures lasting more than 15 min
        - Multiple febrile seizures in 24 hr
        - Postictal paralysis
        - Previously abnormal neurologic exam
        - Family history of epilepsy in parents or siblings

- Prophylactic anticonvulsants should be considered if the child has recurrent febrile seizures, is less than 1 yr of age or has major risk factors for nonfebrile seizures. Options are continuous or intermittent (when febrile) medication.
  1. Continuous: phenobarbital 3-5 mg/kg/day
  2. Intermittent (when febrile), maximum one dose only
     - Diazepam 0.5 mg/kg PR (max: 5 mg <5 yr, 10 mg ≥5 yr), or
     - Lorazepam 0.05 mg/kg PR (max: 4 mg), or
     - Paraldehyde (if available) 0.3 ml/kg PR (300 mg/kg) diluted in equal amount of vegetable or olive oil (max: 10 g)

Acute Ataxia

History

- Recent headache, vomiting, viral illness (e.g., varicella), head trauma
- Presence of vertigo, focal neurologic findings, seizures
- Drug or toxin exposure—e.g., phenytoin, alcohol
- Recurrent acute ataxia—e.g., with migraine, metabolic disorders, or benign paroxysmal vertigo
- Risk factors for strokes (see p 383)
- Family history (migraine, familial ataxia, metabolic disorders)

Examination

- Raised ICP
- Decreased or altered level of consciousness
- Nystagmus, opsoclonus (conjugate jerking of eyes in random directions)
- Weakness or abnormal tone
- Myoclonus
- ENT exam for otitis media, mastoiditis
- Differentiate limb ataxia from truncal ataxia

Investigations

- Depend on history and physical exam
- CT scan (or MRI)
- Lumbar puncture (if no elevation of ICP)
- Electrolytes, glucose, CBC, NH_4, LFTs, plasma amino acids
- Toxic screen (blood, urine) if there is a specific history
- Titres for varicella, mumps, coxsackievirus, echo, influenza A and B, mycoplasma (see p 637)
- EEG
- Urine catecholamines, amino acids, organic acids
- May need further metabolic investigations

Stroke

History
- Past history of strokes, migraine, seizures
- Underlying medical problems such as cardiac disease, bleeding diathesis, leukemia, febrile illness, dehydration
- Medications likely to affect coagulation—e.g., aspirin, or intravenous use of nonprescribed drugs
- Recent trauma, including intraoral trauma

Examination
- Evidence of increased ICP (see p 539)
- Meningismus
- Cranial bruits
- Focal neurologic findings
- Cardiovascular exam: cardiac murmur, heart rhythm, blood pressure
- Evidence of a bleeding diathesis
- Sepsis: scalp or facial lesions, mastoiditis, retropharyngeal abscess, fever
- Presence of a neurocutaneous disorder or hemangioma suggestive of an arteriovenous malformation

Investigations
- CT scan or MRI are investigation of choice (include cervical spine if there are features of a vertebrobasilar stroke). If CT scan reveals:
  1. Space-occupying lesion: may require urgent angiogram prior to neurosurgery
  2. Evidence of cerebral bleeding or infarction: may require angiogram 24-48 hr later. MRI scan may be useful as thrombosis may totally occlude a vessel, preventing visualization on angiogram.
  3. Normal: lumbar puncture may reveal evidence of subarachnoid bleed. Angiogram may subsequently be required.

- CBC; platelets; ESR; blood cultures; sickle cell anemia screen; glucose, electrolytes, acid-base status; bleeding and clotting screens—i.e., PTT, PT, bleeding time, thrombotic screen (fibrinogen, plasminogen, thrombin clotting time). Consult hematologist if detailed work-up is indicated
- Further investigations as indicated (e.g., lactate, serum and urine amino acids, urine organic acids, antinuclear antibodies, lipids)
- ECG; 2 DEcho
- EEG if history and physical exam consistent with postictal event
- Other neuroimaging e.g., SPECT scan

Management

- Monitor for raised ICP, which may be maximal a few days after onset of the stroke
- Correct underlying etiology where possible
- Anticoagulation generally not indicated initially; may be required in specific situations after initial investigations done

Blocked CSF Shunt

History

- Progressive history of increasing lethargy, vomiting, and headache
- May be associated with abdominal pain or fever
- Most useful indication of shunt malfunction is prior similar history with proven malfunction
- Consider shunt infection

Investigations

- Determine shunt patency by depressing subcutaneous pump, usually located in occipital scalp regions: should depress easily and refill within 5-15 sec
- CT scan or MRI to compare ventricular size with that found on previous CT scans. If ventricular size is unchanged but symptoms persist, consider a radionuclide shunt scan

- X-ray of skull, chest, abdomen ("shunt series") to rule out shunt tube disconnection
- If symptoms intermittent or associated with abdominal pain and fever, sample CSF through subcutaneous reservoir for culture

Acute Spinal Cord Lesion

- *A neurosurgical emergency*
- Back pain
- Deteriorating gait with weakness in lower extremities
- Alteration in bladder (increased or decreased urination) or bowel (constipation) function

Physical Examination

- Altered pinprick sensation, in lower extremities, including perianal area. If there is altered sensation, determine the sensory level by moving from area of reduced sensation to normal areas. In a young child, observe the facial expression in response to the stimuli.
  Helpful dermatomes (see Fig. 18-1):
  1. Nipples T4-5
  2. Umbilicus T-10
  3. Dorsal aspect of big toe L-5
  4. Perianal area S-4, S-5, coccygeal
- Hypotonia and depressed reflexes followed by hyperreflexia
- In an older child, examine position and vibration sense in the lower extremities, after establishing that reliable responses are given with upper limb testing
- Bladder may be enlarged and palpable
- Palpate spine for tenderness or a fluctuant mass over the spine
- Spinal bruits

Investigations

- Urgent myelogram (including CSF exam) or MRI
- If myelogram and MRI are normal, consider transverse myelitis (increased WBCs in CSF), cord leukemic infiltration (leukemic cells on cytologic exam) or cord infarction

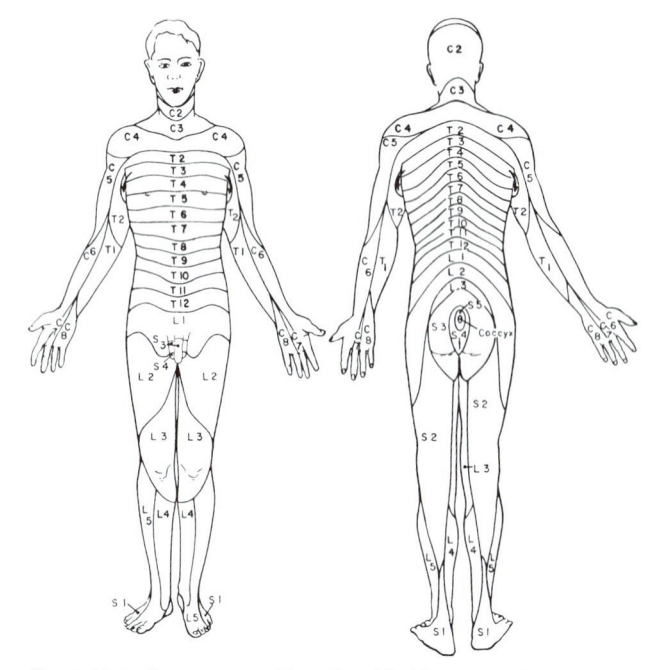

Figure 18-1 **Dermatomes.** (From Barr ML, Kiernan JA. The human nervous system. 5th ed. Philadelphia: Harper and Row, 1988.)

Myelomeningocele

Initial Evaluation and Management
- Initial stabilization (ABC)
- Keep NPO for possible surgery; establish maintenance IV of 5% dextrose and 0.2 saline
- Determine size of lesion, distal motor paralysis of legs and sphincters, associated neurogenic foot deformities, knee and hip contractures, evidence of hydrocephalus, associated congenital anomalies
- Transport for neurosurgical management: keep infant prone with moistened sterile saline dressings applied to open defect (must be kept wet at all times and changed as necessary)
- Initial diagnostic assessment includes head U/S or CT to assess hydrocephalus

Treatment
- Operative repair ± ventriculoperitoneal shunt
- Multidisciplinary team including pediatrician, neurosurgeon, urologist, orthopedic surgeon, physiotherapist
- Assess important neurologic levels re: future function (variable):
  1. Below S1-2 (ankle jerk, L5-S1): independent ambulation ± braces if L5
  2. L3-4: knee function
  3. Above L3: loss of knee function, hip flexion preserved
  4. L1-2: weak hip flexion only
- Urologic: even very distal lesions (S2) will have some degree of neurogenic bladder, often a combination of upper and lower motor neuron (see p 151)
- Orthopedic: legs extended with lesions as low as L-3. Scoliosis increases with more proximal lesions; universal above L-2.

Headache

- Tension headache
  1. Continuous pain throughout the day
  2. Often feels like a tight band around the head (sharp or pressure sensation)
  3. Does not usually interfere with sleep
  4. Often associated with ongoing anxiety or depression
- Headache due to raised ICP
  1. Recent onset (usually weeks)
  2. Increasing severity of headache
  3. Lethargy, drowsiness
  4. Morning vomiting
  5. May be increasing unsteadiness of gait
  6. May be a recent history of significant head trauma
- Migraine
  1. Classic (with aura)
  2. Common (no aura)
  3. Complicated (hemiplegia, ophthalmoplegia, basilar symptoms, or acute confusional state)
  4. Cluster (associated with conjunctival injection, tearing, nasal discharge)
  5. Presence of at least three of the following:
     - Intermittent throbbing headache
     - Complete relief with sleep
     - Aura
     - Unilateral pain
     - Nausea, vomiting, or abdominal discomfort
     - Family history of migraine

Examination
- Fundi for papilledema
- Cranial nerve abnormalities, especially abnormalities of cranial nerve VI with diplopia on lateral gaze
- Hypertension
- Enlarging head circumference, cranial bruit
- Evidence of sinusitis, otitis media, mastoiditis
- Presence of ataxia, weakness, or spasticity, especially in lower limbs
- Skin stigmata of neurocutaneous syndrome or nonaccidental injury

Investigations
- If abnormal neurologic exam or history suggestive of increased ICP obtain CT scan or MRI
- If CT scan or MRI abnormal, consult neurosurgeon. If normal: lumbar puncture, including measurement of opening pressure, CSF for cytology, culture, microscopy, virology, latex agglutination
- If normal neurologic examination with no history consistent with increased ICP: no investigations required, but follow-up essential

Specific Management for Migraine
- Acute management: acetaminophen, dark quiet environment. May use dimenhydrinate (PO or PR) if severe vomiting. Chlorpromazine or meperidine if severe or prolonged (in Emergency Department only)
- History of complicated migraine: use acetaminophen in prodromal stage
- Classic migraine in adolescents only: use sublingual ergotamine in prodromal stage (contraindicated in complicated migraine)

- Prophylaxis (individualized) approach
  1. Propranolol: contraindicated in asthma or cardiac failure; useful for basilar migraine; dosing empiric; range, ~ 10 mg PO tid-qid for most children in 8-15-yr age group (long-acting form available)
  2. Cyproheptadine: causes drowsiness (contraindicated in asthma)
  3. Pizotyline: causes drowsiness and weight gain (contraindicated in children <12 yr)
  4. Others: amitryptaline (adolescents only)
  5. Continue prophylaxis for at least 6 mo provided that there are no major side effects. Include drug holiday in management plan.

Guillain-Barré Syndrome

- Airway protection and ventilation: monitor respiratory parameters (e.g., forced vital capacity [FVC]) with respiratory therapist on daily or twice-daily basis during acute phase
- Intubation (airway protection) and ventilation necessary if
  1. Bulbar involvement (dysphagia, dysarthria, hoarseness, weak cough) with inability to protect airway
  2. Worsening respiratory parameters
  3. Cardiovascular instability
- Monitor for
  1. Cardiac arrhythmias, BP instability
  2. Bowel and bladder hypofunction
- Specific management (in consultation with neurologist)
  1. Plasmapheresis
  2. Gammaglobulin infusion

NINETEEN

Nutrition

Breast Feeding

- Proper positioning: baby horizontal and anteriorly against mother; mouth at the level of the nipple; thumb on top of breast, fingers underneath, well away from nipple
- Proper latching: open mouth wide by running nipple along lower lip; use arm holding baby to push him or her onto breast; may need to pull baby's chin down with index finger during the feed to bring lower lip out
- Complications such as sore nipples or insufficient milk may be corrected with proper positioning or the use of a lactation device if necessary; oral candidiasis may be a contributing factor in sore nipples
- Lactation device: bottle with enlarged nipple hole and 8 French feeding tube; run tube along breast and nipple such that baby nurses from breast and device simultaneously; tube should not pass end of nipple; bottle should not be higher than baby's head
- Breast milk jaundice: do not discontinue breast feeding
- Breast abscess or mastitis: treat with antibiotics (cover *Staph aureus*) and continue to breast feed unless incision and drainage required

Bottle Feeding

- Cow's-milk–based formulas ("Humanized") preferable
- Whole cow's milk not suitable for infants less than 9-12 mo; do not give 2% or skim milk before 12 mo
- Goat's milk must be pasteurized; not recommended for infants <9 mo of age
- Specific situations requiring supplementation

Goat's milk	Folate; Vitamins C, D, and A
Breast fed infants	Vitamin D (10 μg/day)
Breast- or bottle-fed infants at 6 mo (3-4 mo if premature) if no iron-fortified solids	Iron (iron fortified formula should be chosen once formula is initiated)
Water supply <0.3 ppm fluoride	Fluoride (Table 19-1)

TABLE 19-1 Daily Fluoride Supplement for Breast- and Formula-Fed Infants*

Fluoride Content of Drinking Water (ppm)	2 wk-2 yr	2-3 yr	3-16 yr
<0.3	0.25 mg	0.5 mg	1.0 mg
0.3-0.7	0	0.25 mg	0.5 mg
>0.7	0	0	0

*2.2 mg sodium fluoride contains 1 mg fluoride.
Modified from Canadian Pediatric Society Nutrition Committee Fluoride Supplementation. Contemp Pediatr 1987; 3(2):50-56.

Introduction of Solids

- Avoid raw vegetables, hot dogs, nuts, small candies, raw peas, and beans in children <3 yr due to risk of choking and aspiration
- Peanut butter should not be given alone (sticky bolus can compromise airway)
- Discourage bedtime bottle in crib to avoid Nursing Bottle Syndrome (tooth decay)

TABLE 19-2 Timing of Introduction of Various Food Groups

Age	Food	Comments
0-4 mo	Breast milk, formula	Will meet nutritive needs exclusively until 6 mo of age The solely breast fed infant may require a vitamin D supplement during winter months
3-6 mo	Iron-enriched cereal	Introduce rice cereal first (least allergenic) Delay gluten (i.e., wheat cereals) until 6 mo of age
4-7 mo	Puréed vegetables	Yellow-orange vegetables first, green last (more bulk). Do not give high nitrate–nitrite containing vegetables (beets, spinach, turnips) before 12 mo of age. Introduce vegetables before fruit (less chance of "sweet tooth")
6-9 mo	Puréed fruits and juices	Avoid "desserts" and fruit mixtures
6-9 mo	Puréed meats, fish, and poultry; egg yolk	Do not give egg white until 12 mo of age (risk of allergy)
9-12 mo	Finger foods, peeled fruit, cooked vegetables, cheese	Should be without added sugar, fat, salt, or seasonings. Introduce varied food texture and encourage chewing.

Vegetarian Diet

- High in bulk; low in calories, vitamin B_{12}, vitamin D, iron, and possibly protein
- Ca, Zn absorption may be impaired by phytates
- Dietitian's supervision advisable
- Not recommended for preschool children

Failure to Thrive

- Definition: weight <3rd percentile, or a fall in weight over two major percentile lines
- Broad categories
  1. Inadequate intake, persistent regurgitation or vomiting
  2. Inadequate absorption and assimilation
  3. Failure of utilization
  4. Increased metabolism

Investigations

- Careful history (including detailed diet history) and physical exam will be suggestive in >90% of organic FTT
- Determine ideal weight for height as follows: Ideal weight for height is the weight on the same percentile for age and gender as that for height, e.g., height on the 10th percentile, then ideal weight is on the 10th percentile. If height is <3rd percentile, use 3rd percentile weight as a guide.
- Dietary history and socioeconomic status
- CBC, ESR, electrolytes, BUN, creatinine, venous gas, Ca, PO_4, Mg, thyroid function tests, glucose, protein, albumin, Zn, PT, PTT
- Specific vitamin levels if indicated by history and physical findings
- Urine for pH, culture, specific gravity, metabolic screen, reducing substances

- Stool for microscopy (fat, white cells), occult blood. Consider ova and parasites; reducing substances; cultures, including *Giardia*.
- 3-5 day stool collection for fecal fat
- Sweat chloride
- Search for sepsis
- Anthropometry – weight, height, head circumference, skinfold thickness, midarm circumference
- Radiologic investigations may include bone age, skull x-ray, CXR, abdominal and head U/S
- Depending on clinical situation: immunoglobulins, chromosomes, liver function tests, HIV

Treatment

- Trial of high calorie formula or diet may be sufficient to achieve desirable weight gain
- May require hospital admission
- Rehydrate (if necessary) with oral electrolyte rehydration or maintenance solution; may require IV rehydration
- Treat infection, parasites

Diet

- Calories: 150-170 kcal/kg/day (↑ slowly).
- Protein and other nutrient needs are met if high energy formula is used.

Complications

- Diarrhea, infections, bleeding, hypothermia, hypoglycemia

Total Parenteral Nutrition

- TPN indicated when unable to meet nutrient needs via the enteral route
- In most instances, ordering standard TPN solutions at maintenance fluid rates provides adequate nutrient intake.
- To determine caloric requirements, rule of thumb: 1000 kcal + 100 kcal/yr of age, or refer to Table 19-3
- To start, volumes may be calculated based on protein requirement (see Table 19-3), increasing to 4 g/kg/day depending on age and clinical situation, and known protein concentration of selected standard TPN solutions
- Remainder of calories may be provided with lipid solution starting at 1 g/kg/day, and gradually increasing to 4 g/kg/day (N.B.: 10% lipid = 1 g/10 ml = 1.1 kcal/ml; 20% lipid = 2 g/10 ml = 2.0 kcal/ml)
- 20% lipid may be given by peripheral IV
- Special solutions (e.g., additional protein, carbohydrate, minerals, electrolytes) are available; generally mixed on individual basis depending on clinical situation
- For additional fluid requirements, ordinary dextrose and saline solutions should be used
- Must provide lipids to avoid essential fatty acid deficiency
- When weaning off TPN, decrease rate in a stepwise fashion over 1-2 hr to avoid hypoglycemia
- Certain IV drugs are not compatible with TPN. *Check with pharmacy.*
- Plan TPN in advance to allow adequate preparation

Carbohydrates

- May require 25-30% solutions under specific circumstances (e.g., fluid restriction)
- Glucose intolerance
  1. Decrease rate
  2. Decrease concentrations
  3. Rule out sepsis
  4. Rarely require insulin

TABLE 19-3 Summary Examples of

Age	Sex	Energy (kcal/kg/day)	Protein (g/kg/day)
Months			
0-2	Both	120-100	2.15
3-5	Both	100-95	1.46
6-8	Both	95-97	1.41
9-11	Both	97-99	1.37
Years			
1	Both	101	1.21
2-3	Both	94	1.16
4-6	Both	100	1.06
7-9	M	88	1.03
	F	76	1.03
10-12	M	73	1.01
	F	61	1.01
13-15	M	57	0.98
	F	46	0.95
16-18	M	51	0.93
	F	40	0.88
19-24	M	42	0.86
	F	36	0.86
Pregnancy (additional) (kcal/day) (g/day)			
First Trimester		100	5
Second Trimester		300	15
Third Trimester		300	24
Lactation (additional)		500	22

*Recommended Nutrient Intakes Health and Welfare,
†With the exception of energy, all recommended in subsisting on a variety of common foods available in
‡The figures for energy are estimates of average re- amounts are recommended: thiamin, 0.4 mg/1000 doxine, per gram of protein.

Recommended Nutrient Intakes for Canadians*†‡

Fat-Soluble Vitamins			Water-Soluble Vitamins		
Vitamin A (RE/day)	Vitamin D (μg/day)	Vitamin E (mg/day)	Vitamin C (mg/day)	Folate (μg/day)	Vitamin B$_{12}$ (μg/day)
400	10	3	20	50	0.3
400	10	3	20	50	0.3
400	10	3	20	50	0.3
400	10	3	20	50	0.3
400	10	3	20	65	0.3
400	5	4	20	80	0.4
500	5	5	25	90	0.5
700	2.5	7	25	125	0.8
700	2.5	6	25	125	0.8
800	2.5	8	25	170	1.0
800	5	7	25	180	1.0
900	5	9	30	150	1.5
800	5	7	30	145	1.5
1000	5	10	40	185	1.9
800	2.5	7	30	160	1.9
1000	2.5	10	40	210	2.0
800	2.5	7	30	175	2.0
100	2.5	2	0	300	1.0
100	2.5	2	10	300	1.0
100	2.5	2	10	300	1.0
400	2.5	3	25	100	0.5

Canada: 1990.
takes are designed to cover individual variations in essentially all of a healthy population Canada.
quirements for expected patterns of activity. For nutrients not shown, the following kcal; riboflavin, 0.5 mg/1000 kcal; niacin, 7.2 NE/1000 kcal; vitamin B$_6$, 15 μg, as pyri-

TABLE 19-3 Summary Examples of Recommended Nutrient Intakes

		Minerals		
Age	Sex	Calcium (mg/day)	Phosphorus (mg/day)	Magnesium (mg/day)
Months				
0-2	Both	250	150	20
3-5	Both	250	150	20
6-8	Both	400	200	32
9-11	Both	400	200	32
Years				
1	Both	500	300	40
2-3	Both	550	350	50
4-6	Both	600	400	65
7-9	M	700	500	1008
	F	700	500	100
10-12	M	900	700	130
	F	1100	800	135
13-15	M	1100	900	185
	F	1000	850	180
16-18	M	900	1000	230
	F	700	850	200
19-24	M	800	1000	240
	F	700	850	200
Pregnancy (additional) (kcal/day) (g/day)				
First Trimester		500	200	15
Second Trimester		500	200	45
Third Trimester		500	200	45
Lactation (additional)		500	200	65

for Canadians*†‡ (Cont'd)

Minerals (cont'd)

Iron (mg/day)	Iodine (μg/day)	Zinc (mg/day)
0.3	30	2
0.3	30	2
7	40	3
7	40	3
6	55	4
6	65	4
8	85	5
8	110	7
8	95	7
8	125	9
8	110	9
10	160	12
13	160	9
10	160	12
12	160	9
9	160	12
13	160	9
0	25	6
5	25	6
10	25	6
50	6	

Lipids

- Relative contraindications
  1. Neonatal indirect hyperbilirubinemia (free fatty acids compete for binding on albumin)
  2. Thrombocytopenia (may interfere with platelet function)
  3. Respiratory distress (may interfere with gas exchange)
  4. Sepsis (may develop lipid intolerance): withhold lipid for 24 hr

Electrolytes, Vitamins and Minerals

- Requirements vary with age and disease
- Ca, P, Mg, Zn, Cu, Mn, Cr, I, and Se must be present in TPN. For special TPN, new orders must be filled out.
- Iron must be included except for in premature infants <1 mo
- Multivitamins must be supplemented.

Monitoring

- Fluid balance
- Daily urine glucose
- CBC, BUN, P, Ca, Mg, albumin, bilirubin, LFTs and creatinine (baseline and weekly determinations)
- Electrolytes, glucose (baseline and twice weekly)
- Lipid levels twice weekly and with sepsis and solution change; generally keep <1g/L.
- Growth parameters

Complications

- Catheter: thrombosis, infection, leakage, uncoupling, dislodgement, extravasation
- Metabolic: hyperglycemia, hypoglycemia, aminoaciduria, aminoacidemia, electrolyte imbalance, cholestasis (see p 226)
- Infection: thrombophlebitis, bacteremia, fungemia

Indications for Central Venous Line

- Unable to meet requirements through peripheral TPN
- TPN >2 wk (variable)
- Venous access difficulty
- Osmolality of solution (>12.5% glucose solution)

TABLE 19-4 Composition of VAMIN-N Based Standard Solutions (per L)*†

	Premature Infants				Infants, Children, and Adolescents			Fluid Restricted Patients
	P-5	P-7.5	P-10	PI-10	I-10	I-20‡	C-30
Protein (g)	15.0	15.0	20.0	20.0	30.0	30.0	50
Glucose (g)	50.0	75.0	100.0	100.0	100.0	200.0	300.0
Energy (kcal)§	248.0	340.0	455.0	455.0	495.0	870.0	1320.0
Na (mmol)	20.0	20.0	14.3	30.0	30.0	30.0	30.0
K (mmol)	20.0	20.0	18.9	30.0	30.0	30.0	30.0
Cl (mmol)	21.1	21.1	15.7	31.3	32.1	32.1	32.1
Ca (mmol)	9.0	9.0	9.0	9.0	9.0	9.0	9.0
P (mmol)	9.0	9.0	9.0	9.0	9.0	9.0	9.0
Mg (mmol)	3.0	3.0	4.0	4.0	4.0	4.0	4.0
Zn (µmol)	46.0	46.0	46.0	46.0	46.0	46.0	46.0
Cu (µmol)	6.3	6.3	6.3	6.3	6.3	6.3	6.3
Mn (µmol)	1.8	1.8	1.8	1.8	5.0	5.0	5.0
I (µmol)	0.47	0.47	0.47	0.47	0.47	0.47	0.47
Cr (µmol)	0.076	0.076	0.076	0.076	0.076	0.076	0.076
Se (µmol)	0.25	0.25	0.25	0.25	0.25	0.25	0.25
Fe (µmol)#	—	—	—	—	18.0	18.0	18.0

*Modified from Guidelines for total parenteral nutrition. Toronto: The Hospital for Sick Children, 1986.
Fat emulsion, 10%—1100 kcal/L, 100 g fat/L, 47 g linoleic acid/L (1.1 kcal/ml).
Fat emulsion, 20%—2200 kcal/L (2.2 kcal/mL).
†"P" solutions are standard for premature infants who are not fluid restricted. "I" solutions are for premature infants who are fluid restricted and for children and infants.
‡I-20 is intended for central venous line therapy only.
§Energy unit: 1 kcal = 4.2 kJ. The energy content includes the potential energy from the protein as well as that from the glucose.
#Iron can be included in the "P" solutions in neonates who have been receiving TPN for 1 mo or more and should therefore be ordered.

Enteral Nutrition

- No more than 4-8 hr supply of enteral feeds should be hung at one time to prevent bacterial contamination
- Although nasoenteric feeding has been successfully used for up to 18 mo, tube enterostomy is usually indicated if long-term enteral feeding is anticipated
- Discontinue tube feeding when oral intake improves to ⅔-¾ of estimated caloric and protein requirements
- Symptoms of intolerance include abdominal distension, cramping, nausea, vomiting, diarrhea, constipation

Intermittent Feeding
- Gravity flow over 30-45 min (minimum q3-6h; more physiologic but higher risk of aspiration; rarely used for direct intestinal feeds (boluses poorly tolerated)

Continuous Feeding
- Continuous via pump; better for direct intestinal feeds; overall decreased risk of gastroesophageal reflux and aspiration but overnight feeds should be avoided in those <1 yr

Tubes
- Nasoenteric: 5- to 6-French for small infants; 6- to 8-French for older children and adolescents
- Silicone or polyurethane: flexible; guidewire for insertion, replace q2-4 wk. Polyvinylchloride: stiffer; replace q4-7 days due to risk of intestinal perforation.
- Enterostomy: 12- to 18-French; available as rubber catheter with mushroom tip (replace q1.5 yr), silicone catheter with inflatable balloon tip (replace q6-8 mo), or silicone catheter with external "button" device.

Choice of Formula
- <1 yr of age: expressed breast milk, or commercial infant formula if breast milk unavailable
- >1 yr of age: Pediasure for 1-6 yrs of age, or see Table 19-5. For normal digestive and absorptive capacities, use protein isolate formula (e.g., Isosource, Isocal, Osmolite, Pediasure). For impaired pancreaticobiliary function, small bowel obstruction, or direct delivery into small intestine use an "elemental" formula (e.g., Pregestimil, Tolerex, Vital).

Increasing the Energy Content of Formulas
- Concentrate the formula in stepwise fashion to 1 kcal/ml (max 4 g protein/kg); increased intestinal osmolality and renal solute load.
- Add fat (corn oil, microlipid, MCT oil) or CHO (glucose polymers such as Caloreen and Polycose)
- Protein supplements rarely indicated
- Energy Content of Formulas:

Kilojoules/liter	Kilocalories/100 ml	Kilocalories/ounce
2800	68	20
3300	80	24
3800	90	27
4200	100	30
4600	110	33

1 kJ = 4.2 kcal

TABLE 19-5 Composition of Milks and Formulas per

	Energy (kcal)†	Protein (g)	Protein Type	CHO (g)	CHO Type
Milks					
Human, mature	720	11	Lactalbumin, casein	72	Lactose
Cow's, whole	636	32	Lactalbumin, casein	48	Lactose
Cow's, 2%	512	36	Lactalbumin, casein	48	Lactose
Cow's skimmed	360	36	Lactalbumin, casein	52	Lactose
Goat's, whole	712	36	Lactalbumin, casein	44	Lactose
Human Milk Fortifier					
Similac Natural Care	680	22	Whey, skim milk	86	Lactose, glucose polymers
Milk-based formulas					
Alactamil	670	15	Skim milk	69	Corn syrup solids
Enfalac/Enfalac with iron	680	15	Whey, skim milk	69	Lactose
SMA/SMA with iron	680	15	Skim milk, whey	72	Lactose
Good Start	670	16	Whey	74	Glucose polymers, lactose
Similac/Similac with iron	680	15	Skim milk	72	Lactose
Unilac	680	16	Skim milk	70	Lactose
Soy-based formulas					
Isomil	680	18	Soy	68	Glucose polymers, sucrose
ProSobee	670	20	Soy	68	Glucose polymers
Premature infant formulas—for premature infants weighing <2000 g					
Enfalac premature					
20 kcal/oz	680	20	Whey, skim milk	74	Glucose polymers, lactose
24 kcal/oz	805	24		89	
Similac special care					
20 kcal/oz	680	18	Skim milk, whey	72	Glucose polymers, lactose
24 kcal/oz	810	22		86	
SMA "Preemie"					
20 kcal/oz	675	20	Skim milk, whey	70	Glucose polymers, lactose
24 kcal/oz	810	20		86	
Special formulas					
Lamb base-for multiple intolerances	808	23	Lamb	82	Glucose polymers
Lofenalac (low phenylalanine—for PKU)¶	677	22	Hydrolyzed casein	88	Glucose polymers

*Owing to changes in formulation, all data are subject to change. The most current
†1 kcal = 4.2 kJ. Renal solute load can be estimated using the following formula: renal
‡Without iron/with iron.
¶Following instructions on the label will create a 1000 kcal/L formula with a different
MCT = medium chain triglycerides; tr = trace.

Liter Normal Dilution

Fat (g)	Type	Ca (mg)	P (mg)	Vit D (μg)	Fe (mg)	Na (mmol)	Cl (mmol)	K (mmol)	Osmolality (mOsm/kg H$_2$O)
39	Human butterfat	280	140	0.6	tr	8	12	13	290
36	Butterfat	1230	930	9	tr	22	27	40	315
20	Butterfat	1260	950	9	tr	22	28	41	315
44	Butterfat	1270	950	9	tr	23	29	44	N/A
44	Butterfat	1380	1110	0.6	tr	22	37	54	N/A
44	MCT (50%) soy, coconut oils	1700	850	30	3.0	17	20	29	300
37	Coconut, soy oils	550	420	10	12	8	13	19	165
38	Coconut, soy oils	500	330	10	1/13‡	8	12	18	300
36	Beef, coconut, safflower, soy oils	420	280	10	2/12‡	7	11	14	300
34	Palm, safflower, coconut oils	430	240	10	10	7	11	17	235
36	Soy, coconut oils	520	390	10	2/12‡	10	14	17	290
36	Soy, coconut oils	550	375	10	2	10	19	24	301
37	Soy, coconut oils	700	500	10	12	13	15	18	250
36	Coconut, soy oils	630	500	10	13	13	14	20	200
34	Soy, MCT (40%) coconut oils	1100	550	11	2	12	16	17	240
41		1320	660	13	2	14	19	20	280
37	MCT (50%)	1100	600	11	3	13	15	21	250
44	Soy, coconut oils	1320	720	13	3	15	18	26	300
35	Beef, coconut, safflower, soy, MCT (12.5%) oils	750	380	13	3	14	15	19	268
44		750	400	13	3	14	15	19	280
44	Corn oil and lamb	839	320	N/A	2	18	15	25	214
26	Corn oil	630	480	11	13	14	13	18	360

composition is found on the product label.
solute load (mmol/L) = 4 × protein (g/L) + Na (mmol/L) + K (mmol/L) + Cl (mmol/L).

composition.

Continued.

TABLE 19-5 Composition of Milks and Formulas per

	Energy (kcal)†	Protein (g)	Protein Type	CHO (g)	CHO Type
Alimentum—for fat and protein malabsorbtion or protein intolerance	676	19	Hydrolyzed casein	69	Sucrose, glucose polymers
Nutramigen—for intolerance to intact protein	670	19	Hydrolyzed casein	91	Glucose polymers
Portagen¶—for fat malabsorption	680	24	Casein	78	Glucose polymers, sucrose
Pregestimil—for fat and protein malabsorbtion or intolerance to intact protein	670	19	Hydrolyzed casein	91	Glucose polymers
RCF (carbohydrate free)—for carbohydrate intolerance	405	20	Soy	0	
Similac PM 60/40	680	15	Whey, caseinates	69	Lactose
Complete enteral feedings					
Enrich (with fiber)—for constipation	1100	40	Casein, soy	163	Glucose polymers, sucrose, soy polysaccharides
Ensure—oral supplement or tube feeding	1060	37	Casein, soy	145	Glucose polymers, sucrose
Ensure Plus—high calorie oral supplement	1500	55	Casein, soy	201	Glucose polymers, sucrose
Isosource—standard tube feeding	1060	34	Casein, soy	133	Glucose polymers
Pediasure—oral supplement in tube feeding for children 1-6 yr old	1000	30	Whey, casein	110	Glucose polymers, sucrose
Complete "defined" feedings—low residue, lactose-free feeding, requiring minimal					
Vital high nitrogen	1000	42	Hydrolyzed whey, meat, soy; amino acids	186	Glucose polymers, sucrose
Tolerex	1000	21	Amino acids	227	Glucose polymers
Incomplete feedings					
Citrotein (supplement suitable as a clear fluid)	660	41	Egg white	122	Sucrose, glucose polymers
Modular components—for increasing calories or protein in formulas and feedings					
Carbohydrate (per 100 g)					
Polycose powder	380	0	—	94	Glucose
Fat (per 100 ml)					
Corn oil	810	0	—	0	—
MCT	765	0	—	0	—
Microlipid	450	0	—	0	—
Protein (per 100 g)					
Promod	424	76	Whey	<10	Lactose

Liter Normal Dilution (Cont'd)

(g)	Fat Type	Ca (mg)	P (mg)	Vit D (μg)	Fe (mg)	Na (mmol)	Cl (mmol)	K (mmol)	Osmolality (mOsm/kg H$_2$O)
38	MCT (50%) safflower oil	710	510	10	12	13	15	21	370
26	Soy and Corn oils	630	420	9	12	14	16	19	320
33	MCT (85%), corn oil	630	480	5	13	14	16	22	220
26	Corn, MCT (42%) oil	630	420	11	13	14	16	19	350
36	Soy, coconut oils	700	500	10	2	13	12	19	64
38	Corn, coconut oils	380	190	10	2	7	11	15	260
38	Corn oil	720	720	7	13	37	41	40	480
37	Corn oil	500	500	5	10	30	31	31	450
54	Corn oil	600	600	4	14	48	45	49	600
44	Soy, MCT (21%) oils	640	530	5	9	23	30	34	300
50	Safflower, soy, MCT (20%) oils	970	800	9	14	16	28	33	310
digestion and absorption									
11	Safflower, MCT (45%) oils	670	670	7	12	20	25	34	460
2	Safflower oil	556	556	6	10	20	27	30	550
2	Soy oil	1020	1020	7	16	30	26	18	495
0	—	≤30	≤5	0	0	≤5	≤6	tr	N/A
92	Corn oil	0	0	0	0	0	0	0	0
93	Modified coconut oil	0	0	0	0	0	0	0	0
50	Safflower oil	0	0	0	0	0	0	0	80
<9		<670	<500	0	0	≤10	≤1	≤25	N/A

Obesity

- Definition: >120% of ideal weight for height
- Majority are primary. Secondary causes include endocrine, some genetic syndromes (Prader-Willi, Laurence-Moon-Biedl). Most endocrine abnormalities are *secondary* to obesity.
- History: caloric intake, activity, medications (e.g., steroids), psychosocial
- Investigations:
  1. thyroid function tests
  2. fasting blood glucose, HbA1c
  3. ±lipid profile
  4. ±pituitary function (GH, FSH, LH), adrenal tests (cortisol, 17-OH progesterone)
  5. ±chromosomes
- Follow clinically blood pressure, skin (intertrigo), pubertal development, hips (↑ risk of slipped capital femoral epiphysis), menstrual function, blood lipids, glucose tolerance

Management

- Dietary mainstay: involve dietician, family
- Treat underlying cause if secondary—still requires above monitoring

TWENTY

Ophthalmology

Routine Procedures and Screening

PERINATAL

- Ophthalmia neonatorum prophylaxis consists of erythromycin ointment, tetracycline ointment, or silver nitrate 1% drops to both eyes in the immediate perinatal period. N.B.: *Chlamydia* conjunctivitis and gonococcal conjunctivitis may occur despite prophylaxis.

PREMATURE NEONATES

- Neonates <1500 g and/or <32 wk gestation should have first retinal examination at 4-6 wk postpartum. Neonates >1500 g or >32 wk exposed to high doses or long-term oxygen are also at increased risk.

INFANT (<1 yr)

- All newborns and older infants should have periodic external eye exam for anatomic eye defects, ocular movements, ocular alignment (after 4 mo), ocular inflammation, and the ability of each eye individually to fixate on and follow colored objects at close range. Infants should be able to fixate on the face of the caretaker while feeding. Assessment of the red reflex by ophthalmoscopy should be performed at each routine postnatal visit.

1-5 YR

- In general, all children should be seen by an ophthalmologist by 3 yr of age, or earlier if there are systemic risk factors or a family history of ocular disease or visual symptoms. Another routine ophthalmologic examination should be scheduled at age 5-6 yr. Thereafter, visual acuity screening by letter, picture, or E game chart should be conducted by the primary care physician or school yearly until 10 yr of age, after which screening should continue every 2-3 yr.

Basic Principles

- A useful tip in examining the neonate's eyes is to hold the baby in the upright position for reflex eye opening.
- When a patient has glasses, visual acuity should be tested when the patient is wearing the glasses.
- Abnormal vision corrected by viewing through a pinhole indicates a need for glasses as opposed to trauma or ocular pathology—a useful test on the patients who have no glasses or have not brought their glasses to the examination. With glasses on, an improvement of vision through a pinhole indicates the need for recheck of the glasses prescription.
- Amblyopia refers to subnormal vision in an eye, not caused by internal eye disease. It may or may not be associated with strabismus. Amblyopia can be unilateral or bilateral.
- The only contraindication to using a drop of topical anesthetic (proparacaine or tetracaine) is the suspicion of a ruptured globe. A lid speculum may facilitate examination. Similarly, if a ruptured globe has been ruled out, there is virtually no contraindication to dilating the pupils for maximum visibility on fundoscopic examination. If there is a concern about impaired pupillary reactivity for neurologic assessment, use short-acting mydriatics (phenylephrine 2.5%, cyclopentolate 1% or tropicamide 1%).

- The direct ophthalmoscope may be used as a hand-held illuminated magnifier to view the ocular surface and iris by dialing in the higher black numbers as one gets closer to the patient
- Ophthalmology consultation is recommended in all cases of decreased visual acuity (poor fixation of an eye during the preverbal years, <20/40 (6/12) in the verbal preschool child, <20/20 (6/6) in the school-aged child).
- Topical steroids, topical atropine or homatropine, topical miotics, glaucoma treatments, or topical antivirals should not be used without ophthalmologic consultation.
- Topical sodium cromoglycate should not be used as acute treatment of conjunctivitis; only indicated as chronic prophylaxis for confirmed allergic conjunctivitis.

Eyelids

HORDEOLUM (STYE) AND CHALAZION:

- Obstruction of the eyelid glands, on eyelid margin (stye) or within body of lid (chalazion). Stye may have discharge. Chalazion may be chronic mobile lump. Treatment: warm compresses, baby shampoo eyelash scrubs, erythromycin or polysporin ointment. Refer if nonresolving chronic chalazion.

TRAUMA

- May result in ptosis, ecchymosis, edema, or laceration. Upper lid eversion and complete dilated eye examination should be performed to rule out injury to the globe or foreign body. Opthalmologic consultation required for ptosis that persists after ecchymosis and swelling have resolved; laceration of eyelid margin or canthus; deep lacerations with or without ptosis.
- Ptosis (drooping of an upper eyelid) can be unilateral or bilateral, congenital or acquired. It can be an isolated abnormality or associated with a neurologic or orbital disease. Severe ptosis can cause amblyopia in young children.

Nasolacrimal Duct Obstruction

- Generally due to congenital failure of complete canalization of lower end of nasolacrimal duct. Recurrent mild discharge and tearing without conjunctival injection; worse in morning, outdoors, and during respiratory infection.

Treatment
- Massage skin downwards from medial aspect of eye, along side of nose, several times per day. Administer 1-wk courses of antibiotic drops during periods of increased discharge. Majority of cases resolve spontaneously by 6-9 mo; otherwise, refer.

Conjunctivae

- Neonatal conjunctivitis
  1. Chemical: purulent conjunctivitis, lid edema. Occurs in first 24 hr following instillation of silver nitrate prophylaxis. Treatment involves frequent saline lavage and erythromycin or polysporin ointment.
  2. *N. gonorrhea* purulent conjunctivitis, lid edema. This is a vision-threatening emergency. Usually occurs in first week of life but may occur any time in first few months. Gram stain shows intracellular gram-negative diplococci. Must have culture confirmation to rule out nonpathogenic diplococci but begin treatment based on Gram stain. Requires IV course of penicillin or ceftriaxone in addition to topical treatment with erythromycin or polysporin. Frequent ocular lavage with normal saline may be beneficial.
  3. Chlamydia: milder conjunctivitis, less discharge and edema. Usually occurs in first or second week of life but chronic carriage with delayed symptoms may occur. Culture should be performed but immunofluorescent or ELISA procedures on eye swab are acceptable. Gram stain and cultures are negative. Giemsa stain of conjunctival scrapings. Consider presence of chlamydia pneumonia. If neonate is well, treat with oral erythromycin 40-50 mg/kg/day for 14-21 days, in addition to topical erythromycin. Treat parents for genitourinary *Chlamydia*.
  4. Other: conjunctivitis may be caused by various other bacteria and viruses in the neonatal period. Herpetic keratoconjunctivitis is diagnosed with dendritic ulcer on fluorescein stain, and should be referred to ophthalmology. Hemophilus conjunctivitis requires topical and systemic antibiotics. Other bacteria should be treated with appropriate antibiotics.
- Conjunctivitis beyond the neonatal period (see Table 20-1)

TABLE 20-1 Differential Diagnosis of Conjunctivitis

	Bacterial	Viral (nonherpes)	Herpetic	Chlamydial	Allergic
Discharge	Purulent	Clear or mildly purulent	Clear	Purulent	Clear or mucus
Lid swelling	Moderate to severe	Mild to severe	Mild	Mild	Mild to severe
Onset	Acute	Subacute	Acute	Acute or chronic	Acute
Injection	Severe	Moderate to severe	Moderate	Moderate to severe	Mild to severe
Cornea fluorescein staining	Nonspecific	Nonspecific	Dendrite	Nonspecific	None
White corneal infiltrates	—	—	Possible	Multiple peripheral	Rare
Unilateral/bilateral	Uni/bi	Uni/bi	Uni	Bi	Bi
Contact history	Common; STD	Common	Rare	Common; STD	Rare
Preauricular node	Common	Common	Common	Occasional	None
Other associations	Otitis media	Otitis media	Skin lesions	Genital	Chemosis

STD = sexually transmitted disease symptoms or contact.

Ophthalmology

- Subconjunctival hemorrhage: caused by blunt trauma, Valsalva maneuver, forceful cough, bleeding diathesis, severe hypertension. Infants, young children with large (180°-360°) hemorrhages should have full ocular examination to search for nontraumatic causes. Treatment is generally limited to artificial tears for comfort. Blood resorbs over 7-14 days.
- Chemosis: blister-like swelling of the conjunctivae due to conjunctival inflammation, allergy, generalized systemic edema, or venous obstruction (e.g., cavernous sinus thrombosis). Treatment: artificial tear ointments to avoid dessication.
- Burns
  1. Thermal, electrical: most often epithelium only; can be highlighted by fluorescein staining. May require ophthalmologic consultation but can usually be treated as corneal abrasion.
  2. Chemical: copious lavage (5% dextrose with or without saline) is essential. Use 2 L over 20 min (early management at home: tap water or shower). Topical anesthetic prelavage if readily available. Monitor pH of affected eye if prelavage pH testing is available. Lavage should continue until pH is equal to that of the nonaffected eye. Upper lid eversion and, if required, eyelid speculum and restraint or sedation for optimal lavage. After lavage, treat as corneal abrasion. *All alkali or acid burns require urgent ophthalmologic consultation.*

Cornea

- Foreign body: lies on or may be embedded in cornea. Diagnosis by examination with good light and magnification, and fluorescein staining. High-velocity foreign bodies require ophthalmologic consultation and radiologic investigation even with minimal external evidence of injury to rule out penetration into eye. Ophthalmologic consultation generally recommended; after removal, patient is treated as for corneal abrasion.

- Abrasion: an area of absent corneal epithelium. Symptoms are pain and photophobia relieved by topical anesthetic (proparacaine or tetracaine). Corneal fluorescein stain shows area of absent epithelium. If vertical linear abrasion, suspect conjunctival foreign body under upper lid and perform lid eversion, facilitated by having patient look down during procedure. Treat with polysporin or erythromycin ointment plus cycloplegic agent (cyclopentalate 1%); patch affected eye for 24 hr. Refer if still symptomatic after 24 hr.
- Lacerations or ruptured globe: *Requires urgent ophthalmologic consultation.* May be caused by blunt trauma as well as penetration by sharp objects. Clinical features are oval pupil, hyphema, iris prolapsing through cornea, brownish tissue protruding from sclera, 360° subconjunctival hemorrhage, or chemosis. Eyelid edema may prevent adequate exam; high index of suspicion on history alone. When diagnosis is suspected, *stop eye examination immediately.* Shield eye so that there is *no pressure* on the eye. DO NOT PATCH OR INSTILL EYEDROPS.
- Enlarged or "cloudy" cornea may indicate glaucoma or systemic disease; refer promptly.

Anterior Chamber

- Hyphema: blood in anterior chamber (behind cornea and in front of iris). Almost always a sign of severe ocular trauma. Requires urgent ophthalmologic consultation. Treatments include bedrest, shielding, oral antifibrinolytics, topical steroids, and cycloplegics, and occasionally, topical steroids and oral antifibrinolytics. Recurrent hemorrhage and secondary glaucoma may occur.
- Iritis: inflammation in the aqueous humor. Causes include trauma, collagen vascular disease, sarcoid, Lyme disease, leukemia, retinoblastoma, intraocular infection. Iritis may be acute or chronic, and asymptomatic, as in some forms of juvenile arthritis. On inspection, a ring of conjunctival injection behind the edge of the corneal scleral junction may represent the ciliary flush of iritis but slit-

lamp examination is required for diagnosis. Traumatic iritis may be delayed 24-48 hr following trauma. Treatment: topical cycloplegics and steroids after ophthalmologic consultation. Periocular injections, oral, or IV steroids may be needed in severe cases.
- Hypopyon: collection of white cells in anterior chamber. Causes include internal infection, tumors, or severe inflammation; refer promptly.

Pupils and Iris

- Relative afferent pupil defect (RAPD) or Marcus-Gunn pupil: diagnosed by swinging flashlight test. It indicates visual pathway pathology anterior to optic chiasm (vitreous, retina, optic disc, optic nerve) and requires thorough ophthalmic and neurologic assessments.
- Anisocoria: may be difficult to ascertain which pupil is abnormal. Each pupil should be examined for reactivity. A nonreactive pupil is abnormal but if both react briskly, examine the size of the pupils under very dim and bright illumination. If anisocoria is worse in the dark, then the smaller pupil is the abnormal one (Horner syndrome, from sympathetic denervation, or scarring following intraocular inflammation). If anisocoria is enhanced by bright illumination, then the larger eye is abnormal (third nerve palsy, traumatic mydriasis or "tonic pupil"). Most common cause is physiologic anisocoria, which occurs in 20% of the population. In this case, the relative difference in pupil size will be equal in light or dim illumination.
- Coloboma: Notch in pupil or iris. May be associated with eye problems that may preclude normal vision.
- Leukocoria (white pupil reflex): for diagnosis, the examiner should use a direct ophthalmoscope set on a black number between 5 and 10 while sitting in front of the patient at a distance that allows both eyes of the patient to be viewed in focus simultaneously. Generally requires ophthalmologic consultation. Causes can be congenital (e.g., cataract) or acquired (e.g., tumor).

Retina

- Retinal hemorrhages: may be caused by birth, vasculitis, meningitis, cyanotic congenital heart disease, endocarditis, sepsis, blood dyscrasias, head trauma. Sickle cell disease and diabetes do not cause retinal hemorrhages in young children. If above ruled out, retinal hemorrhage beyond 6 wk of age or flame hemorrhages beyond 1 wk of age are suggestive of Shaken Baby Syndrome or other forms of child abuse. Flame-shaped hemorrhages are superficial and transient; intraretinal hemorrhages are dot- or blot-shaped; preretinal hemorrhages may have fluid-blood level and obscure the blood vessels. Hemorrhage may also occur into the vitreous gel. Ophthalmologic consultation is generally required.
- Intraocular candidiasis: appears as fluffy white intraretinal, preretinal, or vitreous opacities. Always accompanied by *Candida* isolated from systemic site. Treatment: IV amphotericin.

Optic Nerve

- Papilledema and papillitis: may look similar on clinical examination. Vision preserved in papilledema, decreased in papillitis. Bilateral papilledema usually due to increased intracranial pressure; papillitis may be due to vasculitis. Optic nerve infiltration with neoplastic cells (e.g., leukemia) is main differential diagnosis. On examination, optic disc is elevated with indistinct margins, peripapillary exudates, and hemorrhages (usually flame-shaped) on or around the disc. Retinal veins may be dilated and tortuous. Presence of spontaneous venous pulsations does not rule out diagnosis. Treatment depends on underlying cause.

- Optic atrophy: Can be congenital or acquired. It requires thorough ophthalmic and neurologic investigations.
- Optic nerve hypoplasia: A congenital anomaly with varying degrees of severity. Mild forms may be compatible with good vision. Most cases are unilateral; bilateral cases require neurologic assessment because of association with CNS abnormalities such as septo-optic dysplasia.

Strabismus

- Abnormal eye alignment (Figs. 20-1 and 20-2): should refer by 4 mo of age. Esotropia most common; exotropia or hypertropia may be suggestive of more serious underlying orbit or neurologic problem. Alignment can be assessed by cover test (Fig. 20-1) or Hirschberg (light reflex) test (Fig. 20-2). Strabismus may cause amblyopia in the eye that is misaligned, but in many cases the eyes retain equal vision despite the strabismus.
- Blow-out fracture: results from blunt trauma pushing eye into socket and causing one or more of the bones of the orbital wall to fracture. Fractures involving inferior or medial wall are most common. Clinically, a restriction of eye movement may occur in the direction away from the fractured orbital wall (e.g., impaired upward gaze following inferior wall fracture). The eye may appear sunken (inferior wall) or proptotic (superior wall); hypoesthesia of the inferior orbital skin may occur in inferior wall fracture. CT scan with coronal views for diagnosis; may be deferred for 1-3 wk as most eye movement restrictions will resolve spontaneously. Ophthalmologic consultation is required. Surgical intervention for severe enophthalmos, orbital roof fracture, failure of conservative management.

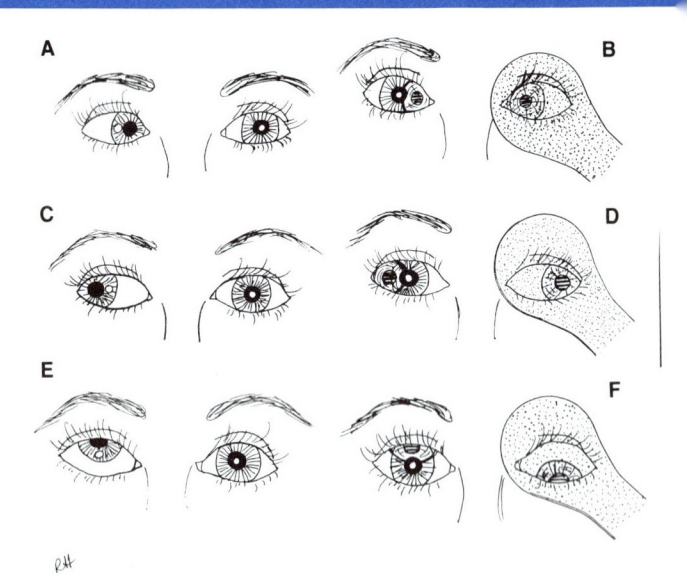

Figure 20-1 Cover-uncover test for tropia. While patient fixates a target (A), the fixating eye is covered and the other eye is observed. If the uncovered eye moves laterally to pick up fixation (B), the patient has an esotropia in that eye. If the uncovered eye moves medially to pick up fixation, then the patient has an exotropia (C and D). Similarly, if the uncovered eye moves downward, hypertropia can be demonstrated (E and F). Upward movement of the uncovered eye would indicate hypotropia. No movement implies that the patient is fixating with that eye but may also mean that severe refractive error or amblyopia is preventing vision in that eye.

Ophthalmology

A

B

0°

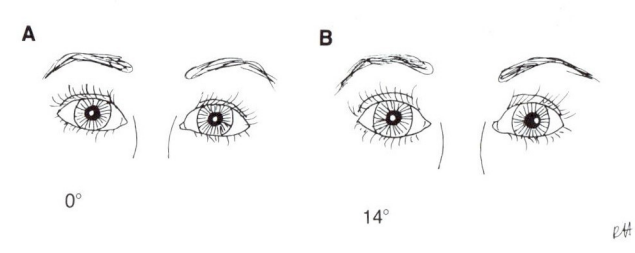

14°

Figure 20-2 **Hirschberg test.** The light reflection on the corneas is observed. Each millimeter the light reflex is located off the center of the cornea represents approximately 7° of deviation. (*A*) Normal; (*B*) Left Esotropia 14°.

TWENTY-ONE

Orthopedics

Lower Limb

INTOEING (Fig. 21-1)

- Establish torsional profile (Fig. 21-2)
  1. Foot progression angle
  2. Measure thigh–foot angle
  3. Measure range of internal and external rotation at the hip
  4. Measure degree of metatarsus varus
- Establish coordination profile
  1. Jumping by age 2 yr
  2. Hopping by age 4 yr

Differential Diagnosis
- Metatarsus varus
- Internal tibial torsion—thigh–foot angle $<-10°$
- Internal femoral torsion—external rotation of hip $<20°$

Management

- Metatarsus varus: neonate: if flexible, observe 3-9 mo; if rigid, refer to orthopedic surgery for casts, Wheaton splints or articulated boot. 9 mo-2 yr: ignore. >2 yr: surgical correction
- Internal tibial torsion: 9-18 mo: observe, rarely consider Denis-Browne night splints × 3-4 mo, or counter-rotation splints
- Internal femoral torsion: splints and shoes ineffective. Correct sitting habits (encourage lotus position); if severe, consider osteotomy at 10 yr for *exceptional* cases.

infants
Metatarsus varus

toddlers
Internal tibial torsion

kindergarten
Internal femoral torsion

normal gait angle is + 10°

EXAMINATION

1

Assess
Gait
Angle

This example shows —30°

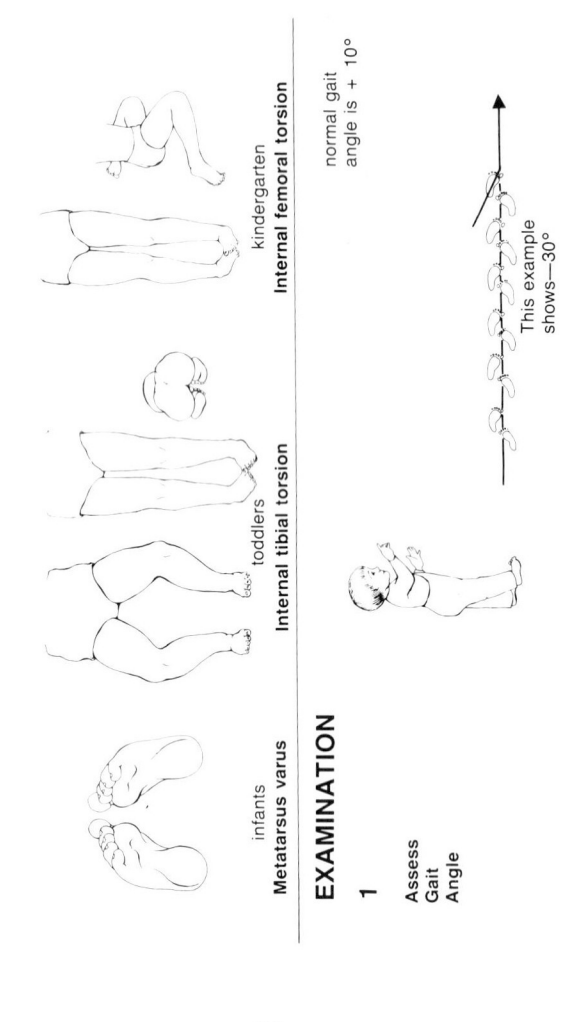

426

2 Assess Thigh Foot Angle

0°–30° ER. metatarsus 10° I.R.
is normal varus = internal tibial torsion

3 Assess Hip Rotation

45°IR 30°ER Normal

90° IR 10° ER internal femoral torsion

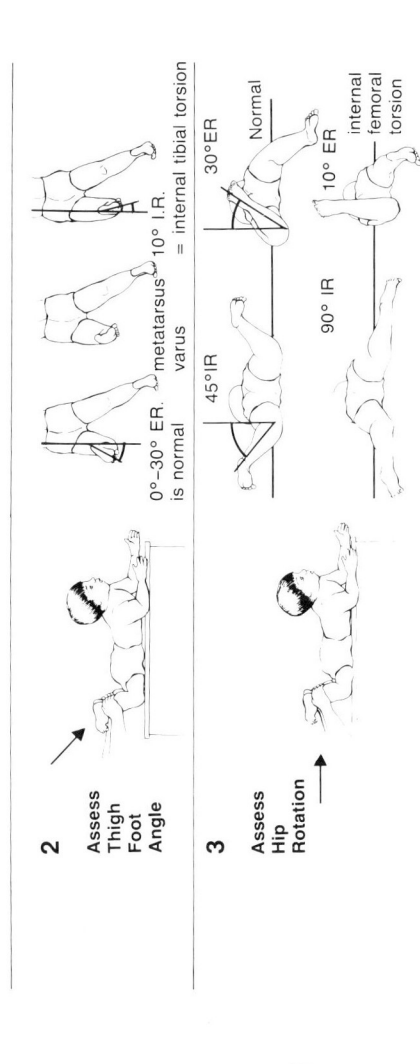

Figure 21-1 **Intoeing varieties.** (From The Easter Seal guide to children's orthopaedics—prevention, screening, and problem solving. Ontario: The Easter Seal Society, 1982.)

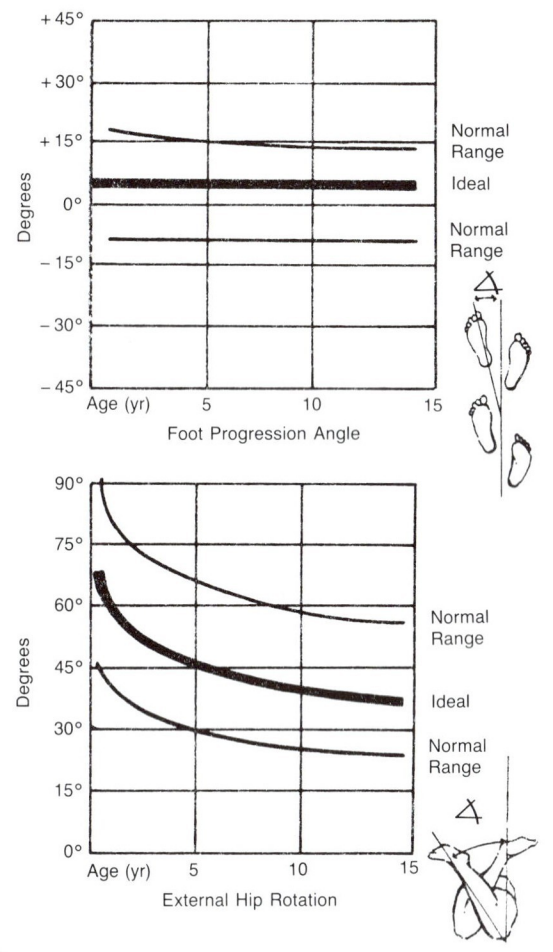

Figure 21-2 **Torsional profile.** (Data based on Staheli LT, et al. Lower extremity-rotational problems in children. Normal values to guide management. J Bone Joint Surg 1985;67A:39-47.)

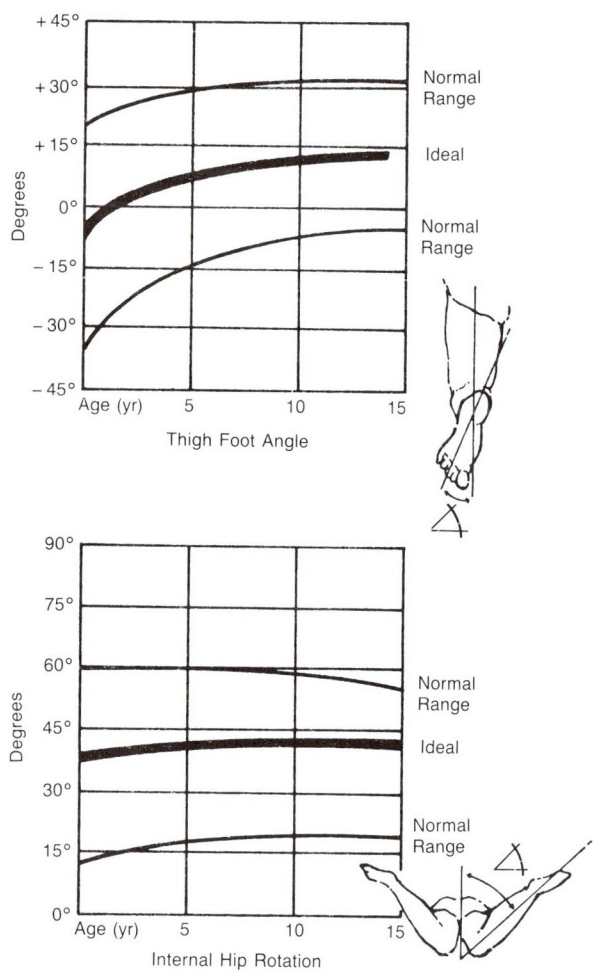

Figure 21-2, continued.

OUT-TOEING

- Usually external femoral torsion; self-correcting when child begins to roll over

FOOT SHAPE CONCERNS

- Must do full neurologic examination (including gait and arch assessment)
- Examine hips carefully

TABLE 21-1 Differential Diagnosis and Management of "Foot Shape" Abnormalities

	Age of Presentation	Frequency	Main Feature	Treatment
Club foot	Birth	1:700	Fixed equino varus	Serial casts at birth; operate on 80% at 3 months
Calcaneo valgus foot	Birth	1:300	Top of foot rests on shin	Always recovers; advise stretching
Metatarsus varus	Birth–3 mo	1:100	Forefoot adduction	Brace at 3 months; after 2 years, requires operation
Vertical talus	Birth–3 mo	1:100,000	Rocker bottom sole	Usually requires surgical correction
Hypermobile flat foot	2 yr +	1:10	Arch appears on tip toeing	Ignore; unaffected by attempts to treat
Pes cavus	10 yr +	1:10,000	Fixed high arch	Investigate: spinal x-ray; nerve conduction studies; possibly myelogram; idiopathic; usually symmetrical; often requires surgery
Toe walking	3 yr +	1:700	Short calf muscle	Exclude dystrophy and cerebral palsy; if persistent, grow muscle with stretching casts

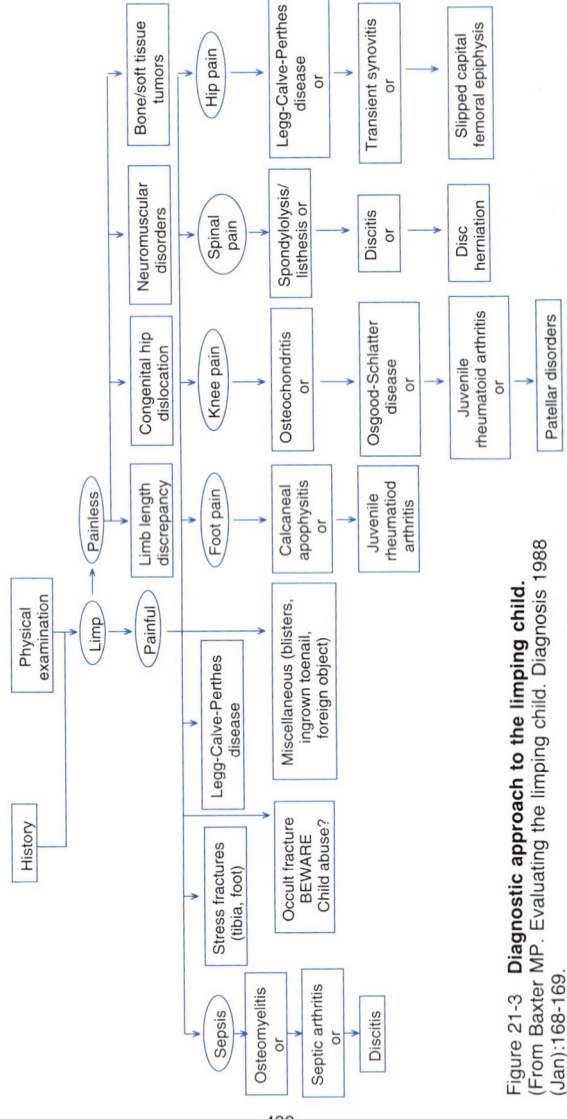

DIAGNOSTIC APPROACH TO THE LIMPING CHILD

Figure 21-3 **Diagnostic approach to the limping child.** (From Baxter MP. Evaluating the limping child. Diagnosis 1988 (Jan):168-169.

KNEE PAIN

- May be referred pain from the hip, e.g., slipped epiphysis
- Meniscal injury *rare* in children

Osgood Schlatter's Disorder (Chronic Stress Fracture of Tibial Tubercle)

- X-ray necessary to rule out other conditions; shows enlarged and fragmented tibial tubercle
- Treatment consists of explanation and reassurance—lasts ~18 mo. Continue sports using a basketball knee protector.

Peripatellar Pain Syndrome

- Most frequent source of knee pain, probably due to overuse
- Pain reproduced by compressing patella against femur
- X-ray normal
- Anticipate protracted course; quadriceps strengthening exercises may help

Osteochondritis Dissecans

- Aching knee pain and "giving way"
- Characteristic x-ray findings
- Observe, occasionally immobilize; rarely—drilling or pinning back. Tends to heal spontaneously in those still growing.

Recurrent Dislocation of the Patella

- May dislocate spontaneously
- Axial x-ray film of patella with knee flexed 40° shows shallow groove
- Treat with quadriceps-strengthening exercises first. Usually requires surgical repair.

HIP PROBLEMS

TABLE 21-2 Clinical Features of Some Common Hip Disorders

	CDH	Transient Synovitis	Legg-Perthes	SFCE	Septic Arthritis
Age	0-4	4-8	3-10	8-15	ANY (0-1 commonest)
ROM	↓ Abduction	↓	↓	↓ Flexion and interior rotation	↓
Pain	None	+ → ++	0 → +	+	++++
X-ray	Dislocation	Normal	Abnormal, varies with stage	Abnormal: slip	Frequently normal

Body temperature	Normal	Normal	Normal	Normal	↑
ESR	Normal	Can be ↑	Normal	Normal	↑ Can be normal in early cases
Treatment	External splint early; surgery late	Rest, gentle ROM exercises	Observation, brace, or surgery depending on age and extent	Surgery	Surgery and antibiotics

CDH = congenital dislocated hip; SFCE = slipped femoral capital epiphysis; ROM = range of motion

CONGENITAL DISLOCATION OF HIP

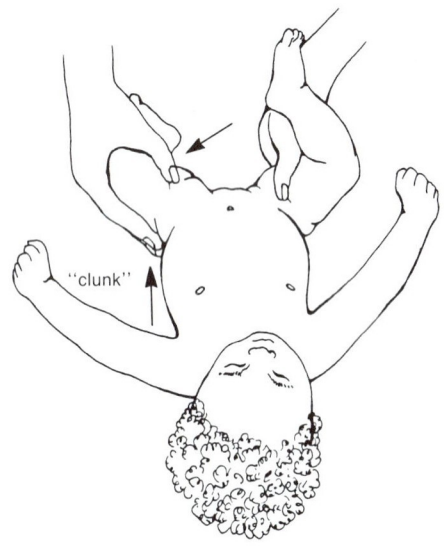

A. Ortolani (reduction) test. With baby relaxed and content on firm surface, the hips and knees are flexed to 90°. Hips are examined one at a time. Examiner grasps baby's thigh with middle finger over greater trochanter, and lifts thigh to bring femoral ead from its dislocated posterior position to opposite the acetabulum. Simultaneously, thigh is gently abdocuted, reducing gently abducted, reducing femoral head into acetabulum. In positive finding, examiner senses reduction by palpable, nearly audible "clunk"

Figure 21-4 **Recognition of congenital dislocation of the hip (CDH).** (Redrawn after Shelov MD, Mezey AP, Edelmann CM Jr, Barnett HL. Primary care pediatrics: a symptomatic approach. Norwalk: Appleton-Centry-Crofts, 1984:489.)

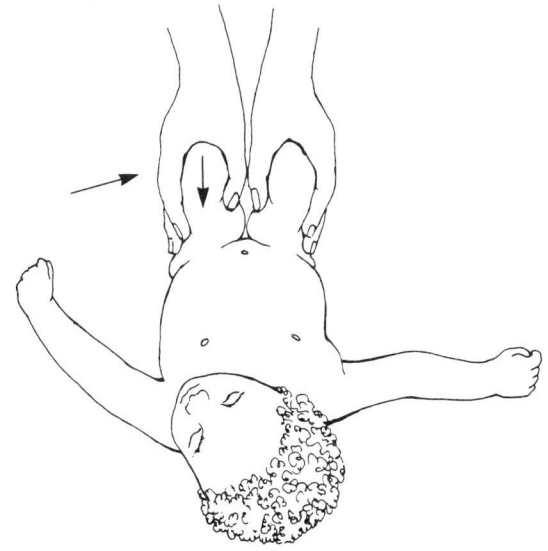

B. Barlow (dislocation) test. Reverse of Ortolani test. If femoral head is in acetabulum at time of examination, the Barlow test is performed to discover any hip instability. Baby's thigh is grasped as above and adducted with gently downward pressure. Dislocation is palpable as femoral head slips out of acetabulum. Diagnosis is confirmed with Ortolani test.

Figure 21-4, continued.

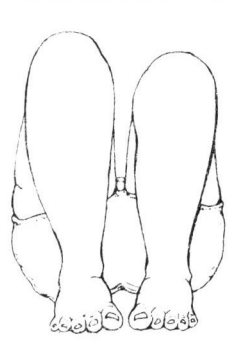

Figure 21-5 **Allis' or Galeazzi's sign: knee is lower on affected side when knees and hips are flexed because femoral head lies posterior to acetabulum in this position.**
(Redrawn after Shelov MD, Mezey AP, Edelmann CM Jr, Barnett HL. Primary care pediatrics: a symptomatic approach. Norwalk: Appleton-Century-Crofts, 1984:490.)

- More common in girls, first-born, left hip, breech presentation
- Stage 1: Dislocatable—hip stays in joint but can be pushed out on Barlow test (Fig. 21-4*B*). Usually recovers spontaneously after a few weeks.
- Stage 2: Dislocated but reducible—positive Ortolani test (Fig. 21-4*A*). Lasts a few weeks before stage 3.
- Stage 3: Fixed dislocation-irreducible—abduction is limited and thigh looks short (Galeazzi's sign, Fig. 21-5): seen after age 3 mo.

Differential Diagnosis

- Synovial click: noise from the hip resembling cracking knuckles. A positive Ortolani sign is not a noise but the feeling of the femoral head jumping into the joint. Clicks require continued followup.
- Congenital adduction contracture in child with "windswept" hips (i.e., adduction contracture of one hip and abduction contracture of other hip)
- Congenital femoral hypoplasia
- Fixed dislocation in arthrogryposis

Investigations

- 3-18 mo: asymmetry of abduction may be only clinical sign; requires full investigation
- Clinical signs best guide for stages 1 and 2
- U/S (investigation of choice) or x-ray (AP + frogleg) for stage 3

Treatment

- Pavlik harness, 0-8 mo
- Traction and closed reduction, 8-18 mo
- Traction, open reduction, innominate osteotomy, 18-30 mo
- Traction, open reduction, innominate osteotomy and femoral shortening, 30 mo-5 yr

Legg-Perthes Disease

- Diagnosis made by x-ray (AP and frogleg); changes usually obvious by the time patient symptomatic
- "Containment" is the underlying principle of treatment. Varies from simple observation to bracing or surgery depending on age of child and extent of disease.
- Bone scan, MRI helpful in occasional cases where diagnosis is unclear

Transient Synovitis

- May be difficult to differentiate from early "septic" hip
- Usually afebrile or low-grade fever, and child looks well

Investigations

- WBC, ESR usually normal; help to distinguish from septic hip or osteomyelitis. X-ray to exclude Legg-Perthes.
- If unable to differentiate from septic hip, refer to orthopedic surgery for joint aspiration.

Treatment

- Bedrest (at home in most cases) ± nonsteroidal anti-inflammatory agent (e.g., naprosyn)
- ± Gentle ROM exercises. Gradual resumption of activity.
- Careful observation to rule out early septic arthritis
- If recurrent or persistent, need to rule out Legg-Perthes

Septic Hip
- See p 247

Slipped Femoral Capital Epiphysis (SFCE)
- 30% bilateral
- Presents most commonly as insidious ache in groin or knee; often mistaken for "pulled" muscle
- May present as acute severe pain and inability to bear weight following trauma

Investigations
- Lateral frogleg of both hips most useful x-ray in mild degrees of slip
- Previous history of SFCE in contralateral hip requires orthopedic consultation even in absence of x-ray abnormalities.

Treatment
- Urgent surgical pinning
- N.B.: association with delayed bone age; rule out endocrine abnormality

Spine

SCOLIOSIS

- Many minimal curves noted in school screening are non-progressive
- Early presentation (infancy and early childhood) suggests underlying skeletal or neuromuscular disorder

Investigations

- 3-foot *standing* PA x-ray of spine: a single film is all that is required to confirm and quantify using Cobb angle (Fig. 21-6). Risser stage refers to stage of skeletal maturation based on degree of ossification of iliac crest.

Orthopedics

Treatment

- Still growing
  1. 10-25°: Check every 6 mo using x-ray exam
  2. 25-45°: Brace
  3. 45°+: Spinal instrumentation and fusion
- Growth complete
  1. <45°: Ignore
  2. >45°: Spinal instrumentation

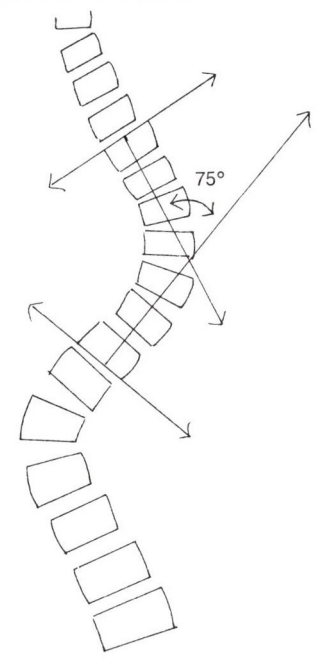

Figure 21-6 **Measurement of Cobb angle in scoliosis. Locate the top vertebra of the curve, i.e., the one whose superior surface tilts to the side of the concavity of the curve. The bottom vertebra is the lowest one whose inferior surface tilts to the side of the concavity of the curve. The Cobb angle is the angle between perpendiculars intersecting the superior surface of the top and inferior surface of the bottom vertebrae of the curve.**

KYPHOSIS

Investigations
- Standing lateral x-ray to measure angle of kyphosis between T-3 and T-12

Treatment
- Still growing
  1. <30°: Normal
  2. 30-45°: Mild; monitor
  3. 45°+: Consider brace
- Growth complete and 50°+: consider surgical correction

BACK PAIN

- More likely to be a definite cause in children than in adults

Differential Diagnosis
- Mechanical: spondylolisthesis, Scheuermann's, thoracolumbar osteochondritis
- Infection: osteomyelitis
- Tumors and tumorlike conditions: eosinophilic granuloma, aneurysmal bone cyst, osteoblastoma, osteoid osteoma
- Injury

Investigations
- X-ray exam, bone scan, ESR
- Consider CT scan or MRI

Upper Limb

PULLED ELBOW

- Common in children 2-5 yr of age
- Produced by tug on outstretched arm; radial head is abruptly pulled distally to become trapped in the annular ligament
- Child will not use arm (pseudoparalysis)
- Fracture is main differential diagnosis

Investigations
- X-ray normal; rule out other injury, fracture

Treatment
- On supination of the forearm, there is a "click" felt, which represents the radial head reducing through the ligament
- Pain disappears within a few minutes
- Occasionally requires a second attempt next day

Neck

CONGENITAL MUSCULAR TORTICOLLIS

- Contracture of sternomastoid
- Physiotherapy to stretch (Fig. 21-7); surgical release in neglected cases
- Examine hips carefully; may be associated with hip dislocation

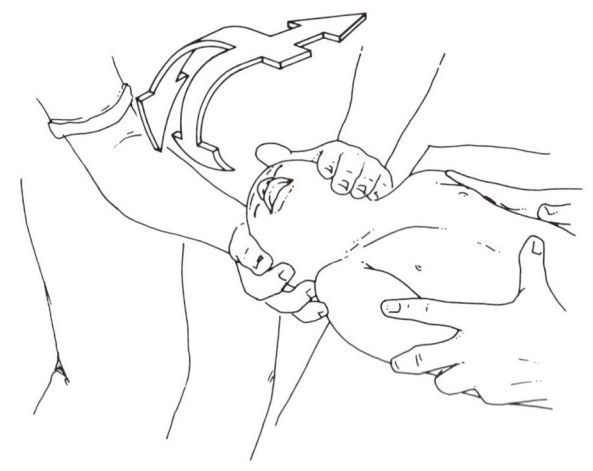

Figure 21-7 **Exercises to stretch out a tight sternomastoid muscle in congenital torticollis. The motion is a combination of rotation toward the affected (right) side, tilting away from the affected side, and extension of the neck.** (From Behrman RE, Vaughan VC, Nelson WE, eds. Nelson textbook of pediatrics. 13th ed. Philadelphia: WB Saunders, 1987.)

Injuries

- Sprains rare in children; usually greenstick, buckle, or epiphyseal fractures requiring x-ray diagnosis
- Fractures in infant <18 mo: high index of suspicion for nonaccidental injury

Management

- Check circulation and nerve function
- Look for skin wound, even puncture wound; NPO in case of potential surgery
- Cover open wounds with sterile dressings, splint, then x-ray

- Undisplaced metaphyseal or diaphyseal fractures: immobilize
- Displaced metaphyseal/diaphyseal fractures: reduce under anesthesia
- Fractures into the joint (type 3 and 4) require open reduction
- Open fractures require urgent debridement, including fractures associated with puncture wounds

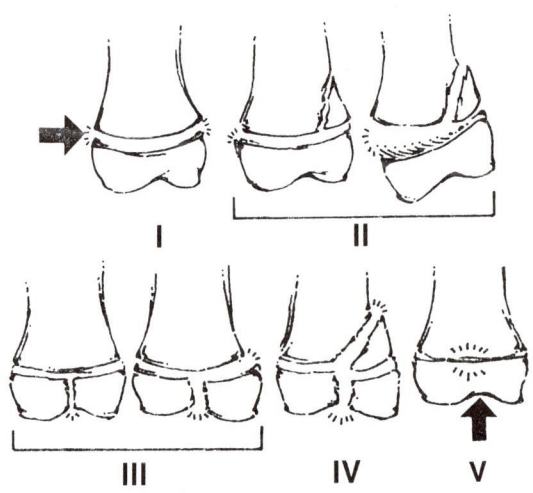

Figure 21-8 **Classification of growth plate injuries.** (From Salter RB, Harris WR. Injuries involving the epiphyseal plate. J Bone Joint Surg 1963;45A:487.)

Infection

- See pp 247-251

TWENTY-TWO

Otolaryngology

Adenotonsillectomy

INDICATIONS FOR ADENOTONSILLECTOMY

Strong Indications
- Obstructive sleep apnea, with or without cor pulmonale
- Dysphagia (warrants tonsillectomy only)
- Possible malignancy (unilateral hypertrophy)
- Peritonsillar abscess (quinsy): one episode (as tends to recur)
- Nasal obstruction (hypertrophied adenoids) producing discomfort in breathing, severe speech distortion, or dentofacial maldevelopment

Possible (Controversial) Indications
- Chronic or recurrent suppurative otitis media
- Conductive hearing loss (serous otitis media)
- Chronic or recurrent tonsillitis: at least three episodes in each of 3 yr, *or* four in each of 2 yr, *or* five episodes in 1 yr, associated with fever, tonsillar or pharyngeal exudate, cervical lymphadenitis, positive culture for group A β-hemolytic Streptococci
- Rheumatic fever in poorly compliant patients
- Mouth-breathing, snoring, or halitosis

CONTRAINDICATIONS

- Medical contraindications to surgery (e.g., bleeding, cardiovascular)
- Velopharyngeal insufficiency

COMPLICATIONS

Hemorrhage
- Primary—occurring within 24 hr postoperatively
- Secondary—occurring between 5 and 8 days postoperatively usually secondary to infection
- Avoid ASA during postoperative period

MANAGEMENT

- Admit patient for at least 1 day for observation if secondary hemorrhage
- Assess fluid status and consider cross-matching and starting IV after CBC
- Make a paste of bismuth subgallate in epinephrine (1:1,000) (yellow powder mixed with epinephrine until pasty) and apply it to pack
- Remove clot and insert pack in nasopharynx or tonsillar fossa for 10 min; postnasal pack may also be required
- Recheck CBC at 8 hrs after control of hemorrhage
- If bleeding persistent or difficult to control, consider checking PT, PTT, and platelets
- Start antibiotic therapy (penicillin)

Foreign Body in Ear

- Visualize with head mirror or headlamp and attempt removal
- Soft material: use loop
- Hard, smooth object: use hook or loop
- Insect: kill it before removal by instilling rubbing alcohol
- General syringing with warm water is helpful, but do not syringe if object is vegetable matter, foam, or paper (it may swell)

Foreign Body in Nose

- Foreign body is the most common cause of unilateral (usually foul-smelling) nasal discharge
- Visualize with head mirror or light
- Anesthetize and shrink nasal mucosa, by inserting cotton packs soaked with cocaine 5% (max dose = 3 mg/kg)
- Suction off discharge
- Attempt removal with:
  1. Forceps: soft material (e.g., paper, cotton)
  2. Hook: solid object

Foreign Body in Larynx, Trachobronchial Tree

- Keep possibility of foreign body (FB) in mind when assessing any child with enigmatic chronic cough, wheeze, chest disease, or dysphagia
- Usually a history of choking or cyanotic episode, but may not have history of acute presentation
- Aphonia + airway distress = laryngeal FB
- Stridor or wheeze, unequal expansion of chest, decreased air entry unilaterally; may have normal examination
- X-ray: inspiratory and expiratory chest films, at least two views
  1. Collapse suggests complete obstruction
  2. Hyperinflation suggests ball-valve obstruction
  3. Tracheal FB (e.g., coin) is seen head on in lateral view; esophageal foreign body seen head on PA view; due to diameters of respective tracts
  4. Fluoroscopy may show unequal diaphragmatic movement

Foreign Body in Esophagus

- History of ingestion, dysphagia, regurgitation, vomiting, or drooling; may be several months' duration
- Examination may be normal or stridor may be present if trachea is compressed
- CXR AP and lateral views (see above)

Management

- Remove FB endoscopically under general anesthesia
- FB in larynx may cause complete obstruction and require urgent bronchoscopy in emergency department. If bronchoscopist not immediately available, endotracheal intubation may be life saving.
- *Stab tracheotomy is a last resort*. Use only for a laryngeal or pharyngeal obstruction.

Otitis Externa

- Localized infection, usually a furuncle, in the outer third of ear canal
- Diffuse infection occurs following aggressive cleaning of the canal, trauma, or swimming
- *S. aureus* commonly causes localized infection; *Pseudomonas aeruginosa* and *Candida* commonly cause diffuse infection

Management

- Cleansing the canal is the single most important part of therapy
- Furuncle may require incision and drainage
- Debridement: gently remove infective and epithelial debris from ear canal (by wet swabbing, gentle irrigation, and suctioning)
- Topical antibiotic drops (e.g., those containing polymyxin, neomycin ± hydrocortisone) for up to 10 days only

- If ear canal occluded by circumferential inflammatory edema, aluminum acetate 1% solution is used: insert moist cotton wick into ear canal; keep it wet with the solution until canal has expanded sufficiently to permit debridement after 1-2 days, then use topical antibiotic drops
- If periauricular swelling, regional adenopathy, and signs of systemic infection present, systemic antibiotics should be used (e.g., cefuroxime or cloxacillin)
- If difficulty in differentiating furuncle of ear canal and mastoiditis with subperiosteal abscess formation, ENT referral indicated

Epistaxis

- Bleeding is usually from Little's area
- More common during acute URIs and in allergic rhinitis

Management

- Mild cases often respond to firm, persistent pressure to nose between fingers for 10 min. Following this, insert cotton plug with petroleum jelly into the nose and leave for 3-4 hr.
- More persistent cases are managed as follows
  1. May be facilitated by sedation PRN (codeine 1 mg/kg IM), visualization (head mirror or light), and suction
  2. Control bleeding with pressure and cotton pledgets moistened with cocaine 5% (max 3 mg/kg)
  3. Cauterize with silver nitrate stick behind bleeding point of vessel
  4. Pack nostrils (Oxycel, Gelfoam, Vaseline gauze) only if cautery ineffective
  5. If bleeding persistent, recurrent, or originating posteriorly, request ENT consult. Persistent bleeding may (rarely) represent a bleeding diathesis. These children should not have cautery with silver nitrate. Control bleeding with Oxycel gauze $\pm$ topical thromboplastin and pressure.

Fractured Nose

- Examine nose for septal hematoma or dislocation (causes nasal obstruction and may result in late nasal deformity). Septal hematoma requires urgent surgical drainage.
- X-ray may aid in diagnosis, but if negative, does not exclude serious pathology
- ENT should be contacted to reduce deformity early (within 2-3 hr of injury) if no swelling. If swelling is present, may observe for 3-4 days. All cases should be referred to ENT clinic for 3-4 day follow-up to check for late septal hematoma, abscess formation, or deformity (noted after swelling subsides).

Corrosive Burns of Upper GI Tract

- Alkaline corrosives common in drain and oven cleaners
- Esophagus may be damaged by the time child arrives in the emergency department
- Degree of visible burns in mouth and pharynx may not be indicative of degree of esophageal involvement
- Presence of two or more symptoms and signs (e.g., dysphagia, oral burns) correlates with esophageal burns

Management

- See also p 478
- Urgent ENT consult
- Determine nature (acid/alkali/other) and form (solid/liquid) of ingested material if possible
- **Do *not* give emetic**
- **Do *not* attempt gastric lavage**
- Promote ingestion of appropriate fluids, unless drooling or signs of mediastinal leak (e.g., chest or back pain, dyspnea) are present
  1. If alkali ingested, give milk or water
  2. If acid ingested, give milk or water
  3. If bleach ingested, give water (first choice) or milk
  4. Ages 1-5, give 250-500 ml; >5 yr, give up to 1 L

- Observe for respiratory distress secondary to laryngeal involvement (hoarseness, stridor, dyspnea)
- Observe for shock; monitor vital signs carefully (see p 546)
- Severe chest and abdominal pain are ominous signs—may be indicative of visceral perforation
- Esophagoscopy is usually performed after oral burns improve (3-5 days), to assess extent of esophageal burn
- Esophageal stricture develops in ~15% of cases of caustic ingestion
- Consider prophylactic steroids (prednisone) and antibiotics (ampicillin) following early endoscopy

Facial Nerve Paralysis

- Common in children: may be secondary to Bell's palsy, trauma (including birth trauma), otitis media, aural neoplasm, or intracranial tumor
- Bell's palsy is a diagnosis of exclusion (does not always resolve spontaneously in children)

Management
- Investigations may include
  1. Audiology
  2. Impedance studies
  3. Nerve-conduction tests
  4. Mastoid tomograms or CT
  5. Schirmer's test (lacrimation)
  6. Salivary-secretion tests
- Therapy:
  1. ENT consult
  2. Treat underlying condition
  3. Steroids may be useful in Bell's palsy

Acute (Suppurative) Otitis Media

- Major organisms include *S. pneumoniae, H. influenzae, Branhamella catarrhalis,* and *S. pyogenes*
- Treatment is initially for 10 days minimum, follow-up is essential (Table 22-1)
- In infants <6 wk, early myringotomy may be warranted for culture
- For perforation with discharge, gentamicin otic drops tid for 10 days is usually recommended in addition to systemic treatment
- Analgesics and antipyretics as indicated
- Decongestants or antihistamines are of no proven efficacy
- Indications for myringotomy
  1. Severe pain—immediately
  2. Bulging drum and severe pain after 48-72 hr of therapy
  3. Otitis media with complication (e.g., meningitis, mastoiditis)
  4. Residual serous otitis 12 wk after an acute otitis despite apparently adequate medical therapy
  5. Immunosuppressed (e.g., chemotherapy)
- If discharge persists after 1 wk of adequate therapy, obtain swabs from deep in external canal for culture.
- Obtain mastoid x-rays only if disease present for ≥3 wk or if acute mastoiditis present (surgery required if air-cell coalescence)
- If symptoms or discharge persist for >1 wk, check cultures for resistant organism and treat appropriately. Daily microdebridement by ENT may be necessary.
- Tympanometry useful pre- and post-treatment to assess presence of and follow-up of effusion

TABLE 22-1 Management of Acute Otitis Media

Antibiotic	Advantages	Disadvantages
Amoxicillin	First choice	
Trimethoprim-sulfamethoxazole	Effective, cheap alternative when there is penicillin sensitivity	Hepatitis Stevens-Johnson syndrome
Cefaclor	Effective against beta-lactamase–producing organisms	Rash, diarrhea 1% risk erythema multiforme and serum sickness Expensive
Erythromycin-sulfisoxazole	As cefaclor, effective against ampicillin-resistant *H. influenzae* and *B. catarrhalis*	Requires qid dosage Expensive
Amoxicillin-clavulinate	Effective against beta-lactamase–producing organisms	Expensive 15% diarrhea
Cefixime	As cefaclor, once-a-day dosage	

Recurrent Otitis Media

- Management includes prophylactic antibiotic (long-term or seasonal) or myringotomy and tympanostomy tube insertion (M and T)
- Amoxicillin or sulfisoxazole are usual choices for chemoprophylaxis. Failure of this method, despite compliance, is an indication for M and T
- *If <6 wk of age, rule out immunodeficiency*

Serous Otitis Media

- Most common cause of hearing loss in children
- Common accompaniment of adenoidal hypertrophy, atopy, and cleft palate
- If undiagnosed or left untreated, *may* result in delayed onset of speech, learning problems, and may lead to chronic ear disease

Management

- Asymptomatic: follow until disappears (tympanometry useful)
- Medical (first choice)
  1. Treat with antibiotics (see "acute otitis media," above) PO × 3-4 wk
  2. Auto-insufflation—Valsalva maneuver
- Surgical
  1. Indicated for symptoms present for >6 mo at time of diagnosis, bilateral hearing loss >20 db, behavior or speech problem secondary to hearing loss, or if medical therapy fails.
  2. Assess each patient individually for required surgical procedure, e.g.,
     - Adenoidectomy ± tonsillectomy with myringotomy ± insertion of middle-ear ventilation tubes have been frequently performed, but are of unclear benefit
     - Insertion of ventilation tube only

3. Note that these procedures are not free of complications, e.g., tympanostomy tubes may lead to permanent structural damage to tympanic membrane, and *may themselves* induce cholesteatoma formation
4. Drainage from tympanostomy tubes may be treated with gentamicin otic drops

Traumatic Perforation of Tympanic Membrane

- Urgent ENT consult, as emergency exploration and repair may be required
- Water should be kept out of ear

Mastoiditis

- Consult ENT
- If subperiosteal abscess formation is present, surgical drainage usually required
- If erythema behind ear and no radiologic evidence of coalescence: cloxacillin 200 mg/kg/day and ampicillin 200 mg/kg/day IV
- Wide myringotomy necessary
- Chronic mastoiditis with chronic otorrhea may be demonstrated by mastoid air cell loss and coalescence on x-ray. Surgery may be necessary to stop otorrhea.

TWENTY-THREE

Plastic Surgery

Abrasions

- Scrub area to remove embedded dirt and prevent tattooing. Use saline or povidone-iodine to avoid irritation caused by stronger detergents; mechanical debridement most important aspect.
- If wound is extensive, scrub wound under general anesthesia
- Review tetanus immunization status

Lacerations

HAND LACERATIONS

- Examine and test flexor and extensor tendons, intrinsic muscles, nerves, joints, bones, vascular supply. Consult plastic surgeon for glass, puncture wounds, or diagnosis in doubt.

FACIAL LACERATIONS

- Use small bites or subcuticular suture to avoid stitch marks. Consult appropriate surgical specialty for free borders of mouth, nose, eye or eyelids, ears.

Management

- Cleanse adjacent skin and infiltrate area with 1% lidocaine (Xylocaine). Do not use epinephrine in appendages
- Flush with normal saline only
- Close fascia and deep dermal layers of mucosa with 4-0 or 5-0 absorbable sutures (e.g., catgut or Dexon)
- Close skin using 5-0 or 6-0 nonabsorbable sutures (e.g., nylon or polyethylene); use 6-0 suture to close skin on face; use small bites to avoid large stitch marks
- Tetanus immunization
- Removal of skin sutures: face, 5 days; elsewhere, 7-10 days

Facial Fractures

- Examine for
  1. Contour deformity
  2. Pain on deep palpation or mastication
  3. Areas of anesthesia
  4. Crepitus, malocclusion
  5. Subconjunctival hemorrhage, eye movement, visual acuity
- Caution: x-ray may be negative

Cleft Lip and Palate

- Requires immediate consultation with multidisciplinary team, plastic surgeon
- Examine child carefully to rule out other malformations (especially cardiac)
- Lip repair at 3 mo, palate repair at approximately 1 yr; may require revision of lip or nasal deformity at 5 yr
- Special attention to *airway* and *feeding* difficulties

Burns

- See p 545 for management of smoke inhalation
- Prevent severe immersion burns by keeping home water at recommended setting of between 49° C (120° F) and 54° C (130° F)
- Cold water immersion of burned area may be helpful immediately after burn or within first hour
- Careful history (including social) and physical examination noting degree, location, and extent of burn
- Beware of nonaccidental injury

TABLE 23-1 Water Temperature and Duration of Exposure Producing Third-Degree Burns

°C	°F	Duration of Exposure
49	120	More than 5 min
52	125	1.5-2 min
54	130	30 sec
57	135	10 sec
60	140	5 sec
63	145	Less than 3 sec
66	150	1-2 sec
68	155	~1 sec

TABLE 23-2 Severity of Burn

Degree	Level of Burn	Characteristics
First	Epidermis	Erythema, painful
Second		
Superficial	Superficial dermis	Blisters, painful
Deep	Deep dermis	Eschar, painful
Third	Subcutaneous tissue	Leathery eschar, painless

TABLE 23-3 Criteria for Hospitalization of Patients with Burns

Extent
  Under 2 yr: ≥6% of body surface area (combination of 2nd and 3rd degree)
  Over 2 yr: ≥10% of body surface area (combination of 2nd and 3rd degree)

Location: burns of face, neck, hands, feet, perineum

Type: chemical, electrical

Associated injuries: smoke, head injury, fractures, soft tissue trauma

Complicating medical problems: diabetes

Social situation: abuse, self-inflicted, psychologic

Management: Outpatient

- Diagram burn area, noting degree (Fig. 23-1)
- Cool the part; eliminate the agent (copious irrigation with water if a chemical burn)

Plastic Surgery

- Cleanse with saline (use sterile gloves)
- Leave intact blisters alone
- Debride broken blisters and loose debris
- Apply Polysporin and then Sofra-Tulle
- Dress with dry gauze and secure with Kling bandage
- Review tetanus immunization status
- Analgesics prn for pain
- Re-evaluate in 2-5 days

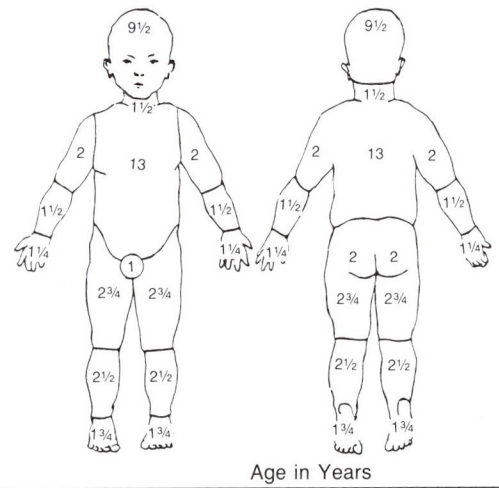

Area	0	1	5	10	15	Adult
Head area	19	17	13	11	9	7
Trunk area	26	26	26	26	26	26
Arm area	7	7	7	7	7	7
Thigh area	5½	6½	8½	8½	9½	9½
Leg area	5	5	5	6	6	7

Age in Years

Total 3rd degree burn____
Total 2nd degree burn____

TOTAL BURNS____

Figure 23-1 **Estimation of burn area.**

Management: Inpatient
- Resuscitation
  1. Establish airway and ventilation especially if flame burn and patient is confined to smoke-filled space (see p 545)
  2. Start large-bore IV in unburned area
  3. Manage smoke inhalation: monitor ABGs, carboxyhemoglobin level, CXR, high FiO_2
  4. CBC, BUN, electrolytes, protein, and albumin
  5. Insert urinary catheter
  6. Record accurate hourly input and output
  7. NPO, nasogastric tube in severe burns, H_2 blocker
  8. Ringer's lactate IV: 4 ml/kg/% burn over first 24 hr, replacing half in first 8 hr postburn and half in subsequent 16 hr postburn. Colloids (e.g., albumin, plasma) may be used as part of replacement fluid after first 8 hr.
  9. In addition to above, in children under 2 yr of age give maintenance fluids as 3.33% dextrose and 0.33% saline
  10. Above formula is only a guide and must be reassessed and adjusted according to hourly urine output (>2-3 ml/kg/hr), general hydration state, hemoglobin, BUN, serum electrolytes
- Burn management
  1. Evaluate + document burn size, location, and depth
  2. Cleanse in burn bath (lukewarm salt water: ~38° C or 100° F) and debride loose tissue and broken blisters; leave intact blisters alone
  3. Take swabs for culture and sensitivity from nose, throat, and burn wound
  4. Apply silver sulfadiazine cream to burn areas on body, and Polysporin ointment to burns on face
  5. IV penicillin (opinions differ on administration)
  6. Review tetanus immunization status
  7. May require high environmental temperature, e.g., 28-30° C (82-86° F) to prevent heat loss
  8. Observe for hypothermia with large burns

- Circumferential burns
  1. Loss of capillary integrity leads to massive swelling with resuscitation
  2. Circumferential eschar constriction may compromise distal circulation
  3. Consider immediate escharotomy
- After 24 hours
  1. Adjust IV rate according to clinical status
  2. Continue albumin, plasma, or blood PRN
  3. Observe carefully for sepsis
  4. Start feeds (e.g., PO or NG) on second postburn day. May require parenteral nutrition support
  5. Beware of ileus

TWENTY-FOUR

Poisoning

General Management

INGESTED POISON

Dilute Poison
- Dilute nondrug poison by giving water PO
- Do not use milk
- Do not attempt to neutralize poison

Gastric Decontamination
- Do not use salt water as an emetic
- Syrup of ipecac: causes vomiting in 80% of children within 15 min
- Timing
  1. Within half hr for alcohols
  2. Within 1 hr for liquid medications
  3. Within 2 hr for pills
- Dose
  1. 9-12 mo—10 ml; no repeat
  2. 1-10 yr—15 ml; can repeat once after 20 min
  3. >10 yr—30 ml; can repeat once after 20 min
- Contraindications
  1. Coma
  2. Convulsions
  3. Caustics
  4. Petroleum-distillate hydrocarbons
- Gastric lavage
  1. Indicated if ipecac is ineffective or patient is comatose
  2. Protect airway if patient is comatose
  3. Suction out stomach contents first
  4. Use large-bore orogastric tube

Poisoning

5. Contraindications
   - Coma—unless an endotracheal tube in place
   - Caustics
   - Petroleum-distillate hydrocarbons (unless they contain another toxin that mandates gastric decontamination, e.g., pesticides)
- Activated charcoal: adsorbs many poisons, making them unavailable for intake by the gut. Administer as soon as possible after gastric emptying (patients may vomit after charcoal administration).
   1. Note: Do not give charcoal until ipecac-induced vomiting has subsided
   2. Dose: 1 g/kg; mix appropriate amount in 120-240 ml fluid and give PO or by nasogastric tube
   3. Contraindications: caustics, hydrocarbons
   4. Administration of half doses q4-6h may be beneficial for many poisonings
- Cathartics: cause more rapid transit time, resulting in less absorption
   1. Major indications: delayed-release products, decreased GI motility
   2. Contraindications: caustics, hydrocarbons, diarrhea, abdominal trauma
   3. Dose:
      - Sorbitol (70%) 1.5-2.0 ml/kg (maximum 150 ml)
      - Magnesium citrate (5%) 4.0 ml/kg (maximum 200 ml); magnesium may be absorbed: caution in renal failure

UNKNOWN POISONING

- Support vital functions
- Proceed as for ingested poison unless poisoning was by another route
- Save vomitus or lavage aliquots and blood and urine samples for toxicology analysis
- Identify symptom complex (if possible) so that specific diagnosis can be made (Table 24-1)

TABLE 24-1 Common Signs and Causes of Poisoning

System	Sign	Causes
Cardiovascular	Bradycardia	Digitalis compounds Beta-blocking agents
	Tachycardia	Sympathomimetics Anticholinergic agents Theophylline
	Hypertension	Sympathomimetics Phencyclidine
	Hypotension	Hypnotic-sedatives Narcotic analgesics
	Arrhythmias	Theophylline Digitalis compounds Tricyclic antidepressants
Respiratory	Bradypnea	Narcotics Ethanol Hypnotic-sedatives
	Tachypnea	Salicylates Carbon monoxide Methanol
Temperature	Hyperthermia	Salicylates Anticholinergic agents Theophylline
	Hypothermia	Ethanol Phenothiazines
Neurologic	Ataxia	Ethanol Barbiturates Phenytoin
	Miosis	Narcotics Barbiturates Phenothiazines Clonidine Benzodiazepines
	Mydriasis	Sympathomimetics Anticholinergic agents
	Nystagmus	Phenytoin
	Convulsions	Sympathomimetics Anticholinergic agents

TABLE 24-1 Common Signs and Causes of Poisoning (Cont'd)

System	Sign	Causes
Neurologic—cont'd	Convulsions—cont'd	Camphorated oil Lindane (γ-benzene hexachloride) Strychnine Theophylline
	Coma	CNS depressants Anticholinergic agents Narcotics Asphyxiant gases Salicylates
	Psychosis	Anticholinergic agents Sympathomimetics Hallucinogens Salicylates
Oral cavity	Dryness	Sympathomimetics Anticholinergic agents Narcotics
	Acetone smell	Acetone Methanol Isopropyl alcohol Phenol Salicylates
	Alcohol smell	Ethanol
	Almond smell	Cyanide
	Garlic smell	Arsenic Phosphorus Organophosphate insecticides Thallium
	Wintergreen smell	Methylsalicylate
	Petroleum smell	Hydrocarbons
Skin	Cyanosis	Methemoglobinemia
Gastrointestinal	Emesis, hematemesis	Iron Arsenic Colchicine Salicylates Theophylline

INJECTED POISON

- If treatment can be started within a few minutes after injection
  1. Apply a *venous* tourniquet proximally
  2. Do not release tourniquet until patient is in an intensive care setting (shock may occur)

POISON BY RECTAL ROUTE

- Give enema

INHALED POISON

- Remove from source of contamination
- Maintain clear airway; support ventilation and O_2 if necessary

POISON IN CONTACT WITH SKIN OR EYE

- Wash with copious amounts of water for 10-15 min
- Do not use chemical neutralizers
- If eye contamination, obtain ophthalmology consultation for further evaluation and treatment

TOXICOLOGY TESTS

- Tests can be either qualitative or quantitative
- Substances for which it is reasonable to request STAT quantitative values
  1. Acetaminophen
  2. Carboxyhemoglobin
  3. Digoxin
  4. Ethanol
  5. Ethylene glycol
  6. Iron
  7. Lead
  8. Lithium
  9. Methanol
  10. Methemoglobin
  11. Paraquat
  12. Salicylate
  13. Theophylline

- Communicate with lab or send clinical information along with samples of blood, urine, gastric fluid
- Toxic screens are notoriously unreliable
- Rule of thumb: treat the patient, *not* the level

Specific Poisons

SALICYLATE INTOXICATION

- Toxic dose of ASA: >150 mg/kg
- Note: Oil of wintergreen (methyl salicylate): 1 ml = 1.4 g of ASA
- Hyperventilation, vomiting, pyrexia, tinnitus, lethargy, confusion, dehydration (rare); may progress to convulsions, coma, pulmonary edema
- Lab: ↑ or ↓ glucose, ↑ PTT (clinical bleeding is unusual)
- Chronically intoxicated patients generally are sicker than their serum salicylate level would indicate

Management

- Induce vomiting (see p 464) if toxic or unknown dose has been ingested within 4 hr
- Give activated charcoal and a cathartic (see p 465) once any lavage or ipecac-induced vomiting has stopped
- Blood for salicylate level. Nomogram (Fig. 24-1) used *only* for *acute* ingestion; should *not* be used for delayed-release salicylates.
- If patient symptomatic, electrolytes, BUN, and glucose. All patients have a mixed acid-base disturbance (metabolic acidosis, respiratory alkalosis). However, infants and young children tend to be acidemic, whereas older children and adults tend to be alkalemic.
- Fluids (IV):
  1. If patient is in shock, give plasma or albumin 10 ml/kg (see p 546).
  2. Allow for daily maintenance, replacement of estimated deficit and ongoing losses. Fluid diuresis is not necessary.
  3. Add KCl 40 mmol/L, when patient has voided

- Correct metabolic acidosis (see p 98)
- Urinary alkalinization: IV sodium bicarbonate 1-2 mmol/kg over 1 hr and repeat as necessary over the next 8 hr to maintain urinary pH 7.5-8.0. Note: To prevent paradoxic aciduria, it is essential to give adequate KCl also.
  Indications
  1. Marked decrease in plasma HCO_3 (respiratory alkalosis is not a contraindication to bicarbonate use)
  2. High serum salicylate level: "Done" nomogram in toxic range (Fig. 24-1)
  3. Note: Do *not* give sodium bicarbonate if arterial pH >7.5
- Indications for hemodialysis
  1. Renal failure
  2. Aspiration pneumonia or pulmonary edema
  3. Salicylate level >7 mmol/L (100 mg/dl)
  4. Rising or steady salicylate level
  5. Refractory acid-base imbalance
  6. Persistent CNS manifestations

Poisoning

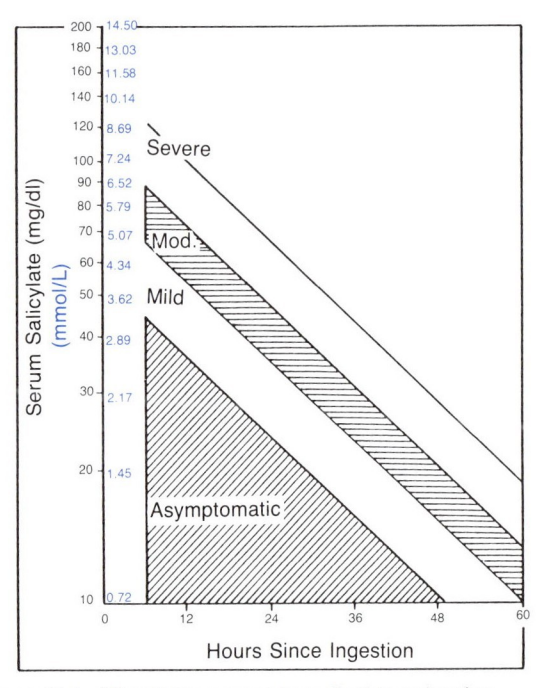

Figure 24-1 **"Done" nomogram for salicylate poisoning.** (Adapted from Done AK. Salicylate intoxication. Pediatrics 1960; 26:805.)

ACETAMINOPHEN (PARACETAMOL) POISONING

- Toxic dose >150 mg/kg
- From 2-24 hr after ingestion: nausea, vomiting, anorexia, pallor, lethargy. No changes in level of consciousness occur at this stage.
- As initial symptoms decrease (24-36 hr), hepatic necrosis develops. Liver becomes enlarged and tender. Liver enzymes begin to rise.
- Days 3-6: jaundice, coagulation defects, hypoglycemia, encephalopathy, renal failure.

Management

- Induce vomiting using ipecac syrup if patient is alert
- *N*-acetylcysteine
  1. Initiate treatment within 10 hr if possible; *may* be beneficial if initiated as late as 24 hr following ingestion
  2. Indications: acetaminophen plasma level in hepatotoxic range (Fig. 24-2). If level not available, start treatment if ingested dose is >150 mg/kg.
  3. Loading dose = 140 mg/kg PO diluted in three volumes of soft drink
  4. Follow with 70 mg/kg q4h PO for total of 17 doses
  5. If vomiting occurs within 1 hr after administration, repeat dose
  6. IV dosing regimen is available; contact poison center for details

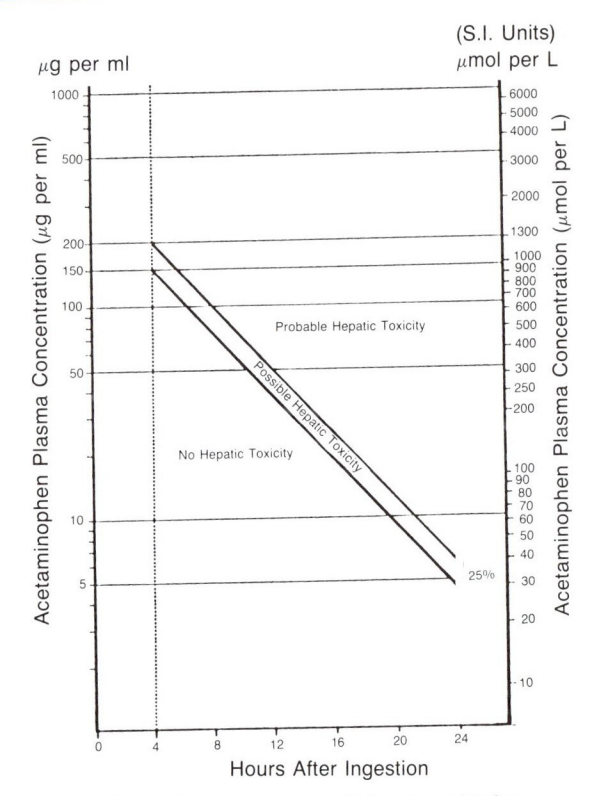

Figure 24-2 **Semilogarithmic plot of plasma acetaminophen levels vs time.** (Originally adapted from Rumack BH, Matthew H. Acetaminophen poisoning and toxicity. Pediatrics 1975; 55:871-876. The adapted form presented here is used with the permission of Micromedex, Inc., Englewood, CO.)

PETROLEUM-DISTILLATE HYDROCARBONS (PDHs)

- Gasoline, kerosene, charcoal lighter fluid, naphthas, mineral seal oils (furniture polish), and benzine (not benzene)
- PDHs are *not* significantly absorbed through the GI tract. Systemic or pulmonary disease occurs *only* as a result of aspiration.

Management of Ingestion

- Do *not* induce vomiting or perform gastric lavage (unless hydrocarbon contains another toxin, such as pesticide, in potentially toxic amounts)
- Do *not* give activated charcoal, oils or cathartics
- Observe for 2 hr; if no respiratory symptoms, may discharge home

Management of Aspiration

- For patients who are not severely ill but have coughing, choking, gagging, or vomiting
  1. History and physical exam
  2. Observe for 6 hr (repeat respiratory rate and chest examination periodically)
  3. CXR at end of 6 hr
  4. If *both* exam AND CXR are normal, may discharge home
  5. If either exam OR CXR is abnormal, hospitalize for further observation and treatment
  6. Symptomatic and supportive care
  7. *No* prophylactic antibiotics or corticosteroids

NONPETROLEUM-DISTILLATE HYDROCARBONS

- Turpentine, xylene, benzene (not benzine) and toluene are the only four nonpetroleum-distillate hydrocarbons
- Significant GI absorption
- If >2 ml/kg is ingested, gastric decontamination using ipecac or lavage (see p 464)
- Treat potential aspiration as for petroleum distillates (see above)

BARBITURATES AND ANTICONVULSANTS

- Drowsiness, ataxia, slurred speech, nystagmus may occur
- Respiratory depression, hypothermia, aspiration pneumonia, bullous skin lesions, and hypotension may occur in severe cases

Management

- In a conscious patient, induce vomiting with ipecac (see p 464), followed by activated charcoal and a cathartic (see p 465)
- In a comatose patient, gastric lavage with an endotracheal tube in place
- Support ventilation and circulation
- Alkaline diuresis (see p 470) only for phenobarbital intoxication (not effective for other barbiturates or anticonvulsants)

PHENOTHIAZINES

- As for barbiturates
- Extrapyramidal reaction: give diphenhydramine 1-2 mg/kg/dose (maximum 50 mg/dose) IV, IM, or PO
- Cardiac arrhythmias: (see p 41)

TRICYCLIC ANTIDEPRESSANTS (e.g., IMIPRAMINE, AMITRIPTYLINE)

- Central and peripheral anticholinergic effects within 6 hr after ingestion
- Anticholinergic effects: fever, mydriasis, urinary retention, decreased bowel activity, flushed skin
- CNS effects: excitation, muscle twitching, hyperreflexia, delirium, hallucinations, confusion, convulsions, and coma
- Cardiovascular effects: tachycardia, conduction defects, extrasystoles, and ventricular arrhythmias

Management

- Maintain ventilation and circulation
- Empty stomach (ipecac or gastric lavage) and follow with activated charcoal and a cathartic (see p 465)
- Cardiac monitor until no arrhythmias for 24 hr
- Limb-lead ECG hourly until 6 hr after ingestion
  1. QRS >0.10 sec = risk of convulsions
  2. QRS >0.16 sec = risk of arrhythmias and convulsions
- Control seizures with either diazepam or phenytoin (see p 378)
- Arrhythmias
  1. $NaHCO_3$ 1-2 mmol/kg IV bolus (may repeat once)
  2. If refractory, lidocaine or phenytoin (see p 49)

ETHANOL

- In children <6 yr 1 ml/kg of absolute ethanol produces a blood concentration of approximately 22 mmol/L (100 mg/dl) 2 hr after ingestion
- Hypoglycemia may occur within 6 hr of ingestion

Management

- Ipecac within 1-1½ hr after ingestion. If patient is obtunded, significant absorption has occurred and gastric lavage will be nonproductive.
- Monitor blood glucose levels
- Avoid CNS-respiratory depressant drugs
- Consider dialysis if ethanol level >110 mmol/L (500 mg/dl)

IRON

- Toxicity is based on the amount of elemental iron ingested
  1. Ferrous fumarate = 33% elemental iron
  2. Ferrous gluconate = 12% elemental iron
  3. Ferrous sulfate = 20% elemental iron
- Toxic dose (elemental iron) >50 mg/kg
- Early phase (½-6 hr of ingestion): vomiting, bloody diar-

Poisoning

rhea, lethargy, hypotonia, hypotension, shock, leukocytosis, and hyperglycemia
- Delayed phase (6-48 hr): patient may appear to improve, but in very ill patients this phase may not be evident. Acidosis, hypoglycemia, shock, hepatic failure, pulmonary edema, and coma may occur

Management

- CBC, electrolytes, glucose, and ABGs
- Serum iron level (STAT)
- Test stool and gastric contents for blood
- Deferoxamine challenge test (useful if serum iron is not available)
  1. Indirect test that detects presence of free circulating iron. Give deferoxamine 25-50 mg/kg (maximum 1 g) IV. If iron level exceeds iron-binding capacity, unbound iron is chelated by deferoxamine and excreted in the urine, producing a "vin rose" color.
  2. Note: A serum iron >53 μmol/L (300 μg/dl) or a positive deferoxamine test is suggestive of serious poisoning and an indication for deferoxamine therapy
- If a potentially toxic dose has been ingested, use ipecac or gastric lavage. An x-ray of abdomen can be used to determine success of gastric emptying.
- Activated charcoal is ineffective but may use cathartic
- Correct electrolyte imbalance and dehydration with appropriate IV fluids; correct shock with blood products
- Monitor urine output and renal function closely
- Deferoxamine: use is determined by serum iron level, tested within 4-6 hr
  1. <53 μmol/L (<300 μg/dl): will recover with above supportive measures
  2. 53-90 μmol/L (300-500 μg/dl): will need brief chelation therapy
  3. >90 μmol/L (>500 μg/dl): vigorous chelation therapy
  4. Deferoxamine initiated at a continuous IV infusion rate not to exceed 15 mg/kg/hr. Therapeutic regimen is complex; contact poison center for details.
- Hemodialysis or exchange transfusion in patients with serum iron >180 μmol/L (>1,000 μg/dl) or if anuria develops

THEOPHYLLINE

- The risk and potential seriousness of theophylline toxicity are directly related to serum concentration. Patients who are chronically overmedicated may develop severe toxicity with serum levels lower than those causing problems in an acute intoxication.
- GI symptoms: nausea, vomiting, hematemesis
- CNS symptoms: restlessness, irritability, convulsions
- Cardiovascular effects: arrhythmias
- Fever (hypermetabolism)

Management

- Ipecac or gastric lavage (see p 464) up to 2 hr following ingestion
- Follow with activated charcoal and a cathartic (see p 465). Charcoal in half-doses should be repeated q4h if theophylline levels in toxic range
- Monitor serum theophylline concentrations
- Treat seizures aggressively: use diazepam and barbiturates, *not* phenytoin
- Treat arrhythmias if they arise (see p 49)
- Hemoperfusion is indicated if
  1. Severe toxicity >440 μmol/L (>80 mg/L) in children. Note: Consider hemoperfusion at lower theophylline levels in situations associated with reduced theophylline clearance (neonates, premature infants, hepatic disease, cardiac failure) or chronic toxicity.
  2. Refractory arrhythmias or convulsions

ALKALINE CORROSIVES

- See p 451 for management of ingestion
- Emesis and gastric lavage *contraindicated*
- Eye contact: wash eyes thoroughly with water
- Skin contact: wash with running water

INSECTICIDES (ORGANOPHOSPHATE TYPE: e.g., MALATHION, DIAZINON)

- Cholinergic signs: vomiting, diarrhea, sweating, salivation, and increased bronchial secretions
- Nicotinic signs: weakness, muscle fasciculations, coma, convulsions, and respiratory insufficiency

Management

- Emesis or lavage if ingested; follow with activated charcoal (see p 465)
- If skin contamination, remove clothes and wash skin with soap and water
- Respiratory problems: treat with suction and assisted ventilation
- If increased bronchial secretions: atropine sulfate 0.05 mg/kg IV; maximum single dose = 2.0 mg. (Atropine dose is larger than that used for routine anesthesia.) Repeat every 5 min until secretions dry.
- If respiratory insufficiency, treat supportively and notify poison center.
- Pralidoxime chloride 25-50 mg/kg up to 2 g IV slowly; repeat in 1 hr if no improvement in muscle activity

NARCOTICS

- Heroin, morphine, pethidine-meperidine, methadone, diphenoxylate, propoxyphene, codeine
- Pinpoint pupils, respiratory depression, coma
- Cyanosis, bradycardia, hypotension

Management

- Maintain ventilation and circulation
- Naloxone 0.03 mg/kg IV. If no response (and diagnosis is certain), naloxone 0.1 mg/kg IV. Doses may be repeated as needed to maintain reversal of narcotic signs. Contact poison center or anesthesia department for continuous naloxone infusion.

LEAD POISONING

- Lead intoxication is a chronic disorder that ranges in prevalence from 18.6% in inner-city children to 1.2% in rural children
- Most serious poisonings are associated with housing renovations or with the ingestion of leaded paint (and putty) from housing built before 1960
- Factors contributing to increased GI absorption of lead include iron deficiency; dietary deficiencies of protein, calcium, zinc, copper; excessive amounts of dietary fats and oils
- Routine laboratory screening for lead poisoning in children less than 7 years is the best way to identify those children who warrant medical intervention

Clinical Features

- Symptoms and signs depend on the blood lead concentration and the child's age
- No pathognomonic subjective complaints or objective physical findings; most patients have little or no clinical symptoms
- Mild-to-moderate poisoning may result in neuropsychologic deficits
- Hypochromic microcytic anemia, elevated blood levels of erythrocyte protoporphyrin (EP), and radiodensity of metaphyseal lines ("lead lines") may be found in more severe cases of lead poisoning
- Severe poisoning characterized by insidious onset of anorexia, apathy, poor coordination, sporadic vomiting, and loss of newly acquired skills (particularly speech)
- Lead encephalopathy characterized by gross ataxia, persistent forceful vomiting, periods of lethargy or stupor, coma, and convulsions. The combination of anemia and convulsions strongly suggests lead encephalopathy. Any one or a combination of encephalopathic signs with an elevated blood lead level constitutes a true medical emergency.

Poisoning

Management

- Screening tests consist of blood lead and erythrocyte protoporphyrin (EP) levels. Elevated capillary blood lead levels should be confirmed using venous blood
- Radiopaque particles in the lumen of the GI tract suggests ingestion of lead within 24-36 hr; cathartics are indicated
- Chelation decisions are based solely on venous blood lead concentrations
- "Acceptable" blood lead levels are currently <25 μg/dl (1.2 μmol/L) but probably will be lowered to <10 μg/dl (0.5 μmol/L)
- Blood lead levels <10 μg/dl (0.5 μmol/L) require no medical intervention
- Blood lead levels 10-15 μg/dl (0.5-0.7 μmol/L): remove environmental lead sources
- Blood lead levels 15-20 μg/dl (0.7-1.0 μmol/L): treat with supplemental iron and removal of environmental lead sources. Consideration should be given to treating with oral chelators (e.g., penicillamine). DMSA (2,3-dimercaptosuccinic acid), another oral chelator, has been effective in therapeutic trials and should be considered for use when it becomes available.
- Blood lead levels >20 μg/dl (1.0 μmol/L): treat with an oral chelator, iron supplementation, and removal of environmental lead sources
- Treatment of symptomatic patients and those with lead levels >70 μg/dl (3.35 μmol/L) is controversial. One approach is to treat with dimercaprol (BAL), 50 mg/m^2 IM every 4 hr, and CaNa$_2$ EDTA (1000 mg/m^2/day as a continuous infusion) started with the second BAL dose. Treatment should be continued for 3-5 days.
- The goal of treatment is the permanent reduction of the blood lead level to an "acceptable" range
- Children who require medical intervention should not return home until the lead source has been identified and removed
- Treated children should be followed with lead and EP levels obtained at intervals until they are at least 6 yr old

Snake Bites

- Rattlesnakes are the only poisonous snakes in Canada and one of several in the United States
- Proper identification of snake is important
- Bites are more serious in children than in adults
- The majority of bites are *not* serious!
- Characteristics include:
  1. Fang marks
  2. Local pain (or numbness) and edema—develop within 4 hr after bite
  3. Local bleeding, ecchymosis
  4. Lymphangitis
  5. Severe pain and swelling—indicates serious envenomation
  6. Paresthesias, diaphoresis
  7. Nausea, vomiting
  8. Bleeding diathesis, hemolysis, disseminated intravascular coagulation
  9. Arrhythmias
  10. Renal failure, convulsions

Management

- First aid
  1. Suction (without cutting) over the fang marks within 30 min after bite
  2. Immobilize extremity
  3. Loose superficial venous-lymphatic tourniquet
  4. Transport to hospital
- Wound therapy
  1. Clean and dress wound
  2. Tetanus prophylaxis (see p 246)
  3. Observe for gram-negative infection

- Systemic therapy (for severe pain or swelling or systemic symptoms)
  1. Measure and record bite area
  2. IV access
  3. CBC, platelets, type and cross-match, PT, PTT, fibrinogen, electrolytes, Ca, BUN, creatinine, glucose, albumin
  4. Urinalysis, ECG
  5. Antivenin: polyvalent crotalidae antivenin is available; contact poison center for management advice

Spiders

BLACK WIDOW

- Mild-to-moderate pain on envenomation
- Muscle spasms within 2 hr
- May cause abdominal pain and rigidity
- Symptomatic supportive care
- Tetanus prophylaxis (see p 246)
- Antivenin is available; contact poison center for management advice

BROWN RECLUSE

- May be no pain on envenomation
- Local vesicles may progress to ulcerations
- Hematologic, cardiovascular, and renal effects may occur
- No antivenin is available
- Many treatment regimens have been proposed, some of which need to be started early after bite; contact poison center for recommendations

TWENTY-FIVE

Respiratory Disease

Alveolar-arterial (A-a) Gradient

- Normal A-a gradient ($P_AO_2 - PaO_2$) $\leq$16 mm Hg
- P_AO_2 = partial pressure of alveolar oxygen; measured based on % inspired O_2. In room air, P_AO_2 ~100 mm Hg.
- PaO_2 = measured in arterial blood
- If patient is hypoxemic and retaining CO_2, relative contribution of *hypoventilation* vs. *impaired gas exchange* should be determined knowing A-a gradient, i.e., normal A-a gradient, correct hypoxemia by ensuring adequate ventilation. All other causes of hypoxemia will ↑ A-a gradient.
- Oxyhemoglobin dissociation curve is illustrated in Fig. 25-1.

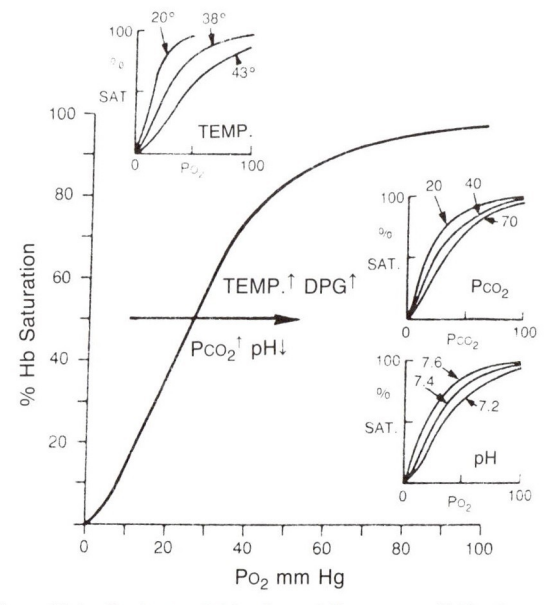

Figure 25-1 **Oxyhemoglobin dissociation curve. Shift of the oxygen dissociation curve by pH, P_{CO_2}, and temperature. As curve shifts to the right, oxygen unloading to tissues is enchanced.** (Modified from West JB. Respiratory physiology: the essentials. 2nd ed. Baltimore: Williams & Wilkins, 1979:73.)

Pulmonary Function Testing (Fig. 25-2)

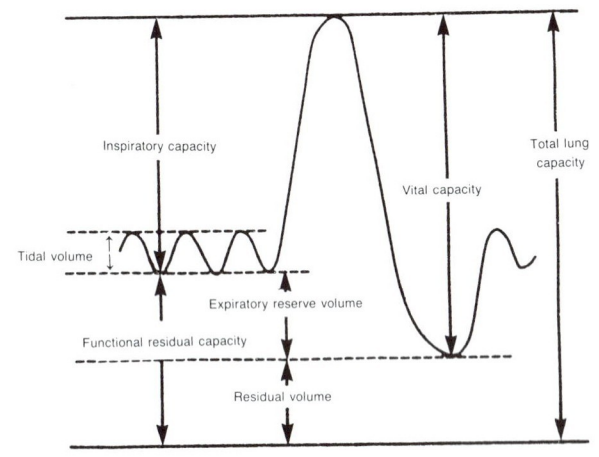

Figure 25-2 **Lung volume subdivisions.**

TABLE 25-1 Normal Values for Peak Flow, FVC and FEV_1*

	Male			Female		
Height (cm)	FVC (L)†	FEV_1 (L)†	PEFR (L/min)†	FVC (L)	FEV_1 (L)	PEFR (L/min)
110	1.311	1.134	160	1.146	0.976	145
115	1.452	1.250	175	1.268	1.078	157
120	1.609	1.378	191	1.403	1.191	170
125	1.782	1.519	208	1.552	1.316	184
130	1.975	1.674	226	1.718	1.454	199
135	2.188	1.845	247	1.901	1.606	216
140	2.424	2.034	269	2.104	1.774	234
145	2.685	2.241	293	2.328	1.960	253
150	2.975	2.470	319	2.576	2.165	274
155	3.296	2.723	348	2.851	2.392	296
160	3.652	3.001	379	3.155	2.642	321
165	4.046	3.308	414	3.491	2.919	347
170	4.482	3.645	451	3.864	3.225	376
175	4.966	4.018	491	4.276	3.562	407
180	5.502	4.428	536	4.732	3.936	441
185	6.095	4.881	584	5.236	4.348	477
190				5.794	4.803	517

*Values obtained with Roxon portable battery-operated turbine spirometer at the Hospital for Sick Children.
†FVC = forced vital capacity; FEV_1 = forced expiratory volume in 1 sec; PEFR = peak expiratory flow rate.

Patterns of PFTs Observed

OBSTRUCTIVE

- Forced vital capacity (FVC) normal or decreased
- Forced expiratory volume in 1 second (FEV_1) decreased
- Forced expiratory flow (FEF) at 75 to 25% lung volume (FEF_{25-75}) decreased
- Ratio of FEV_1 to FVC (FEV_1/FVC) <80% (normal: >80%)
- Total lung capacity (TLC) normal or increased
- Functional residual capacity (FRC) normal or increased
- Residual volume (RV) normal or increased
- RV/TLC normal or increased (normal: 20%)

RESTRICTIVE

- FVC decreased
- FEV_1 decreased
- FEV_1/FVC ≥80%
- TLC decreased
- RV normal or decreased (RV may be slightly increased in some neuromuscular disorders)
- FRC normal or decreased

Respiratory Distress

- Consider pulmonary and extrapulmonary disease (e.g., cardiac, neurologic, sepsis) in the differential diagnosis of respiratory failure—treat underlying cause

Respiratory Disease

Clinical Features
- Tachypnea or bradypnea—apnea
- Grunting, retractions, use of accessory muscles
- Cyanosis
- Decreased or absent breath sounds
- Drooling, stridor (upper airway obstruction)
- Wheeze (lower airway obstruction)
- Decreasing PaO_2, increasing $Pa{CO_2}$
- Restlessness, stupor, obtundation

Management
- Complete respiratory failure—initiate cardiopulmonary resuscitation (see p 530)
- Airway: position jaw, head; insert oral or nasopharyngeal airway
- Ventilation: if spontaneously breathing, provide humidified O_2. If gas exchange inadequate, will require assisted ventilation (bag + mask, endotracheal intubation; see pp 531, 572)
- IV access: In certain clinical situations (i.e., severe upper airway obstruction) risk for exacerbation of respiratory distress to the child by anxiety and pain of IV or phlebotomy must be weighed against need for IV access. Adequate hydration is important but use caution in cardiac or renal conditions where fluid overload may exacerbate respiratory distress.
- Consider pneumothorax if sudden onset of respiratory distress. In life-threatening situations there may be an indication for intrapleural needle aspiration on clinical grounds alone.
- Avoid pharyngeal suctioning in upper airway obstruction
- Position head up at 45° C
- CXR, lateral neck x-ray should *not* delay above management strategies
- Adequate cardiac and O_2 monitoring, and temperature control
- ABG; avoid reliance on venous blood gas in respiratory abnormalities; they are useful only if CO_2 is normal

Upper Airway Obstruction

- Prolonged inspiration
- Subcostal, suprasternal, and supraclavicular retractions
- Increased respiratory rate
- Stridor
- Barking cough is suggestive of subglottic or tracheal obstruction
- Aphonia suggests obstruction at level of cords

Management

- Foreign body (see p 448) and infection (Table 25-2) are major differential diagnoses in acute situation
- Investigations may include AP and lateral soft tissue x-rays of neck and chest. Obtaining radiologic investigations should *never* delay the establishment of an artificial airway in severe airway obstruction.
- Laryngoscopy and bronchoscopy may be required
- Barium swallow useful in detecting vascular compression in nonacute situation; CT scan for other extrinsic causes of airway obstruction

TABLE 25-2 Upper Airway Infection

Factor	Epiglottitis	Croup	Bacterial Tracheitis
Age	Usually older (2-6 yr)	Usually younger (6 mo-4 yr)	Any age
Sex	M = F	M > F	M = F
Agents	Bacterial: *H. influenzae* type b (+++), β-hemolytic strep (+)	Viral: parainfluenza 1 (+++), RSV, parainfluenza 2,3 (+), influenza	Bacterial: *S. aureus* pneumococcus, *H. influenzae*
Seasons	Year round	Late spring, late fall	Any time
Recurrence	Rare	Fairly common	Rare
Clinical	Toxic Severe airway obstruction Drooling, sitting forward Stridor Sternal recession	Nontoxic, but may be restless, cyanotic Not drooling Stridor common Sternal recession common Barking cough, hoarseness, coryza	Toxic Croup-like cough Stridor
Progression	Rapid	Usually slow	Moderately rapid

Epiglottitis

Management
- *Pediatric emergency*
- Diagnose on clinical grounds—"the four Ds": dysphagia, dysphonia, drooling, and distress
- *Do not obtain x-ray, or bloodwork* (child may deteriorate while procedures are being done)
- *Do not try to examine throat or upper airway*
- *Do not agitate child.* Keep NPO. Minimal handling.
- *Contact ENT and anesthesia personnel* immediately
- Controlled intubation done in OR *or*, if necessary, emergency room
- Once child is intubated: IV fluids and antibiotics appropriate for coverage against *Haemophilus influenzae* (cefuroxime usually first line)
- Continue IV antibiotics until child is over acute phase, then continue with oral antibiotics for 7 to 10 days total
- Rifampin prophylaxis recommended for patients and family (see p 236)
- Other *H. influenzae* infections may coexist, e.g., septic arthritis and meningitis

Croup (Acute Laryngotracheobronchitis)

Clinical Features
- See Table 25-2

Management
- Avoid agitation as much as possible
- Mild croup may be managed at home with PO fluids and humidity (bathroom with shower on)
- Warn parents that croup may be worse at night. May clear in cold air outside.

- Stridor at rest, moderate chest wall retractions, decreased air entry, and an anxious, restless child are all indicators of moderate-to-severe disease and signal the need for hospitalization
- A rising respiratory rate correlates well with a falling PaO_2. Hypercapnia occurs late in upper airway obstruction and is a sign of increasing respiratory failure.
- If concerned about degree of respiratory failure, ABG indicated
- Nurse in O_2 and humidity (croupette)
- Racemic epinephrine, 0.5 ml of 2.25% solution in 3 ml normal saline, by nebulizer may provide relief. Effect may last 30-60 min. May repeat q1-2h or, rarely, up to q20min if necessary. A child who has received racemic epinephrine must be admitted for observation.
- If not responding to racemic epinephrine, should be observed in ICU setting and may require intubation
- Use of steroids in severe croup is controversial

Bronchiolitis

Clinical Features (see also Table 25-2)

- Prodrome: upper respiratory tract infection ± fever, poor feeding, and irritability
- Physical signs include fever, dehydration, wheezing, dyspnea, tachypnea (rate, 50 to 80/min), intercostal indrawing with use of accessory muscles, and tachycardia. Rhonchi ± diffuse crepitations on auscultation.
- May see hyperinflation with increased AP diameter and hyperresonance
- Increasing severity indicated by apnea, decreasing PaO_2 (≤65 mm Hg), increasing $PaCO_2$ (≥45 mm Hg), tachy- or bradycardia, increasing tachypnea, cyanosis progressing to respiratory arrest

Management

- CXR examination shows hyperinflation, increased linear markings, and areas of atelectasis
- ABG: hypoxemia initially, then hypoxemia and hypercapnia in more severe cases
- Nasal swab for rapid detection of RSV antigen (fluorescent antibody technique)
- Humidified O_2 to maintain O_2 saturation >92%
- Trial of salbutamol (0.5% solution), 0.01 to 0.03 ml/kg in 3 ml normal saline, by inhalation
- Intubation and ventilation rarely required
- Ribavirin used only in consultation with infectious disease specialist in treatment of hospitalized children with severe RSV infections
- Indications for ribavirin include congenital heart disease, bronchopulmonary dysplasia, chronic lung disease, immunosuppression (chemotherapy, transplant), immunodeficiency, age <8 wk. Additional indications dictated by clinical situation.
- Ribavirin given by small particle aerosol generator (SPAG-2); possible teratogenicity, therefore warn pregnant women. Particles may precipitate on contact lenses.
- Mortality <1%. 30% of patients may have subsequent recurrent wheezing episodes. Recurrent wheeze likely due to asthma.

Pneumonia

Etiology (Table 25-3)

- Viruses most common overall
- Newborn: group B streptococci, *Escherichia coli, Listeria*
- 0-4 mo: consider CMV, *C. trachomatis*
- 0-5 yr: *H. influenza* type B most common; S. pneumoniae; in sick child <2 yr of age consider *S. aureus,* especially if pneumatocele, empyema
- >5 yr: *M. pneumoniae* (most common cause in school-age child); *S. pneumoniae*

- Aspiration: oral bacteria (anaerobes); may be associated with pleural effusion and lung abscesses
- Nosocomial: aspiration (oral bacteria), *S. aureus,* enteric bacilli

Investigations

- CBC, differential count
- Blood culture
- Sputum culture (nasopharyngeal cultures are not representative)
- ABG if patient in respiratory distress
- CXR
- Tuberculin skin test (0.1 ml PPD)
- Cold agglutinin titer, mycoplasma titer, throat swab for *Mycoplasma* culture
- Diagnostic thoracentesis if significant pleural fluid is present

Treatment

- General supportive care, including IV or PO fluids
- Humidified O_2
- IV or PO antibiotics (Table 25-4)
- Empyema requires chest tube drainage
- In compromised patients, broaden coverage to include *S. aureus* (cloxacillin, vancomycin), *P. aeruginosa* (aminoglycosides, piperacillin, ceftazidime), anaerobes (penicillin, clindamycin)
- Flexible bronchoscopy and bronchoalveolar lavage to rule out viral or *P. carinii* infection may be indicated in immunosuppressed patients or in those deteriorating on maximum therapy. Open lung biopsy is occasionally necessary (see p 281).
- Most regimens last 10-14 days total. *S. aureus* usually requires a minimum of 3 wk of therapy.
- Follow patient with CXR at 4-6 wk to document resolution of radiographic changes

TABLE 25-3 Epidemiologic, Clinical, and Laboratory Features of Acute Pneumonia in Normal Infants and Children According to Etiologic Agents

	Bacteria	Virus	Mycoplasma
Temperature	Majority ≥39° C	Majority <39° C	Majority <38° C
Onset	Abrupt, may follow URI	Gradually worsening URI	Gradually worsening cough (days-weeks)
Others in home ill	Infrequent	Frequent, concurrent	Frequent, weeks apart
Associated signs, symptoms	Respiratory distress common; meningitis and septic arthritis occasionally coexist; pleuritic chest pain common	Frequent: myalgia, rash, conjunctivitis, pharyngitis, mouth ulcers, diarrhea	Frequent: headache, sore throat, myalgia Occasional: rash, conjunctivitis, myringitis, enanthem, hacking paroxysmal cough—sometimes productive
Toxicity	+++	+	+
X-ray	Usually infiltrate in distribution of lobe or subsegment of lobe	Interstitial pattern—may be diffuse	May be lobar or diffuse
Pleural fluid	May occur	Infrequent; majority small	Infrequent; majority small

Modified from Long SS. Treatment of acute pneumonia in infants and children. Pediatr Clin North Am 1983; 30:299.

TABLE 25-4 Initial Antibiotic Therapy for Pneumonia

Antibiotics in Uncomplicated Pneumonia

Age	Inpatient	Outpatient
<8 wk	Ampicillin and aminoglycoside	—
8 wk-12 wk*	Ampicillin and cefotaxime	—
3 mo-5 yr	Cefuroxime	Amoxicillin
5-19 yr	Penicillin G or erythromycin†	Penicillin V or erythromycin

Antibiotics in Complicated Pneumonia

Pleural Effusion	Lung Abscess	Aspiration
Cefuroxime	Cloxacillin ± clindamycin	Penicillin or clindamycin + aminoglycoside

*Add erythromycin if *Chlamydia* is a concern.
†Will include *Mycoplasma* coverage.

Acute Asthma

History
- Duration and course of attack, triggering factors (may include viral respiratory tract infections, cold air, exercise, chemical irritants, tobacco smoke, stress, and allergens)
- Determine number of hospital admissions, dependency on steroids, history of ICU admissions, family history of asthma, allergies, medication and adverse drug reaction history
- Rule out cardiac disease, foreign body aspiration, gastroesophageal reflux, bronchiolitis

Physical Exam
- Assess for fatigue, restlessness, altered mental status, inability to speak. *Level of consciousness is major indicator of deterioration.*
- Beware RR >30 breaths/min, HR >110 beats/min in older child
- Look for cyanosis; use of accessory muscles of respiration; asymmetry of air entry; evidence of subcutaneous emphysema, pneumothorax, or pneumomediastinum
- Significant pulsus paradoxus >15 mm Hg. Differential diagnosis includes bronchiolitis, foreign body aspiration, GE reflux.

Investigations
- O_2 saturation monitoring if available
- ABG in moderate or severe cases—beware of patient with a normal, rising, or elevated $PaCO_2$, or with O_2 saturation <92% in room air
- CXR (if clinically indicated) may show hyperinflation, increased peribronchial markings, atelectasis, or evidence of pneumothorax or pneumomediastinum.

- Pulmonary function testing (e.g., peak flow) with portable spirometric device for objective assessment of degree of obstruction. In severe asthma, peak flow rates ~ 20% to 30% predicted value.
- Always obtain theophylline level if child already receiving theophylline preparation

Treatment

- Humidified O_2 to maintain O_2 saturation >92%, by mask or nasal prongs
- Correct fluid deficits if dehydration present and provide maintenance IV fluids and electrolytes. CAUTION: AVOID FLUID OVERLOAD.
- Sympathomimetic drugs: Salbutamol (drug of choice) (0.5% solution), 0.01 to 0.03 ml/kg (maximum 1 ml) in 3 ml normal saline, by aerosol mask. Mild cases: masks q3-4h; in moderate-to-severe cases, may give 0.03 ml/kg in 3 ml normal saline up to q20min.
- Anticholinergic drugs
  1. Ipratropium bromide (Atrovent) useful in treatment of acute asthma when combined with β_2 agents (e.g., salbutamol)
  2. May give 250 µg (1 ml) ipratropium bromide q4h with salbutamol mask; up to q1h in severe cases
- Corticosteroids
  1. Increasingly used early in the management of moderate-to-severe cases, in conjunction with aggressive bronchodilator therapy
  2. IV steroids indicated if child is on maintenance oral or inhaled steroids or if child has needed IV steroids in the last 6 mo
  3. IV hydrocortisone bolus, 4 to 6 mg/kg, then same dose q4-6h
  4. Alternatively, IV methylprednisolone, 0.5-1 mg/kg/dose q6h
  5. If patient improves, convert to oral steroids in 48 hr; taper over following week

- Theophylline
  1. IV drug may be aminophylline (80% theophylline) or theophylline
  2. Effect is dose related; therefore a level in the upper limit of the therapeutic range is best
  3. If child is not taking theophylline, or levels are subtherapeutic, give IV loading dose of 6.0 mg/kg theophylline over 20 min
  4. If child received oral theophylline within 12 hr prior to admission, once theophylline level is known, as a rule of thumb, giving 1.0 mg/kg of theophylline raises the serum level by 10 μmol/L. If level not available, half-load with 3 mg/kg.
  5. Following loading dose, start on maintenance theophylline as intermittent bolus or by continuous drip (see p 732 for protocol to switch from IV to PO in acute phase)
  6. Theophylline metabolism decreased (i.e., levels and potential toxicity increased) by liver disease, congestive heart failure, viral disease, and concurrent erythromycin or cimetidine administration. Conversely, phenobarbital and cigarette smoking increase theophylline metabolism, with potential subtherapeutic levels.
  7. Antibiotics have no role in treatment unless bacterial infection is documented
  8. In refractory cases, ICU care may be necessary for trial of IV salbutamol or possible intubation and ventilation

Chronic Asthma

Management

- Environmental control: eliminate specific environmental allergens or irritants (e.g., *cigarette smoke*)
- Immunotherapy: not generally useful in asthma, considered only if attacks are triggered by specific unavoidable allergens

- Exercise programs: should be encouraged; swimming often is well tolerated even in patients whose asthma is triggered by exercise. Inhalation of β_2 agonists or sodium cromoglycate prior to activity is often beneficial (see below).
- For maintenance therapy, one or more of the following categories of drugs may be necessary. Mild episodic asthma may respond to intermittent sympathomimetic drugs. If symptoms more frequent and persistent, consider maintenance therapy with a prophylactic agent.
- Sympathomimetic drugs
  1. Inhalation route preferred
  2. Salbutamol: give 0.01-0.03 ml/kg (maximum 1 ml) of 0.5% solution in 3 ml normal saline or in 2 ml of 1% sodium cromoglycate by aerosol mask q4-6h. Alternatively, may use metered dose inhaler of salbutamol: 100-200 µg (1-2 puffs) qid, or similar dose using any dry powder system. For children aged 4-7 yr, spacer (aerochamber) attachment useful, or powder inhaler may be tried. For infants and young children, aerochamber with mask may be used.
  3. Oral β_2 drugs in those too young for metered dose inhaler and who have no access to compressor: salbutamol, 0.3 mg/kg/day PO ÷ tid or orciprenaline, 2 mg/kg/day PO ÷ tid (maximum dose, 20 mg)
- Sodium cromoglycate (cromolyn sodium)
  1. Primarily maintenance prophylactic drug
  2. Useful before exposure to cold or in exercise-induced bronchospasm
  3. Usually delivered as dry powder—1 spincap qid or metered dose inhaler delivering 1 mg/puff available, with appropriate dose being 2 mg (2 puffs) qid
  4. May administer 1% solution by nebulizer qid with or without salbutamol

- Corticosteroids (inhalational, oral)
  1. Chronic or intermittent therapy added for patients inadequately controlled with above medications
  2. Beclomethasone, 300 to 400 μg/day (2 puffs 3 to 4 times/day); use of high-dose beclomethasone inhalation (up to 1600 μg/day) shown successful in some adult studies
  3. Adrenal suppression possible with high-dose inhalation
  4. Low-dose side effects include hoarseness and oral candidiasis: suggest rinsing mouth with water after each application; not necessary with aerochamber
  5. Severe asthma may require use of PO steroids for adequate control
  6. Steroid side effects are minimized with alternate day, single morning dose regimen
- Anticholinergic drugs
  1. Ipratropium bromide (Atrovent) available in metered dose inhaler: 20 μg/puff, 2 puffs qid
  2. Slower but more prolonged bronchodilation compared to β_2 drugs
- Theophylline
  1. Sustained-release oral preparations available for bid-tid dosing
  2. GI and CNS (irritability) side effects are main limiting factors
  3. See p 733 for monitoring of levels
- Ketotifen: newer oral prophylaxis. Used in combination with other agents. No effects prior to ~8-12 wk of therapy. Major side effect: mild sedation and weight gain are seen rarely. Dose: 1 mg PO bid >3 yr of age.

Cystic Fibrosis

Diagnosis

- Quantitative analysis of sodium chloride content in sweat using urecholine or pilocarpine iontophoresis is most reliable method of diagnosis

- Minimum of 100 mg of sweat should be collected
- May be difficult to obtain enough sweat in first weeks of life—this is the limiting factor in testing very young infants
- Sweat chloride >60 mmol/L in 98% of cases of cystic fibrosis (CF)
- False-positive results seen with poor laboratory technique, nephrotic syndrome, Addison's disease, malnutrition, nephrogenic diabetes insipidus, G-6-PD deficiency, glycogen storage disease, ectodermal dysplasia, and hypothyroidism
- Pancreatic dysfunction determined by use of 3- to 5-day fecal fat collection

MANAGEMENT

Respiratory

- Frequent sputum samples for culture and sensitivity
- Physiotherapy: postural drainage bid to tid in conjunction with bronchodilator therapy
- Inhalational therapy: used mist alone no longer
- Bronchodilators (salbutamol) often helpful, especially when given prior to physiotherapy as high percentage of CF population have component of hyperreactive airway disease
- Inhalational tobramycin (2 ml tid with salbutamol) is occasionally used in chronic maintenance therapy for up to 1 yr
- Long-term daily oral antibiotics are tailored to sputum C + S results, e.g., cloxacillin, cotrimoxazole, or oral cephalosporins
- Antenatal diagnosis now available: gene localized to long arm of chromosome 7. ΔF508 mutation is a 3-base-pair deletion present in 70% of CF chromosomes. Genetic counseling is advised.

Acute Chest Exacerbation
- Manifested by fevers, increased cough, shortness of breath, sputum production, anorexia, and weight loss
- Increased WBC and ESR may be seen, especially with *P. cepacia* infection
- Check for deterioration in PFTs, ABGs, and CXR
- Mild exacerbation: 2-3 wk trial of oral antibiotic if sputum grows *P. aeruginosa* and patient >13 yr, consider ciprofloxacin
- More severe: hospitalization, IV antibiotics appropriate for sputum C + S, inhalational therapy, physiotherapy, ± O_2, nutritional support

Nutrition

TABLE 25-5 Nutritional Management for Cystic Fibrosis

Calories	120 to 150%
Protein	RDA*
Essential fatty acids	3 to 5% total calories
Vitamin A	5,000 to 10,000 IU/day
Vitamin D	400 to 800 IU/day
Vitamin E	100 to 300 IU/day (water-soluble form)
Vitamin K	5 mg twice weekly for infants 5 mg daily for children and older
Vitamin Bs	RDA × 2
Vitamin C	RDA × 2

Pancreatic enzymes

Infants:	Add one regular cotazym capsule or 1/3 tsp powder to 4 oz of formula (8,000 U lipase/120 ml formula)
Children and adults:	Regular capsules = 6/meal (48,000 U lipase/meal); 2/snack (16,000 U lipase/snack) Enteric-coated microspheres (cotazym ECS) = 3/meal (24,000 U lipase/meal); 1/snack (8,000 U lipase/snack)

N.B.: Enteric-coated capsules are not to be used in children who cannot swallow capsules whole, as mucosal ulceration may develop.

*Recommended daily allowance.
Modified from MacLusky I, McLaughlin FJ, Levison H. Cystic fibrosis. Part II. Curr Prob Pediatr 1985; 15(7):11.

Pleural Effusion

- See Table 25-6
- Send fluid for cytologic examination (cell differential, RBC, WBC, and malignant cells), biochemistry (protein, glucose, pH, LDH, fat content if chylous), microbiology (Gram stain, C + S, acid-fast staining, virology), and immunologic investigations when appropriate (e.g., complement studies)
- Transudates associated mainly with congestive heart failure, nephrotic syndrome, acute glomerulonephritis, cirrhosis, myxedema
- Exudates commonly caused by infection (bacterial, viral, *Mycoplasma*, mycobacterial, fungal), collagen vascular diseases, malignancy, pancreatitis, and subdiaphragmatic abscess
- See p 565 for thoracocentesis. Chest tube generally indicated for empyema, severe respiratory distress, or rapid reaccumulation of pleural fluid.

TABLE 25-6 Constituents of Pleural Effusions

Test	Transudate	Exudate
Protein	<3 g/dl	>3 g/dl
Pleural to serum ratio, protein	<0.5	>0.5
Pleural to serum ratio, LDH	<0.6	>0.6
WBC	<1000/mm^3; usually >50% lymphocyte or mononuclear cells	>1000/mm^3 >50% PMN = acute inflammation >50% lymphocytes = TB, neoplasm
pH	>7.3	7.3 (inflammatory)
Glucose	= serum	↓
Amylase		↑ in pancreatitis

Pneumothorax

- Common causes include asthma, trauma, cystic fibrosis, iatrogenic or hyaline membrane disease, infection
- Incidence of spontaneous pneumothorax is highest in tall, thin, young adult males (approximately 1:10,000). Usually due to rupture of apical pleural blebs.

Clinical Features

- Dyspnea, chest pain, or shoulder tip pain
- May see marked respiratory distress and cyanosis on physical examination
- Chest wall movement decreased on affected side
- Percussion note on affected side tympanitic
- Larynx, trachea, and mediastinum may be shifted contralaterally
- Cardiac function may be compromised if pneumothorax is under tension

Management

- Small pneumothorax (<5%) requires only observation; usually spontaneous resolution within 1 wk
- Small pneumothoraces resolve more quickly with 100% O_2, which will increase N_2 gradient between pleural gas and blood. Beware CO_2-retaining patient depending on hypoxic drive. Avoid hyperoxia in premature infants.
- Larger pneumothoraces require chest tube drainage to underwater seal (see p 566)
- To prevent recurrences in patients at risk, consider chemical pleurodesis (e.g., quinacrine), possible open thoracotomy, and pleural bleb excision or plication and stripping of apical pleura

TWENTY-SIX

Rheumatology

Approach to the Child with Arthritis

History
- Early morning stiffness—often prominent with chronic arthritis
- Interference with activity
- Heel pain—may indicate enthesitis
- Associated fever or rash
- Older child—sexual activity
- Family history—psoriasis, inflammatory bowel disease, ankylosing spondylitis, or chronic back pain

Physical Examination
- *All* joints, including spine
- Gait—walking and running
- Muscle wasting
- Limb length discrepancy
- Bony tenderness
- Tenderness over entheses (sites of insertion of tendons and ligaments to bone)
- Tendon thickening

Investigations

- CBC + differential, ESR
- Blood cultures and antibody titers as indicated
- Antinuclear antibody (ANA)—especially if pauciarticular juvenile arthritis (JA)
  1. Rheumatoid factor (RF)—especially if polyarticular JA
  2. HLA B27—if ankylosing spondylitis psoriatic arthritis or arthritis associated with IBD
- Immunoglobulins, baseline liver function, renal function, urinalysis, and C3 and C4 if SLE is suspected
- X-ray of involved joints, if trauma, infection, malignancy, or chronic arthritis is suspected
- Ophthalmologic assessment—slit-lamp examination to detect uveitis, particularly in a young child with pauciarticular arthritis
- Bone scan, if osteomyelitis is suspected
- Arthrocentesis, if septic arthritis is suspected

TABLE 26-1 Synovial Fluid Analysis

	Normal	Inflammatory	Infectious
Color	Colorless to straw	Yellow	Variable
Turbidity	Clear	Clear to turbid	Turbid
White cell count	$<0.2 \times 10^9$/L (<200/mm^3)	2.0-75.0×10^9/L ($2,000$-$75,000$/mm^3)	Often $>100 \times 10^9$/L ($>100,000$/mm^3)
Neutrophils, %	<25	>50	>75
Glucose	Nearly equal to blood glucose	<2.8 mmol/L below blood glucose	>2.8 mmol/L below blood glucose
Culture	Negative	Negative	Often positive

Modified from Kelley WN, Harris ED, Ruddy S, Sledge CB. Textbook of rheumatology. Vol. 1, 2nd ed. Philadelphia: W.B. Saunders, 1985:562.

Juvenile Arthritis (JA)

Diagnostic Criteria
- Arthritis in one or more joints for at least 6 wk
- Onset <16 yr
- Exclusion of other rheumatic diseases
- Classification (based on clinical presentation in first 6 mo after onset of disease)
  1. Systemic: fever, rash, hepatosplenomegaly, lymphadenopathy, serositis, leukocytosis, anemia
  2. Polyarticular: ≥5 joints
  3. Pauciarticular: ≤4 joints

Management
- Education of patient and family
- Drug therapy
  1. First line
     - Nonsteroid anti-inflammatory drugs, e.g., naproxen (Naprosyn), tolmetin sodium (Tolectin), indomethacin (Indocid). If ASA is used, levels should be monitored and influenza vaccine should be administered annually.
  2. Second line
     - Hydroxychloroquine
     - Gold salts
     - D-Penicillamine
     - Sulfasalazine

3. Corticosteroids
   - Local: eyes (for uveitis); intra-articular
   - Systemic: indicated for systemic JA with life-threatening complications or fever unresponsive to nonsteroidal anti-inflammatory drugs; chronic uveitis unresponsive to topical therapy; severe polyarticular JA
4. Immunosuppressive agents, e.g., methotrexate
- Physical and occupational therapy
  1. Exercise to maintain range of motion of joints and muscle strength
  2. Activities such as swimming and bicycle riding
- Splints to help prevent deformity
- Heat (e.g., warm bath)—helps to relieve pain and stiffness, may be useful in early morning
- Multidisciplinary approach: physiotherapy, occupational therapy, social worker, school, orthopaedic surgery, ophthalmology

TABLE 26-2 **Subgroups of Juvenile Arthritis***

	Pauciarticular Type I	Pauciarticular Type II	Polyarticular RF-Negative	Polyarticular RF-Positive	Systemic Onset
% of JRA patients	30	15	25	10	20
Sex	80% girls	90% boys	90% girls	80% girls	Male = female
Age at onset	Early childhood	Late childhood	Throughout childhood	Late childhood	Throughout childhood
Joints	Large joints—knee, ankle, elbow	Large joints—hip girdle	Symmetric—any joints	Symmetric—any joints	Usually polyarticular—any joints
Sacroiliitis	No	Common (late)	No	Rare	No
Iridocyclitis	30% chronic iridocyclitis	10% acute iridocyclitis	Rare	No	No

RF	Negative	Negative	Negative	100%	Negative
ANA	60%	Negative	25%	75%	Negative
Association with HLA-B27	No	Yes	No	No	No
Ultimate morbidity	Ocular damage	Subsequent spondyloarthropathy	Severe arthritis 10-15%	Severe arthritis, >50%	Severe arthritis, 25%
Extra-articular		Psoriasis, colitis, enthesitis			Lymphadenopathy, fever, hepatosplenomegaly, rash, serositis, leukocytosis, anemia

*Classification based on clinical presentation within first 6 mo after onset of disease. RF = rheumatoid factor; ANA = antinuclear antibodies.

Modified from Schaller JG. Chronic arthritis in children. Clin Orthop 1984; 182:79-87.

TABLE 26-3 Differential Diagnosis of Arthritis in Childhood

Trauma
Infection
- Bacterial: *S. aureus, H. influenzae*, meningococcus, gonococcus, mycobacteria
- Viral: Rubella, hepatitis, parvovirus, EBV (may precede hepatitis)
- Other: Mycoplasma
  Lyme arthritis—*Borrelia burgdorferi*

Malignancy: Leukemia, neuroblastoma, bone tumor
Hematologic disease: Hemophilia, sickle cell disease
Rheumatic disease

Type	Important features
Juvenile arthritis	Pauciarticular or polyarticular arthritis
Juvenile ankylosing spondylitis (JAS)	Asymmetrical, pauciarticular arthritis, lower limbs, usually boys >10 yr
Psoriatic arthritis	Commonly asymmetrical pauciarticular arthritis; may have polyarticular arthritis or dactylitis ("sausage" digit characteristic); typical rash often absent at time of diagnosis
Arthritis with inflammatory bowel disease	Commonly, peripheral pauciarticular arthritis; GI symptoms may be subtle
Reactive arthritis Rheumatic fever	See revised Jones criteria, p 51 ; migratory pauciarticular arthritis, large joints
Postinfections arthritis	Following gastrointestinal or genitourinary infection, e.g., *Salmonella*, *Shigella*, *Yersinia*, Reiter's syndrome
Vasculitis syndromes Henoch-Schönlein purpura	Usually transient arthritis, large joints; palpable purpura ± renal and GI involvement
Kawasaki disease	Usually transient arthritis (see p 518)

Henoch Schönlein Purpura

- Clinical diagnosis; most managed as outpatients. Major differential diagnosis is thrombocytopenia or infectious causes of purpura.
- For most, baseline renal function and urinalysis is adequate
- More severe impairment of renal function; 24-hr urine studies
- May have associated ↑ IgA
- If hospitalized (severe GI, renal, CNS): treatment is mainly supportive (hydration, nutrition). Steroid use is controversial but advocated by some for GI hemorrhage, testicular torsion, CNS; no proven value in renal disease.
- Surgical consultation if intussusception, testicular torsion suspected

Kawasaki Disease

- 80% of affected children are <4 yr
- Most common in children of Asian descent; more common in blacks than whites
- Most common cause of acquired heart disease in children

Diagnostic Criteria

- Fever lasting ≥5 days
- Presence of four of the following five conditions
  1. Bilateral nonpurulent conjunctival injection
  2. Oral mucosal changes: may have any one of erythema, dryness or fissuring of lips, strawberry tongue, erythema of oropharynx
  3. Peripheral extremities: may have any one of edema or erythema of palms or soles, desquamation of tips of fingers or toes
  4. Rash: commonly truncal; polymorphic, nonvesicular
  5. Cervical lymphadenopathy >1.5 cm
- Illness unexplained by another disease

Associated Clinical Features
- Irritability, arthritis, aseptic meningitis, hydrops of the gallbladder, hepatic dysfunction, anterior uveitis, diarrhea, pneumonitis, urethritis, serous otitis media

Cardiovascular Manifestations
- Acute phase (febrile):
  1. Myocarditis, pericarditis, endocarditis
  2. Arrhythmias
  3. ECG abnormalities
- Subacute phase (afebrile, but elevated ESR and platelet count): coronary artery aneurysms in approximately 20% of untreated cases

Laboratory Features (Nonspecific and Nondiagnostic)
- Increased WBCs, neutrophilia
- Mild-to-moderate anemia
- Elevated ESR
- Increased platelets in subacute phase

Treatment
- All treatment should be in consultation with rheumatologist and cardiologist
- Acute phase: ASA 100 mg/kg/day and IV gammaglobulin 2 g/kg × 1 dose
- Subacute phase: ASA 3-5 mg/kg/day ± dipyridamole

Incomplete (Atypical) Kawasaki disease
- May not fulfill all diagnostic criteria
- Difficult to diagnose in very young infants
- Maintain high index of suspicion in any prolonged febrile illness

Follow-up
- ECG and 2D-ECHO at 3 wk, 2 mo, 6 mo, ± 1 yr after disease onset

TWENTY-SEVEN

Surgery

Neonatal Abdominal Emergencies

- Vomiting of bile-stained fluid in the first few days of life indicates intestinal obstruction until proven otherwise
- Sepsis must be ruled out
- Consider surgical problem if: polyhydramnios, excessive salivation ("mucousy"), cyanosis, choking with feeds, abdominal distention, passage of meconium more than 24 hr after birth (meconium may be passed from bowel distal to an obstruction), large gastric aspirate in the delivery room

General Management Principles
- NPO
- Cross match ~100 ml packed red cells at time of admission
- Hemodynamic ± ventilatory support
- Correct electrolyte and acid-base abnormalities
- A No. 10 nasogastric tube should be passed in any suspected intestinal obstruction in newborns >2000 g; No. 8 if <2000 g. Usually open-ended; occasionally to low Gomco suction.
- Chest, abdominal x-rays (AP, lateral decubitus)
- Radiocontrast enema to rule out malrotation, volvulus, and colonic atresias. If normal, follow by upper GI and follow-through contrast studies.
- Rule out other congenital anomalies

ESOPHAGEAL ATRESIA

- Polyhydramnios, excess salivation, choking with feeds ± cyanotic spells
- Diagnosis made by inability to pass a No. 10 nasogastric tube into the stomach, and demonstration of its tip in air-filled dilated proximal esophagus (usually T3-5) on CXR
- An air-contrast outline of the pouch can be obtained by taking a CXR while insufflating the pouch with air through the tube

Management

- See general management principles (p 520)
- Surgery to correct atresia with fistula usually done within 24 hr of diagnosis. May be delayed if
  1. Aspiration pneumonitis
  2. Severe associated cardiac (or other) anomalies
- While awaiting surgery, the infant should be kept head-up, supine, or prone, with suction tube in proximal pouch to avoid further aspiration

DUODENAL ATRESIA OR STENOSIS

- Not associated with distended abdomen; jaundice may be present. If obstruction proximal to ampulla of Vater, vomitus is *not* bile stained (less than 10% of cases).
- See general management principles (p 520)
- Abdominal x-ray: "double bubble" pattern classically
- Acid-base and electrolyte status ($\downarrow K^+$, $\downarrow Cl^-$, metabolic alkalosis)
- Urgent contrast enema to rule out malrotation, volvulus, and colonic atresias. Usually followed by upper GI contrast studies.

SMALL INTESTINAL ATRESIA

- May be associated with cystic fibrosis
- See general management principles (p 520)
- Abdominal x-ray: intestinal distention and multiple air-fluid levels
- Contrast enema: helpful in defining level and cause of obstruction and ruling out a more distal second obstruction

MALROTATION WITH MIDGUT VOLVULUS

- Presentation may be similar to that of necrotizing enterocolitis ± hematochezia ± peritoneal signs
- Presentation may be delayed or subacute
- See general management principles (p 520)
- Abdominal x-ray: multiple air-fluid levels or a relatively gasless abdomen; occasionally, the film is compatible with duodenal obstruction
- Urgent radiocontrast enema and upper GI study necessary to confirm the presence of malrotation or duodenal obstruction
- Delays associated with high morbidity and mortality 2° to gangrenous small bowel

MECONIUM ILEUS

- >95% associated with cystic fibrosis. Complicated meconium ileus may present with signs of peritonitis (± intra-abdominal calcifications) 2° to intrauterine volvulus or perforation of the gut.
- See general management principles (p 520)
- Abdominal x-ray: distended bowel may have "ground glass" appearance; air-fluid levels may be absent, ± intra-abdominal calcifications

- In uncomplicated meconium ileus, gastrograffin or Hypaque Muco-myst enema is used to relieve the obstruction in an attempt to avoid surgery. Repeated attempts are often necessary to produce complete resolution.
- Surgery is required in ~50% of patients
- Sweat chloride >1-2 mo of age (see p 502)

NECROTIZING ENTEROCOLITIS

- Should be strongly considered in the presence of abdominal distention, feeding intolerance, bloody stools, bilious aspirates
- In the acute stages, frequent assessments including abdominal x-rays q6-8h are necessary to exclude pneumoperitoneum
- Abdominal x-ray variable; thickened bowel loops ± free peritoneal fluid; pneumatosis intestinalis or gas in the portal vein
- Reddened edematous abdominal wall
- CBC, differential (may have decreased platelets, decreased WBC)
- Full septic screen including CSF, urine, blood, and stool cultures
- Barium enema is contraindicated during the acute episode, unless diagnosis is in doubt
- See general management principles (p 520)
- IV antibiotics (e.g., ampicillin, gentamicin, and clindamycin) × 7-10 days
- Indications for surgical intervention include
  1. Perforation
  2. Increasing abdominal wall erythema
  3. Failure of medical therapy
  4. Persistent fixed loop on consecutive abdominal films
- Complications include late strictures (3-4 wk) usually of the large bowel, may be asymptomatic; "short-gut" syndrome with malabsorption

HIRSCHSPRUNG'S DISEASE

- May present as neonatal enterocolitis. Rectal examination often results in explosive passage of liquefied meconium and air in previously obstructed infant.
- Barium enema may not be diagnostic in the first few days of life but *is* useful in excluding other causes of bowel obstruction. Barium is not cleared in a delayed film 24 hr later in Hirschsprung's disease.
- Rectal biopsy necessary to confirm absence of ganglion cells
- Decompressing colostomy initially; later, definitive pull-through surgery

DIAPHRAGMATIC HERNIA (BOCHDALEK)

- CXR diagnostic (e.g., bowel loop in thoracic cavity)
- Cardiorespiratory monitoring essential
- See general management principles (p 520)
- Consider early sedation and paralysis for optimal cardiorespiratory support
- Poor prognostic signs
  1. Respiratory distress in first 12 hr of life
  2. Hypoplastic lungs, persistent pulmonary hypertension, and "high" ventilatory requirements

HYPERTROPHIC PYLORIC STENOSIS

- Jaundice and constipation are frequent accompanying features
- Diagnosis made by palpating the pyloric "tumor." To facilitate examination
  1. Insert No. 10 nasogastric tube and connect to suction to empty the stomach
  2. Allow baby to drink a solution of warm dextrose water while flexing legs at the hips to relax the abdominal wall

3. As the baby relaxes, the hypertrophied pylorus is felt midway between the xiphisternum and the umbilicus in the middle position of the upper abdomen
4. Structures that can be mistaken for the pylorus include left lobe of liver and right kidney
- Consider congenital adrenal hyperplasia (neonate with vomiting, dehydration, and electrolyte abnormalities) in differential diagnosis
- If the diagnosis is in doubt, abdominal U/S or upper GI series
- Laboratory: decreased Cl^-, decreased K^+, metabolic alkalosis
- Mild-to-moderate dehydration is present in most cases; can be severe if the diagnosis is made late
- Correct fluid and electrolyte deficits prior to surgery. A useful approach is 0.45% normal saline with KCl, 20 mEq/L, to correct deficit; provide for maintenance and ongoing losses. May initially require colloid
- Surgery is definitive treatment, early refeeding postop

Miscellaneous Emergencies in Older Children

INTUSSUSCEPTION

- The classic presentation of colicky abdominal pain, currant jelly stools, and palpable abdominal mass is often not seen.

Investigations and Management

- See general management principles (p 520; neonatal principles apply to older children)
- Air-contrast enema will confirm diagnosis and may be used to reduce intussusceptions in ~85% of cases. (Barium enema an alternative)
- ~10% incidence of recurrence after successful hydrostatic reduction; early surgery in these cases
- Hydrostatic reduction of an intussusception contraindicated when there is clinical evidence of peritonitis or far-advanced intestinal obstruction (danger of perforation)

APPENDICITIS

Management
- See general management principles (p 520)
- Antibiotics (usually ampicillin, gentamicin, and clindamycin) are used for all cases of ruptured appendicitis and continued for 5-7 days
- A dose of an antibiotic, usually cefoxitin, is given preoperatively for prophylaxis in unruptured appendicitis
- When the diagnosis is not certain, hospitalize and observe

INGESTED FOREIGN BODY

- Long, sharp objects in the stomach may be removed endoscopically or with a magnetic probe under fluoroscopy. Once past the pylorus, they may be allowed to advance spontaneously unless symptoms of persistent abdominal pain develop, or if impaction of the object against the intestinal wall results in arrest of distal migration, in which case laparotomy is indicated.
- Enemas or cathartics *should not* be used to evacuate most foreign bodies. Exception: enemas may be used to increase evacuation of micro batteries used for cameras and calculators. After 48 hr, leakage of corrosive fluids contained within the battery can result in bowel perforation.

INGUINAL HERNIAS

- High incidence of incarceration below age 1 yr, with danger of testicular artery thrombosis as well as intestinal obstruction
- Reduction of previously incarcerated hernia should be followed by repair within 24-48 hr.
- In premature infants, repair usually delayed until a weight of 2500 g is attained

CRYPTORCHIDISM

- Most undescended testes will descend during first year of life.
- Hormonal treatment (β-HCG) best in retractile high scrotal testes. Not usually successful in true undescended testes but may increase size, which will make surgery easier. Side effects related to increased production of testosterone.
- Orchidopexy at ~age 18 mo-2 yr

BILIARY ATRESIA

- Associated developmental anomalies may coexist: situs inversus, dextrocardia, polysplenia
- Differential diagnosis usually includes neonatal hepatitis or metabolic diseases resulting in hepatic dysfunction (see p 216)
- Liver biopsy and liver scan (DISIDA) are the most useful tests for discriminating between neonatal hepatitis and biliary atresia
- Portoenterostomy (Kasai procedure) is most successful in relieving jaundice if done before the age of 2 mo
- Liver transplantation is the treatment of choice if diagnosis is made after 3 mo due to poor results of late Kasai

UMBILICAL GRANULOMA

- Results from chronic infection at the site of umbilical cord separation
- Treatment: cautery with silver nitrate sticks
- Must be differentiated from omphalomesenteric duct remnants (look for fecal or serous discharge), which may require excision and abdominal exploration

TWO

EMERGENCIES

Cardiopulmonary Resuscitation

- See inside cover for quick guide to resuscitation drugs
- Unlike adults, the precipitating factor in the majority of pediatric cardiac arrests is not a cardiac event but hypoxia secondary to respiratory failure and hypovolemia
- Arrhythmias in arrests: asystole following bradycardia (80%) or bradyarrhythmias (10%). Ventricular arrhythmias (10%) predominantly in underlying congenital heart disease or direct cardiac trauma.
- Preceding history critical to definitive management

BASIC LIFE SUPPORT

- Determine unresponsiveness
- Call for help
- Open the airway
  1. Head extension to neutral position
  2. Chin lift
  3. Jaw thrust
- Check breathing
  1. Look, listen, and feel
  2. If patient is breathing, check for cause of coma
- Ventilate
  1. Mouth to mouth
  2. Mouth to nose
- If chest not moving, consider airway obstruction: see p 531
- If central pulse is slow (<80/min neonate; <50/min older infant and child), start cardiac compressions
  1. Infant: on sternum just below intermammary line, 100/min; depress 1.5 to 2.5 cm, using two or three fingers
  2. Child: lower sternum, 80-100/min; depress 2.5 to 4 cm, using heel of hand

ADVANCED LIFE SUPPORT

- Airway, Breathing
  1. Endotracheal intubation (see p 572)
  2. Provide 100% O_2 if possible. Non-rebreathing bag-valve-mask apparatus delivers 70-90% O_2; anesthetic bag delivers 100% O_2.
- Circulation: establish parenteral access
  1. Attempt peripheral IV once or twice, then try intraosseous infusion (see p 563)
  2. Cut down on long saphenous vein, antecubital fossa, or femoral vein. In abdominal and lower extremity trauma, sites on upper body are preferred.
  3. Percutaneous access to central veins if experienced personnel are available
- Drugs
  1. See Table 1 for recommended therapy
  2. If IV access is not established early, endotracheal route may be used for epinephrine, atropine, isoproterenol, or lidocaine (same doses as IV)
- IV fluids
  1. For intravascular volume expansion, suitable fluids include isotonic crystalloid (Ringer's lactate, normal saline) or colloid (5% albumin). Fresh frozen plasma may be used when available. Type of solution not as critical as volume administered.
  2. Generally use 20 ml/kg as an initial bolus and 10-20 ml/kg during the subsequent hour; response to volume reflected as changes in heart rate, peripheral perfusion, capillary refill, and blood pressure
- Defibrillation (for ventricular fibrillation)
  1. One paddle on upper right chest below the clavicle and the other paddle at the level of the left nipple in the anterior axillary line
  2. Initially, 2 joules/kg (2 watt-sec/kg)
  3. If unsuccessful, then 4 joules/kg
  4. Repeat once more, if necessary, 4 joules/kg
  5. If unsuccessful, correct hypoxemia, acidosis, other metabolic abnormalities and hypothermia; administer epinephrine and repeat defibrillation at 4 joules/kg as necessary

TABLE 1 Drug Therapy in Cardiopulmonary Resuscitation

Diagnosis	First-Line Therapy	Secondary
Asystole, bradycardia or normal rate with no pulse	O_2, $NaHCO_3$, epinephrine, fluid bolus	Atropine, isoproterenol, dextrose, ± calcium
Ventricular fibrillation	O_2, defibrillation	Lidocaine, $NaHCO_3$, epinephrine, ± bretylium
Sinus tachycardia	O_2 Fluid bolus	
Tachyarrhythmias	See pp 48-49	

CONTINUING SUPPORT

- Monitor and correct abnormalities in ABG, electrolytes, glucose, and calcium
- Continue with elective ventilation even if spontaneous respiratory effort returns. Posthypoxic encephalopathy can be minimized by maintaining effective cerebral perfusion and oxygenation in the postarrest period. Sedation and muscle relaxation may be required.
- Avoid hypothermia (common)

Anaphylaxis

- Treat patient at first sign of anaphylaxis. Do not wait for symptoms and signs to evolve.
- ABCs
- Discontinue any ongoing parenteral medications or blood products
- O_2 by mask
- Medications
  1. Epinephrine 1:1000 (1.0 mg/ml) 0.01 ml/kg (min 0.1 ml/dose; max 1.0 ml) SC, or epinephrine 1:10,000 (0.1 mg/ml) 0.1 ml/kg (min 1 ml/dose; max 10 ml) IV. May repeat once in 5 min.
  2. Diphenhydramine 1-2 mg/kg (max 50 mg) IM or IV
  3. If severe reaction, hydrocortisone 5-10 mg/kg IV
- If BP is falling, treat as for shock (see p 548)
- If bronchospasm is present, treat as in asthma (see p 498)
- Observe patient for recurrence of symptoms (that may be life threatening) over the next 24 hr
- See p 14 for management of anaphylaxis once acute episode is resolved

Choking

- If good air exchange (forceful cough, wheezing inspiration, and loud cry), allow child to continue with spontaneous efforts to clear the airway. Poor air exchange (very weak or nonexistent cough, no cry) or total airway obstruction requires definitive management.

CHILD >1 YR

- Six to 10 abdominal thrusts (Heimlich maneuver), administered in standing position in the older conscious child, or by placing the heel of one hand on the abdomen between the umbilicus and the rib cage with the child in a recumbent position. Thrusts should be directed inward and upward.

- If above maneuvers unsuccessful, use head extension and tongue-jaw lifts (anterior displacement of the mandible, using fingers behind the mandibular ramus or by gripping the mandible anteriorly and lifting forward). If a foreign body is visualized, finger sweeps may be used to remove it. Blind finger sweeps may further impact the foreign body and should be discouraged.
- When the child is unconscious, continue with basic CPR and attempts at ventilation. If ventilation is not possible, repeat above maneuvers.

INFANT

- In the choking infant, abdominal thrusts may be traumatic and should be avoided if other means are effective
- Place the infant in 60° head-down position, lying on the rescuer's forearm
- Administer four back blows between the shoulder blades with the heel of the rescuer's hand
- If unsuccessful, turn the infant over and administer four chest thrusts (as with cardiac compression)
- Attempt to visualize foreign body in mouth; if seen, remove with finger sweeps
- Open airway with tongue–jaw lift technique
- Attempt to ventilate
- Repeat the above maneuvers until ventilation is possible
- If unsuccessful, abdominal thrusts may be attempted

Coma and Altered Level of Unconsciousness

- The most common pattern of coma in children is a diffuse impairment of cerebral hemisphere function
- A useful mnemonic to remember the important causes in children is AEIOU & TIPS (see Table 2)
- Clinical features: most patients are stable at presentation but may have a rapidly progressive process and require simultaneous investigations and therapy. Occasionally, patients require emergency resuscitation with few initial investigations.

TABLE 2 Causes of Coma: AEIOU & TIPS

A	Alcohol	T	Trauma, tumor
E	Encephalopathy, endocrinopathy, electrolytes	I	Infection
I	Insulin, intussusception	P	Psychiatric
O	Overdose	S	Seizure, stroke
U	Uremia		

Adapted with permission from Advanced Pediatric Life Support. Copyright ©1989, American Academy of Pediatrics (Elk Grove Village, Ill.) and American College of Emergency Physicians (Dallas, Tex.)

Management

- Initial assessment (ABCDE)
  1. Airway, breathing
     - Frequently overlooked in unconscious children
     - Ensure airway patent
     - Assess adequacy of respiratory effort
  2. Circulation
     - Check vital signs, perfusion
     - Monitor; start IV
     - Chemstrip: give glucose 0.25 g/kg (25% dextrose 1 ml/kg), expectantly, or if Chemstrip low
  3. Disability (neurologic status)
     - Glasgow Coma Scale (Table 3)
     - Check pupils; give naloxone (0.03 mg/kg) if small or pinpoint
  4. Exposure
     - Measure temperature
     - Check for obvious evidence of trauma
- Secondary survey
  1. History
     - History of known underlying illness, acute fever, trauma, ingestion
  2. General and neurologic examination (Table 4)
     - Look for evidence of infection, intoxication, and metabolic and traumatic causes
     - Oculomotor movements
     - Motor responses (focal signs)
     - Breathing patterns
     - Fundi (retinal hemorrhages), fontanelle, nuchal rigidity, bruits

TABLE 3 Modified Glasgow Coma Scale*

	Score	<1 yr	>1 yr	
Eye opening	4	Spontaneously	Spontaneously	
	3	To shout	To verbal command	
	2	To pain	To pain	
	1	No response	No response	
Motor response	6	Obeys	Obeys	
	5	Localizes pain	Localizes pain	
	4	Flexion with drawal	Flexion with drawal	
	3	Decorticate	Decorticate	
	2	Decerebrate	Decerebrate	
	1	No response	No response	
	Score	0-23 months	2-5 yr	>5 yr
Verbal response	5	Smiles, coos, cries	Appropriate words and phrases	Oriented and converses
	4	Cries	Inappropriate words	Disoriented, converses
	3	Inappropriate cry or scream	Cries or screams	Inappropriate words
	2	Grunts	Grunts	Incomprehensible sounds
	1	No response	No response	No response

*ICU, Hospital for Sick Children.

TABLE 4 **Distinguishing Diffuse Versus Focal Causes of Coma**

	Diffuse	**Focal**
History	Previous illness	± Previous illness
Consciousness	Gradual ↓	Rapid ↓
General physical exam	Breath, odor, skin color	Trauma
Progression	Affects different levels simultaneously	Rostral-caudal changes
Breathing	↑ than ↓ RR	Ataxic
Pupils	Small, equal and reactive	Unequal and/or unreactive
Focal signs	Less common	Common
Motor	Myoclonic jerks Multifocal seizures Symmetrically decorticate or decerebrate Grasping rigidity	Focal oculomotor changes Facial asymmetry Monoparesis or hemiparesis ↓ Cough or gag

Investigations

- Will depend on knowledge of etiology and clinical condition
- Determine need for CT
  1. Diffuse causes (majority): infection, ingestion, metabolic; CT not essential immediately
  2. Focal cause (usually trauma): CT essential
- Blood: CBC, culture, ABG, glucose, electrolytes, BUN, creatinine, calcium, magnesium, liver enzymes, NH_4, clotting screen. Blind toxic screen without specific history NOT generally useful except for acetaminophen ingestion, as most other ingestion injuries will present with specific clinical picture.
- Urine: urinalysis, culture, latex agglutination
- CSF: cell count, protein, glucose, Gram stain, culture, latex agglutination. Opening pressure may be useful but is difficult to measure accurately in infants and young children. LP contraindicated if profoundly comatose, evidence of raised ICP, or hemodynamic instability.
- Gastric fluid: toxic screen if specific history
- Radiology: head CT; plain x-rays of chest, cervical spine, abdomen; skeletal survey
- Other: ECG

Continuing Support

- Treat underlying problem
- Increased ICP (see below)
- Seizures
- Homeostasis: O_2, CO_2, fluids, acid-base, electrolytes, nutrition

Raised ICP

- Clinical features
  1. Early: headache, vomiting, decreased level of consciousness, full fontanelle
  2. Advanced: decreased HR; increased BP; unequal or unresponsive pupils; papilledema; cranial nerve III, IV, VI palsies; other evidence of herniation

- General management
  1. Careful handling
  2. Elevate head of bed 30° and keep head in midline to decrease pressure on jugular veins
  3. O_2 (PaO_2 >100 mm Hg)
  4. Intubate and hyperventilate ($PaCO_2$, 25-30 mm Hg). Premedication with lidocaine may prevent rise in ICP associated with intubation. Intubation in this situation should only be attempted by experienced personnel skilled in the use of anesthetic agents.
  5. Maintain cerebral perfusion pressure (mean arterial pressure >60 mm Hg)
  6. Fluid restriction (30-50%)
  7. Normothermia
- Pharmacologic management
  1. Mannitol 0.2-0.5 g/kg/dose (1-2.5 ml/kg/dose of 20% solution over 10-30 min), q2h PRN. Monitor urine output.
  2. Dexamethasone 0.1-0.25 mg/kg q6h may be of benefit
- Other
  1. ICP monitoring: useful only if risk of rapid increase in ICP
  2. Surgical decompression for severely increased ICP; only effective if space-occupying lesion or Reye's syndrome

Environmental Illnesses

HYPERTHERMIA AND HEAT ILLNESSES

- Fluid and electrolyte loss and exertion in a hot climate are major factors in environmental heat illnesses
- Often not associated with significant core temperature elevation
- Guidelines
  1. <41° C: seldom harmful, although discomfort may occur >39.5° C and neurologic symptoms secondary to temperature alone can develop >40.5° C
  2. 41-42° C: can tolerate for brief periods
  3. >42° C: usually harmful; cellular damage will occur >42.2° C

- Heat exhaustion is characterized by temperature of ≥39° C and water depletion with lethargy, thirst, headache, vomiting, increased HR, decreased BP, hemoconcentration, hypernatremia, increased urine specific gravity
- Salt depletion may predominate with similar features to above as well as weakness, fatigue, muscle cramps, hyponatremia, increased urine Na
- Heat stroke is characterized by core temperature ≥41° C with
  1. More severe neurologic dysfunction: combativeness, delirium, convulsions, and coma when temperature >43° C
  2. Vomiting and diarrhea
  3. Hot skin; sweating may stop
  4. Risk of rhabdomyolysis, acute tubular necrosis, and DIC
  5. Circulatory collapse
  6. Na normal or increased, CPK increased, Ca increased

Management

- Mild hyperthermia: remove from heat source; remove clothing; antipyretics; fluid replacement (PO or IV); cool with ice packs to head and trunk
- More severe: requires rapid cooling (consider immersion in ice bath), O_2, and cardiovascular support. Promote diuresis with furosemide or mannitol if myoglobinuria.
- Malignant hyperthermia: treat with dantrolene and supportive measures in intensive care setting

HYPOTHERMIA

- Definition: core temperature <35° C. Hypothermic patients with absent vital signs are not considered deceased until rewarmed to >33° C with no subsequent response to resuscitation.
- Cardiorespiratory system
  1. Immediate increase in BP, HR, then decreased HR with prolonged cooling. Complete vasomotor paralysis occurs at ∼ 30° C. ECG shows prolongation of all phases of the cardiac cycle, and a J wave (elevation of the ST segment) may be seen at 33-32° C.

2. Sinus bradycardia or atrial fibrillation at 30° C. Ventricular fibrillation from 28-26° C; slow sinus rhythm may be maintained.
  3. Immediate hyperventilation, then normoventilation from 35-33° C
  4. Hypoventilation or apnea (especially in premature neonates) at lower temperatures
- Neuromuscular
  1. Early shivering thermogenesis, followed by abolishment of shivering, progressive rigidity, and pupillary dilation from 33-30° C. Coma occurs at 30-28° C; fixed dilated pupils, <25° C.
- Renal: "cold diuresis," acute tubular necrosis, hypokalemia, or hyperkalemia
- Metabolic: lactic acidosis

Investigations

- CBC, electrolytes, BUN, creatinine, glucose (especially in neonates), amylase, blood gases, drug screen, coagulation screen, thyroid function, CXR, ECG
- Monitor core temperature, blood pressure, ECG, urine output, and temperature of inspired gases

Management

- ABCs; note that arrhythmias may be resistant to cardioversion until rewarming occurs
- Correct metabolic acidosis
- Rewarming
  1. Mild hypothermia (33-35° C): passive slow external rewarming, i.e., remove from exposure, remove wet clothing, cover with warm blankets
  2. Moderate hypothermia (30-33° C): add active external rewarming, i.e., heated water mattress, immersion in warm water (37-40° C; not often practical), radiant heater. Also, active core (airway) rewarming: give warm humidified O_2 (40-45° C by mask, or 40° C if intubated).

3. More severe hypothermia: additional core rewarming, i.e., warm (37° C) IV fluids, gastric lavage, or colonic irrigation with warm normal saline. Peritoneal dialysis, hemodialysis, or cardiopulmonary bypass in refractory cases.

Prevention

- Avoid prolonged exposure during procedures and transport
- Nurse in the thermoneutral range
- Warm IV fluids when large volumes given
- Monitor temperature frequently

FROSTBITE

- May accompany hypothermia or may occur independently; usually restricted to head and extremities—frozen part is white and firm.
- After the core temperature has returned to normal, immerse the injured extremity for about 20 min into water kept 37-40° C (do not start to thaw an extremity if there is any chance of the patient being re-exposed to the cold)
- Refer patient to plastic surgeon if extensive area of involvement

NEAR DROWNING

- Hypothermia often present; may improve prognosis but hinders cardiac resuscitation. Reliable prognostication not possible until patient rewarmed to >33° C and trend of hemodynamic and neurologic status determined.

Management

- Pre-hospital care
  1. Immediate mouth-to-mouth resuscitation in the water
  2. Remove from water with cervical spine control, as there may be other injuries
  3. Full CPR, if necessary, once on a solid surface. Do not use Heimlich maneuver.
  4. 100% O_2 as soon as available
- Hospital care
  1. ABCs with cervical spine control
  2. 100% O_2
  3. Monitoring: frequent vital signs including temperature, cardiac monitor, O_2 saturation, urine output
  4. IV, NG tube
  5. Investigations: ABG, CXR (may be deferred initially)
  6. Indications for immediate intubation
     - Apnea
     - Tachypnea at rest
     - FiO_2 requirement > 0.5 to achieve $PaO_2 \geq 90$ mm Hg
     - $PaCO_2 > 40$ mm Hg
     - Inability to protect airway
     - Significantly altered level of consciousness
  7. Secondary survey
     - History: consider possible neglect or abuse, substance abuse
     - Physical exam: Glasgow Coma Score, complete neurologic exam, look for other injuries
     - Investigations: CBC, electrolytes, BUN, creatinine, coagulation ± specific drug levels if indicated by history
  8. Treatment
     - Fluid bolus (10-20 ml/kg isotonic crystalloid or colloid)
     - $NaHCO_3$ (1-2 mmol/kg prior to initial gas if prolonged asphyxia)
     - Bronchodilators and diuretics as indicated
     - Treatment of CNS injury: prevention and treatment of increased ICP (see p 539)

9. Criteria for hospitalization (any of the following)
   - Submersion >1 min
   - Loss of consciousness at any time
   - Cyanosis at any time
   - Apnea at any time
   - Requirement for any resuscitation at the scene

SMOKE INHALATION

- Always give 100% O_2 from time of rescue until proven unnecessary
- Consider in *all* fire victims, but especially when history of exposure in a confined space, loss of consciousness at the scene, or history of deaths at the scene. Physical markers include facial burns, singed nasal hairs, hoarse voice, carbonaceous sputum
- Multiple mechanisms of injury: thermal (upper airway edema, obstruction), particulate matter (tracheobronchitis), toxic fumes (alveolitis if distal airways reached). Carbon monoxide and cyanide can enter the blood and poison cellular respiration.

Management

- Investigations
  1. ABG: metabolic acidosis common; PaO_2 does NOT reflect available oxygen in the presence of carboxyhemoglobin
  2. Carboxyhemoglobin level (COHb): elevated levels require treating with 100% O_2; reduces half-life to approximately 60 min
  3. CXR: essential as baseline but may be normal in the first 24 hr in up to 40% of patients

- Treatment
  1. Airway patency (N.B.: delayed development of edema)
     - Endotracheal intubation for O_2, humidification, tracheobronchial hygiene, continuous positive airway pressure (CPAP), or intermittent positive pressure ventilation (IPPV) with positive end-expiratory pressure (PEEP)
     - Relatively high ventilation pressures and PEEP may be required because of the alveolar capillary leak, reduced compliance, and possible pulmonary edema
  2. Supplemental O_2: high FiO_2 (100% if possible) until COHb levels are <0.05 (5%), or 5-6 hr of therapy. Hyperbaric O_2 therapy may be considered if available.
  3. Bronchial hygiene: humidification, suction, physiotherapy, bronchoscopy (rare) to remove tracheal debris
  4. Fluids: aim for urine output 1 ml/kg/hr. N.B.: risk of Adult Respiratory Distress Syndrome (ARDS); careful monitoring essential.

Shock

- Early recognition critical. Classical symptoms and signs often absent due to compensatory mechanisms. May see only mild increase in HR and decrease in BP before complete cardiovascular collapse. Concurrent hypothermia further masks signs and symptoms, as well as hinders therapy.
- Early symptoms: poor feeding, fever, lethargy or irritability, decreased urine output; history of underlying illness
- Early signs:
  1. Resting tachycardia, tachypnea
  2. Normal systolic blood pressure but
     - decreased pulse pressure suggests hypovolemia
     - increased pulse pressure suggests sepsis
  3. Mottling, cool extremities, increased capillary refill time (normal, ≤2 sec)
- Early laboratory: metabolic or mixed acidemia with elevated lactate, hyper- or hypoglycemia
- Some forms of shock have specific clinical features
  1. Septic shock: early hyperdynamic "warm" phase
  2. Neurogenic shock: hypotension without tachycardia or decreased peripheral perfusion
  3. Cardiogenic shock: gallop rhythm with hepatomegaly, cardiomegaly, or dilated neck veins
  4. Obstructive shock: muffled heart sounds or increased resonance with chest percussion
- Manifest shock
  1. Hypotension: systolic BP <5th %ile for age (<80 mm Hg systolic from 6 wk to 6 yr old) (see pp 360-365) or documented decrease of 30% from pre-shock state
  2. Tachycardia
  3. Decreased peripheral perfusion: weak peripheral pulses, cool extremities, mottled skin, increased capillary refill time
  4. Decreased urine output (<1 ml/kg/hr)
  5. Altered mental state: lethargy, confusion, combativeness, coma

TABLE 5 Types of Shock

Type	Primary Circulatory Derangement	Common Causes
Hypovolemic	↓ intravascular blood volume	Hemorrhage, trauma Fluid losses, gastroenteritis
Distributive	Vasodilation → venous pooling → ↓ preload Maldistribution of regional blood flow	Sepsis Anaphylaxis CNS or spinal injury Drug intoxication
Cardiogenic	↓ Myocardial contractility	Heart surgery Congenital heart disease Arrhythmias Hypoxia, ischemia
Obstructive	Mechanical obstruction to ventricular inflow or outflow	Cardiac tamponade Tension pneumothorax Coarctation of aorta

Adapted from Witte MK, Hill JH, Blumer JL. Shock in the pediatric patient. Adv Pediatr 1987; 34:139-174.

Management

- Respiratory support
  1. O$_2$ to keep O$_2$ saturation ≥90% or PaO$_2$ ≥60 mm Hg
  2. Low threshold for artificial ventilation; reduces work of breathing and cardiac demands, especially in cardiogenic and septic shock
- Hemodynamic support
  1. Preload (circulating blood volume)
     - Initial: isotonic crystalloid (0.9% normal saline or Ringer's lactate) 10-20 ml/kg, over 15-30 min then assess for response (heart and respiratory rate, capillary refill, sensorium, urine output). May repeat to give 30 ml/kg total.
     - Subsequent (if little or no response to fluids)
       a. Isotonic colloid (5% albumin) or blood products when specifically indicated, alternating with crystalloids for further fluid therapy
       b. CVP monitoring necessary, especially for distributive or cardiogenic shock
       c. Hypovolemic shock: consider CVP monitoring. Further boluses of 10 ml/kg as needed.
       d. Distributive or cardiogenic shock: increase contractility and afterload (see below), avoiding use of large volumes of fluids
  2. Contractility
     - Correct pH and other substrate abnormalities
     - Adequate ventilation
     - NaHCO$_3$ if pH still <7.20 once PaCO$_2$ <40 (give weight [kg] × base deficit × 0.15 mmol). Repeat if necessary.
     - Glucose infusion; ensure calcium and electrolytes are normal
     - Dopamine (Fig. 1) 5-20 μg/kg/min. N.B.: Dopamine should always be administered through a central line when possible because of the risk of tissue necrosis, although in an emergency setting the drug may be administered peripherally (IV or intraosseous) for a short period at low doses and preferably through a separate line. Infusion of inotropes generally requires ICU setting
     - Epinephrine (Fig. 1) 0.1-1 μg/kg/min (rarely needed except in severe shock)
  3. Afterload
     - Will be improved initially with above measures. Later, afterload reduction with vasodilators may be necessary

Amount (mg) to Put into 50 ml Syringe

μg/kg/min	0.15 × wt	0.3 × wt	0.6 × wt	1.5 × wt	3 × wt	6 × wt	15 × wt	30 × wt	60 × wt
	ml/hr	ml/hr	ml/hr						
0.05	1								
0.075	1.5								
0.1	2	1							
0.2	4	2	1						
0.3	6	3	1.5						
0.4	8	4	2	ml/hr					
0.5	10	5	2.5	1					
0.6	12	6	3						
0.7	14	7	3.5						
0.8	16	8	4						
0.9	18	9	4.5		ml/hr				
1	20	10	5	2	1				
1.5		15	7.5	3	1.5	ml/hr			
2		20	10	4	2	1			
2.5				5	2.5				
3			15	6	3	1.5			
3.5				7	3.5				
4				8	4	2			
4.5				9	4.5		ml/hr		
5			20	10	5	2.5	1		
6				12	6	3			
7				14	7	3.5			
8				16	8	4			
9				18	9	4.5			
10				20	10	5	2		
12					12	6			
14					14	7		ml/hr	
15					15		3	1.5	ml/hr
20					20	10	4	2	1
25							5	2.5	

Isoproterenol 0.05 – – Dopamine 1.0 / 2.0 – 25

Nitroglycerin, Salbutamol 0.5 – 10

Epinephrine, Morphine 0.1 – 1.0

		15	3	1.5
		20	4	2
			5	2.5
			10	5
			15	7.5
			20	10

30				
40				
50				
100	6			
150	8			
200	10			
	20			

Figure 1 Table for calculation of drug infusion dilution (1) Select desired drug dosage to be delivered in μg/kg/min (see named bars to right of chart—start at lower end of the dose range and adjust according to response). (2) Select infusion rate of syringe pump in ml/hr from table. (3) Calculate number of milligrams of drug to be mixed in 50 ml syringe: wt = patient's weight (kg). If 250-ml bag is used, add same mass of drug, but run at 5 × rate quoted in table.

For example, a 7-kg infant requires dopamine: from the bars on the right of the chart, the range of dosages for dopamine is 2 to 25 μg/kg/min; start with 2 μg/kg/min. We will opt for a rate of fluid infusion of 1 ml/hr. For 1 ml/hr to give 2 μg/kg/min, we need to put 6 × weight, i.e., 42 mg into 50 ml of solution. (Modified from Shann F. Continuous drug infusion in children: a table for simplifying calculation. Crit Care Med 1983; 11:462-463.)

Investigations

- Blood
  1. CBC, platelets, coagulation screen, ABG, electrolytes, BUN, creatine, calcium
  2. Culture if appropriate
  3. Cross-match if appropriate
- CXR
- Sepsis work-up if appropriate

Monitoring

- Noninvasive monitoring
  1. Vital signs every 15 min initially
  2. Blood pressure
  3. Continuous ECG
  4. Bladder catheterization for urine output
  5. Pulse oximetry for O_2 saturation monitoring
  6. Arterial blood gases if oximetry not available
- Invasive monitoring
  1. Central venous line for CVP
  2. Arterial line for repeated blood sampling, blood pressure monitoring

Further Management

- Specific treatment of underlying illness: antibiotics for sepsis (p 271); surgical treatment of hemorrhage, tamponade, or pneumothorax; corticosteroids for suspected adrenal insufficiency
- NG tube to empty stomach and decrease risk of aspiration
- Diuretics (furosemide) to promote urine output (when euvolemic)
- Observation for development of multiorgan failure and secondary complications (infection)

Child Abuse

Definitions
- Physical injury or deprivation of nutrition, care, or affection in circumstances indicating that such injury or deprivation is not accidental
- Age-inappropriate sexual encounter between a child and another individual. N.B.: Children may be the victims of more than one type of abuse.

Investigations
- History
  1. Allegations made by or on behalf of the child
  2. Guardian(s): social risk factors, substance abuse, mental health, present crisis; history of sexual or physical abuse in guardian
  3. Child: development, past injuries, illness or accidental poisoning, behavior
  4. Presenting complaint: contradictory or no explanation; explore circumstances and home management of the injury; assess appropriateness
- Physical examination (Table 6)
  1. Must be conducted with patience and sensitivity
  2. Complete examination is essential
  3. Plot heights and weights on appropriate charts
  4. Examine fundi of infants; check for retinal hemorrhages
  5. Examine genitalia and anus. Do internal examination only if specific indications. DO NOT use restraining measures: if the child will not cooperate, defer examination or enlist the help of a subspecialist.
  6. Document all visible trauma—size, shape, color, and location
  7. Record child's behavior and reactions
- Laboratory
  1. Suspected physical abuse
     - Hematology—rule out blood dyscrasia
     - Skeletal survey or bone scan in young children—record location and age of fractures; rule out metabolic bone disease

2. Alleged sexual abuse; see also p 149
   - Forensic specimens; some jurisdictions use sexual assault evidence kit
   - Specimens for sexually transmitted diseases
   - Pregnancy test
3. Color photography: record obvious trauma—important legal documentation

Treatment and Further Management

- Most jurisdictions have laws requiring professionals to report *suspected* child abuse to the appropriate authorities *without delay*
- Admit for treatment or protection if indicated
- Treat injuries and other medical problems, e.g., sexually transmitted diseases, as indicated
- Obtain necessary consultations, e.g., social work, psychiatry
- Protection assessment to be carried out by appropriate authorities
- Disposition to be planned with joint medical and social input

TABLE 6 Child Abuse Indicators*

Physical

1. Injuries not explained by history given
2. General care and nutrition
   - Inadequate clothing
   - Poor hygiene
   - Failure to thrive
   - Inadequate medical attention
3. Bruises and welts
   - On face, back, buttocks, thighs
   - At different stages of healing
   - In the shape of an instrument or hand
4. Burns
   - Cigarette burns, especially multiple burns
   - Immersion burns
   - Burns in the shape of an instrument
   - Rope burns
5. Fractures
   - To skull or facial structure
   - Multiple, particularly at different stages of healing
   - Spiral fractures
6. Retinal hemorrhages
7. Genitourinary
   - Pregnancy
   - Sexually transmitted diseases
   - Abnormal dilation of orifices

Behavioral

Child
1. Extreme wariness of parents and adults in general
2. Extremes of behavior, e.g., aggressiveness, withdrawal, compliance, fearfulness
3. Pseudomature behavior
4. Self-destructive behavior, including suicide threats or attempts
5. Changes in school performance
6. Running away from home
7. Sexual acting out or age-inappropriate sexual knowledge
8. Functional complaints, particularly abdominal pain

Guardians
1. Poor self-control, seem under stress
2. Not responsive to child's needs
3. History of physical or sexual abuse as a child
4. Single parent, particularly if young and without support systems
5. Substance abuse
6. Mental illness

*Some of these symptoms and behaviors can be caused by events other than child abuse. Also, almost any physical or behavioral symptom can be the result of child abuse. However, those listed above are indicators that, particularly in combination, should raise the suspicion of the examining physician.

Transport of the Sick Child

- The keys to a successful transport include
  1. Stabilization of the patient at the base facility
  2. Anticipation of likely complications
  3. Availability of qualified transport personnel (usually a nurse, respiratory therapist ± physician)
  4. Adequate fixation of all lines, drains, and tubes prior to performing the transport
  5. Communication with receiving physician and institution
  6. Use of most appropriate transport method
  7. Discussion of transport with receiving physician (trauma team leader, general surgeon, ICU, emergency room)
  8. Receiving hospital should be requested to retrieve patient if transport facilities available
- Land
  1. Quicker to arrange
  2. May be stopped en route to perform tasks or diverted to another hospital if patient suddenly deteriorates
  3. Slower for long journeys; spine fractures a concern re: movement
  4. Requires more fluids, drugs, O_2 for the trip
  5. Paramedic assistance may not be available
- Helicopter
  1. Not always available (already in use; bad weather)
  2. May require land transport to helicopter
  3. Fast for medium-distance transport
  4. Usually well equipped
  5. Paramedic support usually provided
- Fixed wing aircraft
  1. Slow to arrange
  2. May not have equipment or personnel provided
  3. Requires land transport at each end
  4. Useful for long-distance transport to a major facility once patient is stabilized

- In addition, transport by helicopter or fixed wing aircraft involves transport at altitude. The extra problems include
  1. Increased gas volume during ascent, e.g., expansion of pneumothorax, air in stomach, air in inflated cuff of endotracheal tube, air above fluid level in drip chamber of IV line
  2. Fall in the partial pressure of O_2; worse in unpressurized craft
  3. Often increased background noise levels, making auscultation difficult
  4. Vibration of concern in new spine fractures
  5. Confined space, with difficult access to the patient, especially if the aircraft interior is not designed for regular patient transport
- Prior to transport
  1. Check equipment
     - Intubation equipment, including bag and mask
     - Adequate O_2 supply
     - Stable IV access; sufficient fluids for maintenance and resuscitation
     - Drugs available, drawn up, and at hand (e.g., anticonvulsants)
     - Suction equipment
     - Humidification, e.g., small condenser humidifier on endotracheal tube
     - ECG monitor
     - BP cuff or Doppler monitor
     - O_2 saturation monitor if available
     - Precordial or esophageal stethoscope
  2. Ensure that appropriate personnel accompany the child, e.g., M.D., transport-trained R.N., respiratory therapist or paramedic
- Respiratory
  1. Secure the airway: endotracheal intubation if necessary: nasal tube preferable to oral tube (more stable). Use a bite block in orally intubated patients.
  2. Ensure adequate ventilation, oxygenation.
  3. Insert chest tubes if there is pneumothorax and attach to Heimlich valves to avoid clamping chest drains
  4. Use a condenser humidifier (i.e., Swedish nose)

- Cardiovascular
  1. Stabilize the blood pressure and pulse rate before transport
  2. Two intravenous cannulas are advisable. Portable syringe drivers are preferable to hanging fluid bags because of limited head room.
- Other
  1. NG tube to open drainage
  2. Aim to maintain normothermia
  3. Monitor dextrostix for high risk patients (neonates, fasting, liver failure)
  4. Keep record of observations during transport

Triage of the Multiple Trauma Patient

- The history of the mechanism and force of the trauma is important in the anticipation of possible injuries, which may not be initially apparent
- Common life-threatening problems in the immediate period after the traumatic event include acute respiratory failure (e.g., airway obstruction or apnea) and hemorrhagic shock

Immediate Management

- ABCs with cervical spine control
- Additional experienced staff should be alerted
- Consider transfer to a pediatric trauma center after
  1. Stabilization
  2. Organizing the transfer through direct physician-to-physician contact

Stabilization

- Secure a patent airway
  1. Assume that the patient has a fractured cervical spine
  2. Clear the pharynx; position the chin and jaw as for CPR

3. Intubate if
   - Simpler measures of clearing airway fail
   - The patient has a Glasgow coma score of 7 or less (see p 537)
   - There is an airway burn
- Assist ventilation if
  1. Apnea
  2. Inefficient ventilation due to chest trauma
  3. Glasgow coma score of 7 or less
- Intravenous access preferable with two wide-bore cannulas
- Hemostasis and fluid resuscitation
  1. Even in the presence of head injury, give initial bolus of 10-20 ml/kg of crystalloid (Ringer's lactate) or colloid (5% albumin) in a patient with signs of hypovolemic shock after trauma (see p 548)
  2. Have sufficient fluid available to continue resuscitation during transport of the patient
  3. Transfuse with packed red cells if more than 10% of the child's blood volume has been lost (blood volume in a child is approximately 80 ml/kg)
  4. Antishock trousers (MAST) have limited uses and many potential complications (increased vascular resistance, hemorrhage). Should not be used in the presence of pulmonary edema or myocardial dysfunction and only with caution if there is CNS injury or suspected diaphragmatic rupture. Use only if available in pediatric size.
- Examine patient thoroughly for significant injury (see assessment below)
- Place NG or orogastric tube (consider the latter in the presence of facial or basal skull fractures)
- O_2 to all patients initially
- In hospitals with medium level trauma care facilities, baseline investigations should be performed before transport to a pediatric trauma center: ABG, hemoglobin, cross-match, electrolytes, and CXR
- Chest tube(s) in all ventilated patients with documented pneumothorax or hemothorax
- Measures to avoid hypothermia (see p 543)

Further Assessment

- Head
  1. Laceration, bruising, swelling ± fracture
  2. Hemorrhage from nose, mouth, or ears or clear fluid (CSF) from nose or ears
  3. Unequal or abnormally reacting pupils, abnormal extraocular movements, penetrating eye injury, visual acuity disturbances
- Neck
  1. Tenderness
  2. Laryngeal or tracheal injury (abnormal cry, stridor, subcutaneous emphysema)
  3. Assume there is cervical spine fracture during initial exam
- Chest
  1. Flail segment or penetrating wounds
  2. Signs of pneumothorax or hemothorax (tracheal deviation, auscultation for reduced air entry, chest expansion)
  3. Rib fractures, bruising over precordium
- Abdomen
  1. Penetrating wounds
  2. Bowel sounds
  3. Guarding
  4. Peritoneal lavage should not be performed unless discussed with a pediatric surgeon
- Pelvis
  1. Instability or pain on compression
  2. Perineal injury
- Extremities
  1. Fractures-dislocations *(remove clothing)*
  2. Pulses, perfusion
- Back
  1. Tenderness of spine
  2. Bruising of flanks

THREE

PROCEDURES

Venous Access

- For all procedures involving skin puncture, skin should be prepared with appropriate antiseptic, e.g., povidone-iodine × 1 min followed by alcohol
- For difficult or urgent access (dehydration, shock, CPR, trauma), internal jugular vein, femoral vein or cutdown of saphenous vein are alternatives, but should be accessed by skilled personnel, preferably in intensive care or emergency room setting
- Syringe for blood withdrawal should be attached after vein is entered to allow for initial spontaneous blood return ("flashback") into cannula or butterfly needle
- Scalp vein needles with shorter bevels are available
- Proper restraint, positioning, equipment, and lighting are essential
- For access to external jugular vein, needle should penetrate skin in caudal direction where vein crosses sternomastoid muscle
- For access to femoral vein, needle should be inserted medial to femoral pulse, 1-2 cm distal to flexion crease of groin, aiming cephalad and slightly medially until vein is entered
- When starting intravenous infusions using a "butterfly" needle and catheter, the catheter should be flushed with saline prior to insertion into the vein. In general, once inserted, needle or catheter should be flushed with 2-3 ml saline prior to connecting to IV tubing to rule out extravasation
- IV catheters may be left in situ for 72 hr; may allow longer period depending on clinical indications and availability of alternative access
- In intra-abdominal trauma, avoid using lower limb veins for venous access
- For larger-gauge catheters (18G, 16G) consider local anesthetic

INTRAVENOUS CUTDOWN

- Equipment: No. 15 blade scalpel, 4-0 nylon or silk stitch, 4-0 silk ligatures, a fine hemostat, scissors, appropriate-gauge IV catheter (18 G or 20 G), 1% lidocaine, sterile gloves, towels, sponges, disinfectant
- Optimal site: long saphenous vein at angle 1 cm above and 1 cm medial to medial malleolus. The antecubital fossa veins are smaller and vary in distribution
- 1-cm transverse incision is made; visualize vein by using hemostat to separate fat and subcutaneous tissues in a direction parallel to vein
- Pass two 4-0 silk ties around vein, using distal tie to apply downward traction to vein
- A small nick is made on the surface of the vein, followed by gentle insertion and advancement of venous catheter. The proximal 4-0 tie is used to secure the vein to the catheter.
- 4-0 nylon or silk suture is used to close the incision and secure hub of catheter to skin

INTRAOSSEOUS ACCESS

- Used in emergency situations. Landmark is 2 cm inferior and 1 cm medial to tibial tuberosity. Needle is inserted at a 90° angle, using a clockwise "screwing" motion until bony cortex has been penetrated. Remove stylet by counterclockwise "unscrewing" motion.
- May infuse drugs and blood products, flushing with saline after each
- Blood return may not occur; therefore, must ensure that needle is not subcutaneous with test saline infusion
- Often unstable and easily dislodged: may fix using a hemostat clamped to hub and taped to extremity

LONG-TERM CENTRAL VENOUS LINES

- Generally two types: external (e.g., Roka or Hickman catheter) and buried reservoir (e.g., Port-a-cath)
- Buried reservoir requires needle insertion whenever hook-up is required; otherwise remains "invisible"

Advantages	Disadvantages
External	
No pain involved in hook-up	Twice-weekly heparin flush
Double-lumen catheters available for large volumes, chemotherapy, dialysis, TPN	Frequent dressing changes
	No swimming
	Risk of pulling out
Buried	
Little care at home	Incorrect needle placement when hooking up
Heparin flush in hospital q 4-6 wk	Discomfort with hook-up
Normal activities, swimming	

- Complications: infection (especially coagulase-negative *Staphylococcus*), obstruction (blockage, thrombosis), mechanical

Respiratory Procedures

- All needles, catheters, and tubes should be inserted over superior surface of rib to avoid damage to neurovascular bundle

NEEDLE ASPIRATION OF PNEUMOTHORAX

- Indicated for immediate management of cardiovascular compromise (e.g., tension, pneumothorax), using IV catheter, 10-ml syringe, and three-way stopcock
- 20-23 G intravenous cannula is inserted into 2nd interspace in midclavicular line or 5th interspace anterior or midaxillary line
- Remove air using syringe attached via stopcock to catheter to decrease tension while monitoring hemodynamic parameters. Alternatively, catheter can be attached to IV tubing with distal end under water
- Should always be followed by insertion of chest tube under controlled conditions

THORACOCENTESIS

- Positioning: infant held against chest of assistant; older cooperative child leaning forward against pillow or backrest of chair
- Check fluid level by percussion, upright CXR, or U/S
- After appropriate antiseptic and draping, infiltrate with 1% lidocaine to anesthetize skin, muscle, and pleura
- 18 G needle or intravenous catheter attached via tubing to three-way stopcock and 20-ml syringe
- Needle inserted bevel down along posterior axillary line at fluid level (generally 6th to 7th interspace appropriate, but will depend on volume, loculation, etc.)
- Aspirate fluid slowly in 20-30 ml aliquots using syringe and stopcock
- Must obtain follow-up CXR post procedure to rule out pneumothorax

CHEST TUBE INSERTION

- Equipment: 1% lidocaine, chest tube (No. 8 for preterm, 10-12 for infant, 22 for child <40 kg, 24 for child >20 kg or adult), No. 15 blade scalpel, hemostat, Kelly forceps, 2-0 silk suture, Pleurovac or bottle with underwater seal drain (or Heimlich valve if available), tubing for Pleurovac
- Landmarks: 5th interspace anterior or midaxillary line. Slightly more anterior incision favors posterior placement in pleural cavity and vice versa
- Patient should be positioned lying down with affected hemithorax elevated to near vertical position
- After antiseptic preparation and appropriate draping, infiltrate skin with 1% lidocaine
- Measure approximate distance chest tube to be inserted prior to insertion
- 1-1.5-cm incision is made; Kelly forceps (hemostat in smaller infants) are advanced through the chest wall between the 5th and 6th ribs. Spreading of tips once through pleura and inside pleura cavity creates a tunnel. Kelly forceps or hemostat are used to guide tip of chest tube through tunnel and into pleural cavity.
- Chest tube must remain clamped while being inserted before connecting to tubing to prevent inspiration of air into pleural cavity
- Chest tube is advanced to variable distance (generally until resistance is felt, i.e., several cm). Condensation will form inside tube confirming location in pleural cavity.
- Chest tube is then fixed to skin using purse-string silk suture to facilitate subsequent removal of tube and closure of skin defect
- Connect tube to Pleurovac set at suction of 10-20 cm of H_2O or underwater seal
- CXR essential to confirm position of tube and assess effects
- Generally removed after 72 hr if no further escape of free air as evidenced by bubbling in underwater seal, and/or no reaccumulation of intrapleural air with suction off or tube clamped × 24 hr. *Always remove tube at end of inspiration to prevent reaccumulation of pneumothorax.*
- Postremoval CXR should always be done.

TRACHEOTOMY

- Tracheotomy should be performed only by skilled and experienced personnel
- Cricothyroid puncture with 16 G IV catheter attached to 3-ml syringe barrel with plunger removed will allow for emergency oxygenation via a T-piece until more definitive airway management is possible. This set-up allows for insufflation but note that patient actually exhales passively through vocal cords (not through catheter). This procedure carries significant risk of complications and should only be performed after failure of less invasive techniques to establish airway in a life-threatening situation.

Abscess Incision and Drainage

- Equipment: 1% lidocaine, No. 15 blade scalpel, hemostat, povidone-iodine-soaked ¼″ gauze, topical ethyl chloride
- Limited effectiveness of topical anesthesia as pH of pus and surrounding tissue inactivate lidocaine; topical ethyl chloride may be optimal form of anesthesia.
- Small incision is made in overlying skin. After pus is evacuated (gentle probing with hemostat for loculated pus), abscess cavity is packed with povidone-iodine-soaked gauze (Q12h × 4) and covered with clean dressing.

Umbilical Vein Catheterization

- Generally indicated for emergency venous access, exchange transfusions
- Equipment: appropriate umbilical vessel catheter (3.5-5 Fr for artery, 5-8 Fr for vein), three-way stopcock, iris forceps, Hunt probe, syringes, blunt-ended needle, saline, heparin, umbilical tape, silk skin suture, adhesive tape, No. 15 blade scalpel
- The shoulder-umbilicus length should be measured, and the appropriate calculation made (Fig. 1) to determine catheter insertion length
- Umbilical tape is loosely tied at the base of the stump for hemostasis
- After antiseptic preparation and appropriate draping, umbilical stump is cut with scalpel to within 1.0-1.5 cm of the abdominal wall
- Identify exposed vessels (two thick-walled arteries — and one thin-walled, larger vein)
- Insert catheter which is connected to syringe via three-way stopcock ± blunt-ended needle (system filled with heparinized saline: heparin, 1 U/ml of normal saline), while maintaining gentle traction on cord stump
- The catheter is secured with a "pursestring" suture around the stump, followed by a "bridge tape" support (Fig. 2)
- Confirm position of catheter with x-ray (in IVC above diaphragm)
- Main complication is thrombosis and embolism

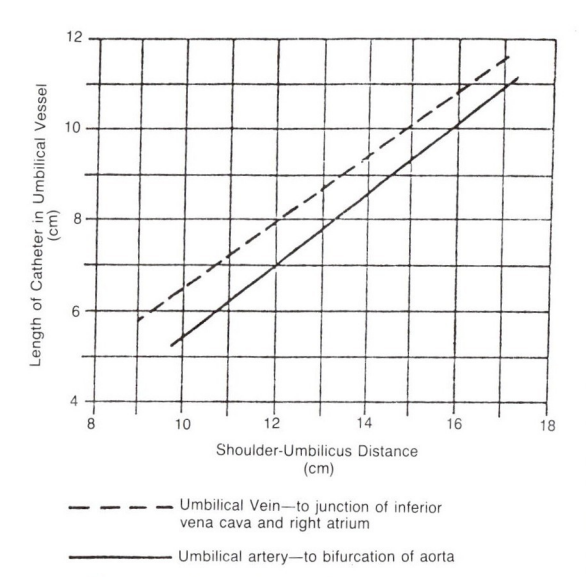

Figure 1 **Determination of length of catheter to be inserted for appropriate arterial or venous placement. The length of the catheter read from the diagram is to the umbilical ring; add length of the umbilical cord stump. The shoulder–umbilicus distance is the perpendicular distance between parallel lines at the level of the umbilicus and through the distal ends of the clavicles.** (From Klaus MH, Fanaroff AA, eds. Care of the high risk neonate. 3rd ed. Philadelphia: WB Saunders, 1986:430.)

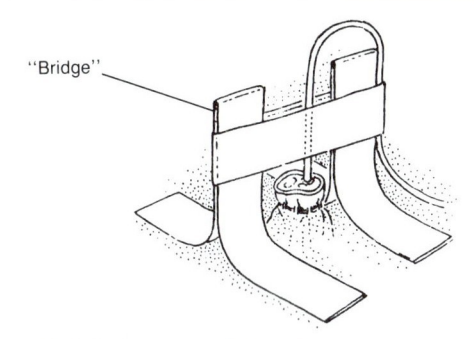

Figure 2 **Umbilical artery catheterization.** (Adapted from Klaus MH, Fanaroff AA, eds. Care of the high risk neonate. 3rd ed. Philadelphia: WB Saunders, 1986:431.)

Umbilical Artery Catheterization

- Similar preparation and equipment as for UVC
- Because of smooth muscle content of arterial wall and potential for spasm, probe or iris forceps are used to increase lumen patency
- 3.5-5 Fr catheter is connected to syringe via three-way stopcock ± blunt-ended needle (system filled with heparin in normal saline, 1 U/ml of normal saline). Insert catheter to desired length (Fig. 1).
- Secure as in umbilical vein
- Confirm position (L3-4) with x-ray
- Complications: blanching of toes, legs, or buttocks requires removal of catheter (warming of contralateral leg may help in some cases). Hemorrhage from loose connections is a major complication. Other complications include renal ischemia (irreversible hypertension), bowel ischemia (perforation or necrotizing enterocolitis), spinal cord ischemia (paraplegia), bleeding, infection, aortic aneurysm.
- Contraindications: acute conditions in area of supply of abdominal aorta (necrotizing enterocolitis, acute tubular necrosis); umbilical complications (omphalitis, omphalocele)
- UAC may be used for saline, dextrose-containing solutions, and TPN or antibiotics if urgent need and no other vascular access

Endotracheal Intubation

- Emergency intubation should be attempted by *only* the most skilled personnel available
- Essential features of pediatric airway include larynx more anterior, floppy epiglottis, relatively large tongue, and narrowest point at cricoid cartilage
- In the apneic patient, positive pressure ventilation by bag and mask with O_2 *must* be administered before attempts at laryngoscopy. Airway obstruction that may appear complete often can be partially overcome by bag and mask technique, allowing correction of hypoxemia and preparation for intubation. Preoxygenation is essential.
- Check equipment (suction, laryngoscope) prior to attempting intubation
- Muscle relaxant and sedating drugs should not be used in patients with upper airway obstruction
- In the acute resuscitation situation, oral intubation is preferred until patient is stabilized. Elective nasotracheal intubation may then be performed.
- Nasotracheal intubation contraindicated in suspected basal skull fracture or severe facial injury
- Selection of appropriate tube size (Table 1): appropriate ETT is the largest one that allows a leak of air around the tube when 25-30 cm H_2O positive pressure is applied
- A rough guide to ETT size (internal diameter) in children older than 1 yr is

$$\frac{\text{age (yr)}}{4} + 4$$

- Use smaller ETT if airway obstruction or syndrome known to be associated with anatomic airway abnormality (i.e., Down syndrome)
- For patients with croup, select 3.0 mm for <6 mo, 3.5 mm for 6-24 mo, and for older patients:

$$\frac{\text{age (yr)}}{4} + 3$$

- Introducer may be required for oral intubation; Magill forceps are required for nasotracheal intubation
- Most tubes have landmarks to indicate appropriate level of placement
- Always confirm position with CXR. Correct position is ETT tip at midtracheal level (1-2 cm above carina). Note that extension of head at time of x-ray exam will cause tube to advance distally and flexion will cause tube to rise away from carina.
- Check clinically for symmetrical chest movement and air entry. If right-sided only, pull tube proximally.
- Complications: trauma, right mainstem bronchus intubation with left-sided collapse, bradycardia secondary to pharyngeal vagal stimulation
- Atropine to prevent brachycardia generally used in older children (0.01-0.02 mg/kg/dose)

TABLE 1 Endotracheal Tube Size

Age	Tube Size	
Neonate		
<1500 g	2.5	
>1500 g	3.0	
1-6 mo	3.5	
7 mo-2 yr	4.0	uncuffed
2 yr	4.5	
3-4	5.0	
5-6	5.5	
7-8	6.0	
9-11	6.5	
12-13	6.5	cuffed
14-18	7.0	

Bladder Catheterization

- Retract prepuce in males if uncircumcised and swab penis to base with appropriate antiseptic
- In females, separate labia and swab periurethral area with antiseptic
- Drape sterile towel above and below urethra
- Lubricate catheter
- Apply caudal traction to penis, or separate labia
- Introduce catheter into urethral meatus, advancing until urine is obtained
- If Foley, inflate balloon with H_2O or saline (variable volume according to catheter used)
- Attach outlet end aseptically to closed drainage system

TABLE 2 Urinary Catheter Sizes

Age	Intermittent Catheterization	Indwelling Catheters
0-5 yr	3½-5 Fr feeding tube	3½-5 Fr feeding tube
5-7 yr	5 Fr feeding tube	5 Fr feeding tube
7-10 yr	8-10 Fr disposable urinary catheter	8-10 Fr Foley (Silastic)
10-14 yr	10 Fr disposable urinary catheter	10 Fr Foley (Silastic)
>14 yr	12-14 Fr* disposable urinary catheter	10-14 Fr Foley (Silastic)

*N.B.: Foleys >14 Fr are latex

Suprapubic Bladder Aspiration

- Any growth of bacteria from a suprapubic urine sample is considered significant
- Infant placed in frog-leg position
- Appropriate antiseptic and draping
- Landmark: 1-2 cm above symphysis pubis in midline; usually corresponds to transverse lower abdominal crease just above symphysis pubis
- Advance needle (23-25 gauge, 2-3 cm) attached to empty 3-5 ml syringe in caudal direction at 10-20° from perpendicular to abdominal wall, aspirating gently while advancing

Lumbar Puncture

- *Be sure to exclude ↑ ICP (by examining fundus, palpating sutures and fontanelles, or using CT scan) prior to performing LP.* Consult neurosurgeon if any suspicion.
- LP contraindicated in bleeding diathesis, thrombocytopenia (<50,000), infection over skin or along needle insertion site
- Proper positioning and adequate restraint of patient is absolutely essential to a successful tap
- Place patient with back fully flexed and either sitting up or lying on one side with hips, knees, and neck flexed
- Patients with cardiorespiratory compromise need close monitoring during the procedure
- Draw an imaginary line between the two iliac crests, and the intervertebral space (L3-4) at, or caudal to (L4-5) this line is located. Avoid L2-3 space in infant (cord lower than in older child).
- Appropriate antiseptic and draping
- In infants and older children (not neonates), may infiltrate skin and subcutaneous tissue with 1% lidocaine

- Select an appropriate needle (21-23 G short needle *with stylet* for infants, and 20-21 G long needle *with stylet* for older children) and insert in midline, just below the spinous process, angled toward the umbilicus, and slowly advance until a "pop" is felt (except in infant) as dura is penetrated. In infants, stylet must be withdrawn frequently to check for CSF flow.
- When fluid appears, a three-way stopcock and manometer (must be available before start of procedure) may be attached and the opening pressure measured (useless in crying child). Normal values, <200 mm H_2O. *Do not aspirate fluid.*
- Collect fluid in appropriate tubes and send for biochemical (glucose, lactate, protein), bacteriologic studies (culture, Gram stain, antigen-detection tests, e.g., CIE or latex agglutination), and cytology (count, morphology), as appropriate
- An extra specimen may be left refrigerated for later testing, e.g., metabolic tests

CSF Cell Count

- Use a dry, clean Fuchs-Rosenthal counting chamber
- Place ½-1 drop of undiluted CSF on chamber A—place a coverslip over top. CSF should cover the entire chamber without overflowing. There should be no bubbles under the coverslip.
- In a separate test tube, place three drops of CSF and one drop of Fujiwara stain. Mix. Place mixture to cover chamber B.
- Examine side A under 40× objective
  1. Count number of RBCs in five large squares (the four corners and one in the center)
  2. Count number of WBCs in similar manner
  3. If count done from Side B, multiply result by ⅓
  4. If more than three WBCs seen, do differential from Side B

- Notes
  1. Each big square contains 16 small squares
  2. Each five big squares = 80 small squares = 1 mm^3 = $\times\ 10^6$/L
  3. If sample heavily blood stained, dilute CSF to 1:20 with sterile normal saline (1 part CSF plus 19 parts saline). After counting number of RBCs in five big squares, multiply the results by 20.
  4. If 0-25 cells are seen in one small square, count all five big squares
  5. If 25-50 cells are seen in one small square, count one big square and multiply by 5
  6. If >50 cells are seen in one small square, count one small square and multiply by 80

Arterial Blood Sampling

- Preferred sites for arterial puncture in older children are radial and posterior tibial arteries
- In infants, may use radial, dorsalis pedis, and posterior tibial arteries
- Avoid femoral artery puncture as it may produce septic arthritis of hip, as well as risk of thrombosis and embolus and distal ischemia
- Use 25 G needle and heparinized syringe. Alternatively, 23 or 25 G butterfly needle may be used with an assistant aspirating into syringe.
- Insert needle in cephalad direction at 60-degree angle, bevel up, adjusting position until blood return, then gently aspirating into syringe
- Must apply direct pressure post removal for ~ 5 min
- Arterial line insertion, done preferably in intensive care setting by experienced personnel

Gram Stain

- Make a thin smear of the material to be studied
- Air dry
- Heat fix by passing the slide through a Bunsen flame two to three times
- Cover with crystal violet (or gentian violet) × 1 min
- Rinse with water
- Cover with Gram's iodine × 1 min
- Rinse with water
- Flush with 95% ethanol, acetone, or acid-alcohol until washings are colorless; not to exceed 10 sec
- Counterstain by flooding the slide with safranin (or carbol-fuchsin) × 1 min
- Rinse with water
- Blot gently—leave to dry
- Place a drop of oil over stained field
- Examine using oil immersion (100×) objective

KOH Preparation

- Scrape scales from affected skin with side of scalpel blade onto black paper. If indicated, also pluck 5-10 hairs or take nail clippings or scrapings of subungual debris.
- Transfer some material to a microscope slide, apply 1-2 drops of 10% KOH (dissolves keratin), apply coverslip (wait 15-30 min), and examine under medium power. A positive test will show hyphae.
- Send the black paper containing the remainder of the collected scales to the lab for fungal culture (culture takes up to 1 mo)

Stool Smear

- Place small drop of feces on glass slide
- Place single drop of normal saline on edge of coverslip and, using this edge, agitate the drop of stool and mix it with the saline
- Lower coverslip over specimen and examine by microscope
- Look for fat, starch, meat fibers, WBC, yeast, and parasites
  1. Neutral fats: 1 drop of stool and 2 drops Sudan red stain on slide; mix with 2 drops saline, then place coverslip and examine slide under microscope. Red-stained droplets = fat globules.
  2. Fatty acid crystals: best seen with polarizing attachment on microscope
  3. Leukocytes suggest bacterial infection or inflammatory bowel disease
  4. Erythrocytes suggest colitis
  5. Parasites: examine stool smear slide under low power to locate and under high power to identify. Add 1 drop 1% potassium iodide stain to 1 drop of stool on slide for easier species identification.

Reducing Substances in Stool (to Detect Carbohydrate Malabsorption)

- Dilute small amount of liquid stool with twice its volume of water in a test tube
- If to detect sucrose (which is not a reducing sugar): add 1 N HCl, instead of H_2O, to stool; boil mixture very briefly
- In another tube, add 15 drops of stool mixture, then one Clinitest tablet, and compare color of resulting solution with Clinitest chart after reaction has ended
- Value <0.25% is normal; >0.5% suggests carbohydrate malabsorption
- Stool should be liquid to warrant performing test

Examination for Pinworms (Enterobiasis)

- Cellophane-tape specimen should be obtained before patient bathes, in AM
  1. Put piece of tape, sticky side out, on end of wooden tongue depressor
  2. Gently apply taped end of stick to perianal area
  3. On a glass slide, put 1 drop xylol, then apply the piece of tape (sticky side down), and search for ova under the microscope

TABLE 3 Maximum Volumes of Enemas to Be Administered Rectally*

Age	Volume
0-3 mo	30-100 ml
3-12 mo	100-250 ml
1-6 yr	250-500 ml
6-12 yr	500-1000 ml

*N.B.: The above volumes are guidelines only. In certain circumstances (e.g., encopresis), larger volumes may be recommended (see appropriate section).

FOUR

LABORATORY REFERENCE VALUES

LAB REF VALUES

Hematology

Hemoglobin, Hematocrit, RBC Count, Reticulocytes

	Hemoglobin (g/L)	Hematocrit	RBC Count ($\times 10^{12}$/L)	Reticulocytes ($\times 10^9$/L)
Birth				
28 wk gestation	110-170	0.30-0.40	3.0-4.5	
34 wk gestation	120-180	0.35-0.50	3.0-5.0	
38 wk gestation	140-200	0.40-0.55	3.5-5.5	
40 wk gestation	150-250†	0.52-0.79†	3.5-6.0	200-300
2 days	150-250†	0.46-0.74†	3.5-6.0	<5.0
2 wk	140-200	0.40-0.74†	3.5-6.0	<5.0
1 mo	115-180	0.35-0.54	3.5-5.5	
2 mo	90-135	0.27-0.40	3.5-5.5	
3-6 mo	100-140	0.30-0.42	3.5-5.0	5.0-250.0
1-5 yr	110-140	0.33-0.42	4.0-5.0	10.0-100.0
6-14 yr	120-160	0.36-0.48	4.5-5.5	10.0-100.0

†If a capillary value is close to the upper limit of normal, a VENOUS sample should be obtained. The venous hemoglobin value should be less than 220 g/L. A venous hematocrit value should be less than 0.65.

Conversion from SI to Traditional Units

Hemoglobin: 120 g/L = 12.0 g/dl
Hematocrit: 0.36 = 36%
RBC Count: $4.0 \times 10^{12}/L = 4.0 \times 10^{6}/mm^{3}$
Reticulocytes: $\dfrac{\text{Reticulocytes } (\times 10^{9}/L)}{\text{RBC count } (\times 10^{12}/L) \times 10}$

= Reticulocytes (% of RBC count)

e.g. $\dfrac{10.0 \, (\times 10^{9}/L)}{4.0 \, (\times 10^{12}/L) \times 10} = 0.25\%$

Red Blood Cell Indices

	MCV*	MCH†	MCHC‡
Birth			
28-37 wk gestation	120		
38-40 wk gestation	110		
1 wk	110		
1 mo	90	24-34	320-360
2 mo	80	24-34	
3-12 mo	70	24-31	
Older	80-94	24-31	

*MCV = Mean corpuscular volume (fl).
†MCH = Mean corpuscular hemoglobin (pg).
‡MCHC = Mean corpuscular Hb concentration (g/L).

PLATELET COUNT

All ages: $150.0\text{-}450.0 \times 10^9/L$

ESR

All ages: 1-10 mm/hr

Hemoglobin Electrophoresis

	Patient Age	Percentage
Hgb F	40 wk gestation	60%-95%
	2 mo	30%-55%
	3 mo	15%-30%
	4 mo	5%-20%
	6 mo	2%-5%
	1 yr	0.2%-2.0%
Hgb A_2	>1 yr	1.2%-3.2%

White Blood Cell Count and Differential ($\times 10^9$/L)

	Birth	1 Wk	2 Wk	3-12 Mo	2-5 Yr	6-10 Yr	Older
Total WBC	20.0-40.0	5.0-21.0	5.0-20.0	5.0-15.0	5.0-12.0	4.0-10.0	4.0-10.0
Differential							
Polymorphs	6.0-26.0	1.5-10.0	1.0-9.5	1.5-8.5	1.5-8.5	1.5-8.0	2.0-7.5
Bands	0-4.5	0-0.8	0	0	0	0	0
Eosinophils	0.02-0.85	0.07-1.1	0.07-1.0	0.05-0.7	0.02-0.5	0-0.5	0-0.5
Basophils	0-0.6	0-0.2	0-0.2	0-0.2	0-0.2	0-0.2	0-0.2
Lymphocytes	2.0-11.0	2.0-17.0	2.0-17.0	4.0-10.5	2.0-8.0	1.5-7.0	1.5-4.0
Monocytes	0.4-3.1	0.3-2.7	0.2-2.4	0.05-1.1	0-0.8	0-0.8	0-0.8

Note: WBC differential counts are reported as absolute numbers.

LAB REF VALUES

Coagulation Values (For Full-Term Newborns and Older)

	Patient Age	
Antithrombin III (AT-III)	<1 mo ≥3 mo	0.48-1.10 U/ml 0.80-1.20 U/ml
Factors V, VIII		0.50-1.50 U/ml
Factors VII, IX, X, XI, XII	<1 mo ≥9 mo	0.20-0.80 U/ml 0.50-1.50 U/ml
Fibrinogen*	<6 mo ≥6 mo	1.5-4.0 g/L 2.0-4.0 g/L
Ivy bleeding time		2-7 min
Partial thromboplastin time (PTT)	<1 mo ≥3 mo	25-60 sec 25-40 sec
Prothrombin time (PT)	<1 mo <3 mo ≥1 mo ≥3 mo	10.5-18.0 sec 10.5-13.5 sec
Ristocetin cofactor		0.60-1.50 U/ml
von Willebrand factor		0.50-1.50 U/ml
INR (see p 697)		

*Fibrinogen is an acute phase reactant.

Blood

Agent or Test	Reference Values (SI Units)		Notes
	Arterial	**Venous**	
Acid-base (blood gases)			Normal values for capillary gas levels range from venous to arterial, depending on how arterialized the sample site is
pH			
Newborn	7.33-7.49	—	
1 day	7.25-7.43	—	
2 days-adult	7.35-7.45	7.32-7.42	
P_{CO_2}			
Birth-2 yr	26-41 mm Hg	—	
2 yr-adult	33-46 mm Hg	40-50 mm Hg	
P_{O_2} (room air)			
Newborn	65-76 mm Hg	—	
Child-adult	80-100 mm Hg	25-47 mm Hg	
	Bicarbonate	**Base excess**	
Newborn	17-24 mmol/L	−10 to −2 mmol/L	
2 mo-2 yr	16-24	−7 to 0	
Child	18-25	−3 to +3	
Adult	18-29	−3 to +3	

Continued.

Blood (Cont'd)

Reference Values

Agent or Test	SI Units	Traditional Units	Notes
Acid phosphatase (total) p-npp at 37° C			Source: spleen, liver, prostate, osteoclasts, red blood cells, platelets
Newborn	7-20 U/L		
2-13 yr	6-15		
>13 yr	up to 11		
Adrenocorticotropic hormone (ACTH)			For adequate interpretation, cortisol should be measured in same sample
Day 1	<88 pmol/L	<400 pg/ml	
Over first few weeks of life the adrenals mature and values decrease to the following: Child and adult (0900 hr—diurnal variation)	<22 pmol/L	<100 pg/ml	
Alanine aminotransferase (ALT, formerly SGPT) At 37° C, with pyridoxal phosphate (Kodak method)			Source: liver, skeletal muscle, kidney, heart
<1 yr	<60 U/L		
1 yr-adult	<40		

Albumin

0-1 yr	32-48 g/L	3.2-4.8 g/dl
Child and adult	33-58	3.3-5.8

Aldosterone

	166-2900 pmol/L	6-104 ng/dl
<1 yr; free diet; varied time of day		
1-4 yr; free diet; varied time of day	<940	<34
5-15 yr; free diet; varied time of day	<600	<22
>15 yr; normal salt; ambulant; at noon	220-420	8-15
>15 yr low-salt diet	550-1220	20-44

Varies widely depending on time of day, posture, and sodium and potassium intake
For adequate interpretation, serum and potassium should be measured in same sample, along with 24-hr urine sodium collection. In hypokalemic hypertension, serum potassium should be normal before aldosterone is measured. Drugs such as diuretics (e.g., furosemide, spironolactone), purgatives, and liquorice derivatives (e.g., carbenoxolone) interfere with results; should be discontinued 3 wk prior to testing.

Alkaline phosphatase
(Kodak method, p-npp at 37° C)

Male
<1 yr	175-600 U/L
1-8 yr	175-400
9-11 yr	180-475
12-15 yr	200-630
16-17 yr	100-455
18-19 yr	80-210
>19 yr	60-150

Source: bone, liver, kidney, intestinal mucosa
Isoenzymes exist for bone, liver, and intestine

Continued.

Blood (Cont'd)

Reference Values

Agent or Test	SI Units	Traditional Units	Notes
Alkaline phosphatase—cont'd			
Female			
<1 yr	185-555 U/L		
1-2 yr	185-520		
3-8 yr	185-425		
9-13 yr	160-500		
14-15 yr	90-400		
16-18 yr	45-140		
>18 yr	25-100		
Alpha-1-acid glycoprotein (orosomucoid)	0.3-1.35 g/L	30-135 mg/dl	Acute phase reactant
Alpha-1-antitrypsin	0.9-2.1 g/L	90-210 mg/dl	Acute phase reactant. Protease Inhibitor (PI) typing: MM—normal (89% of population) MS—normal variant (8%) MZ—heterozygous for deficiency (2.5%) SS and SZ—each <0.2% ZZ—homozygous for deficiency (0.01%)

Alpha-1-antitrypsin clearance
See p 633

Alpha-fetoprotein
Adult normal   <5 μg/L   <5 ng/ml   Very high levels at birth

Aluminum
<560 nmol/L   <15 μg/L

Amino Acids
Purpose: screening is done by chromatography to detect genetic-metabolic disease. If screen is abnormal quantitative values should be obtained. Reference values are age dependent and should be interpreted by a specialist in metabolic disease.

Ammonium (NH_4^+)
Newborn   <100 μmol/L   <180 μg/dl, as NH_4^+

Child and adult   <60   <108

Amylase
<1 yr, poorly defined; lower than in older child

1 yr-adult   20-140 U/L   Source: pancreas, salivary glands

Continued.

LAB REF VALUES

Blood (Cont'd)

Reference Values

Agent or Test	SI Units	Traditional Units	Notes
Androstenedione			Source: ovaries, adrenals. Until puberty in females, and from 5 mo of age to puberty in males, an adrenal-specific androgen
Poorly defined in children			
Male			
1-5 mo	<2.8 nmol/L	<80 ng/dl	
5 mo-adrenarche	<1.6	<45	
Adult	1.7-5.2	50-150	In females, values are higher during the luteal phase of the cycle than during the follicular phase, but should still be within the range shown
Female			
Birth-adrenarche	<1.6	<45	
Adult	1.7-7.0	50-200	
Antihyaluronidase			
See p 637			
Antistreptolysin O (ASO)			
See p 637			

Aspartate aminotransferase (AST, formerly SGOT)
37° C with pyridoxal phosphate
<1 yr   <110 U/L   Source: cardiac and skeletal muscle, liver, kidney, erythrocytes
1-10 yr   <45
11-20 yr   <36

Arginine vasopressin (AVP, antidiuretic hormone)
<10 ng/L   Interpret in relation to plasma osmolality

Beta-1-C globulin
See C3 *complement*

Beta-human chorionic gonadotropin
See *human chorionic gonadotropin*

Beta-hydroxybutyrate
See *3-hydroxybutyrate*

Bicarbonate (actual)
See *acid-base*

Bile salts (radioimmunoassay for glycocholate)
Fasting   <1.3 μmol/L
2-hr pc   <5.5

Bilirubin (direct)
1 mo-adult   0-7 μmol/L   0-0.4 mg/dl

Continued.

Blood (Cont'd)

Reference Values

Agent or Test	SI Units	Traditional Units	Notes
Bilirubin (total)			In general, "physiologic hyperbilirubinemia" clears at approximately 1 wk of age for term neonates and at 2 wk for prematures (see p 334)
Premature			
<24 hr	17-100 μmol/L	1-6 mg/dl	
1-2 days	100-140	6-8	
3-5 days	170-200	10-12	
1 mo–adult	<17	<1	
Term			
<24 hr	34-100 μmol/L	2-6 mg/dl	
1-2 days	100-120	6-7	
3-5 days	70-200	4-12	
1 mo–adult	<17	<1	
Blood gases			
See *acid-base*			
Blood urea nitrogen (BUN)			
See *urea*			
C-Reactive protein	<8 mg/L	<0.8 mg/dl	

C3 complement (beta-1-C globulin)			Acute phase reactant
0-1 yr	0.6-1.7 g/L	60-170 mg/dl	
1 yr-adult	0.8-1.8	80-180	
C4 complement			Acute phase reactant
0-6 mo	0.07-0.26 g/L	7-26 mg/dl	
6 mo-adult	0.10-0.40	10-40	
Calcium (ionized, free)			Acidosis increases free calcium whereas alkalosis decreases it (for a given total calcium)
>1 mo-adult	1.0-1.35 mmol/L	4.0-5.4 mg/dl	
Calcium (total)			Prolonged venous stasis (e.g., prolonged use of a tourniquet) alters the result. Serum calcium levels less than the aforementioned range may be normal if hypoalbuminemia is present. Adjusted calcium should be in the normal range.
Premature (birth-7 days)	1.75-2.5 mmol/L	7-10 mg/dl	
Term (birth-7 days)	1.8-3.0	7.2-12	
Child	2.25-2.74	9-11	
Adult	2.12-2.62	8.5-10.5	

For SI units: Adjusted Ca (mmol/L) = Calcium(mmol/L) − $\frac{\text{Albumin (g/L)}}{40}$ + 1.0

For traditional units: Adjusted Ca (mg/dl) = Calcium (mg/dl) − Albumin (g/dl) + 4.0

Carboxyhemoglobin		Expressed as fraction of total hemoglobin
Newborn (nonsmoking mother)	<0.05	
Nonsmokers	<0.05	

Continued.

Blood (Cont'd)

Reference Values

Agent or Test	SI Units	Traditional Units	Notes
Carcinoembryonic antigen (CEA)			
Adult	<3 µg/L		
Carnitine			
Total	48-72 µmol/L		Normal ratio fraction free/total = 0.75-0.9
Free	35-50		For interpretation consult specialist in metabolic disease
Carotene	0.9-3.7 µmol/L	50-200 µg/dl	
Ceruloplasmin			
Child >6 mo-adult	180-450 mg/L	18-45 mg/dl	Acute-phase reactant
CH$_{50}$-total hemolytic complement	≥1:12		Sample must be sent on ice immediately to laboratory
Chloride		mEq/L	
Premature infant	95-110 mmol/L		
Term infant	96-106		
Child	99-111		
Adult	98-106		

Cholesterol
<3 mo	<4.5 mmol/L	<175 mg/dl
3 mo-2 yr	<4.9	<190
2-17 yr	3.2-4.4	124-170

Values are based on fasting states (before feeds in babies; after a 12-hr fast in older children). Fasting is not essential if total cholesterol is requested without any other lipid determinations.

Cholinesterase-pseudocholinesterase
Cholinesterase	620-1370 U/L
Dibucaine no.	77-83
	(heterozygote, 45-70)
	(homozygote, 15-30)
Fluoride no.	56-68
Chloride no.	4-15
Scoline no.	87-92

Chorionic gonadotropin
See *human chorionic gonadotropin*

Complement
See C3, C4, CH$_{50}$

Copper
Child >6 mo-adult   10.5-23.0 μmol/L   67-146 μg/dl

Continued.

Blood (Cont'd)

Cortisol

Agent or Test	Reference Values SI Units	Traditional Units	Notes
Cortisol			
Poorly defined during first weeks of life			Result at 2000 hr is <50% of the 0800 hr value in 88% of cases.
Child 1-17 yr, in hospital 0800-0900 hr	190-740 nmol/L	7-27 µg/dl	Diurnal variation of cortisol may not develop until about 1 yr of age.
2000 hr	30-300	1-11	In Cushing's disease or syndrome, cortisol levels may be normal, but diurnal variation is lost. Other steroids produced in congenital adrenal hyperplasia or tumors crossreact with cortisol assay; only poor diurnal variation may be evident. Stress or shock can elevate cortisol levels.
Healthy adult, 0800 hr	140-690	5-25	

Creatine kinase (CK)

Kodak method at 37° C
Values below are for healthy school children with no restriction of physical activity

Male
11 days-1 yr	<390 U/L
1-12 yr	<255
13-14 yr	<300
15-16 yr	<570
17+	<435

Female
11 days-1 yr	<390
1-6 yr	<230
7-14 yr	<215
15-16 yr	<180
17+	<170

Source: skeletal and cardiac muscle, smooth muscle, brain
Elevated CK levels occur after physical activity and intramuscular injections
Blacks have significantly higher levels of CK than whites
Bed rest for several days may drop CK levels by 20%-30%

Creatine kinase isoenzymes

Child over 4 yr and adult (as fraction of total CK)
CK-MM	0.94-1.0
CK-MB	0-0.06
CK-BB	0

Source: CK-BB: predominantly brain; CK-MB: cardiac muscle, type II skeletal muscle fibers; CK-MM: skeletal muscle, cardiac muscle
Purpose: To help differentiate skeletal from cardiac muscle disease or trauma. CK-MB is not specific for myocardial damage in first weeks or months after birth

Continued.

Blood (Cont'd)

Reference Values

Agent or Test	SI Units	Traditional Units	Notes
Creatinine			Low concentrations occur in patients with small muscle mass (as with muscle disease or severe malnutrition)
<5 yr	<44 µmol/L	<0.5 mg/dl	
5-6 yr	<53	<0.6	
6-7 yr	<62	<0.7	
7-8 yr	<71	<0.8	
8-9 yr	<80	<0.9	
9-10 yr	<88	<1.0	
>10 yr	<106	<1.2	
Creatinine clearance see p 625			
Cryoglobulins			Normally absent
Dehydroepiandrosterone sulfate (DHAS, DHEA-S)			Source: adrenal glands
Male			
1-5 mo	<4 µmol/L	<1500 ng/ml	
6 mo-7 yr	<0.5	<180	
8-9 yr	<3	<1100	
10-12 yr	<6	<2200	
13-19 yr	3-12	1100-4400	

Female
 1-5 mo   <4 μmol/L   <1500 ng/ml
 6 mo-7 yr   <1.0   <350
 8-9 yr   <3   <1100
 10-12 yr   <8   <3000
 13-19 yr   1-12   350-4400

DHAS
See *dehydroepian-drosterone sulfate*

1,25-Dihydroxyvitamin D   25-100 pmol/L

Estradiol
Poorly defined in children
Male
 Birth   <370 pmol/L   <100 pg/ml
 1 yr-adrenarche   <92   <25
 Adrenarche through
  puberty (rising to
  adult levels)
 Adult   <165   <45

Continued.

Blood (Cont'd)

Reference Values

Agent or Test	SI Units	Traditional Units	Notes
Estradiol—cont'd			
Female			
Birth-adrenarche (as in males)			
Adrenarche through puberty (rising to adult levels)			
Adult			
Follicular phase	110-183 pmol/L	30-50 pg/ml	
Luteal phase	550-845	150-230	
Treated with synthetic estrogens	<165	<45	
FEP			
See *free erythrocyte protoporphyrin*			
Ferritin			
<1 yr	10-300 µg/L	ng/ml	
>1 yr	16-300		
α-**Fetoprotein**			
See *alpha-fetoprotein*			

Folate
RBC folate >270 nmol/L >120 ng/ml
Serum folate >4 >1.8

Follicle stimulating hormone (FSH, WHO 78/549 standard)
Male
 0-4 mo <15 IU/L (most <6 IU/L) mIU/ml
 4 mo-2 yr <3
 2-11 yr <4
 11 yr-adult <7
Female
 0-6 mo <38 IU/L mIU/ml
 6 mo-2 yr <8 (most <5)
 2-10 yr <4
 Puberty—rising to adult level <9
 Adult
  Follicular & luteal values <9
  Ovulatory value <13

Free erythrocyte protoporphyrin (FEP, zinc protoporphyrin)
0-10 yr <0.62 μmol/L of RBC <35 μg/dl   Investigation of lead poisoning, congenital erythropoietic porphyria, erythrohepatic protoporphyria. Increased FEP occurs in iron deficiency anemia and anemia of chronic disease
>10 yr <1.33 μmol/L of RBC <75

Continued.

Blood (Cont'd)

Reference Values

Agent or Test	SI Units	Traditional Units	Notes
Galactosemia screen			Qualitative test of RBC galactose-1-phosphate uridyl transferase activity. A blood transfusion within 3 mo prior to this test may invalidate the results. Other screening tests may be available (depending on center) that may not be invalidated by RBC transfusion, but results of these may be falsely negative if the child was not ingesting galactose-containing foods when the blood was taken.
Galactose-1-phosphate uridyl transferase			Quantitative assessment of RBC galactose-1-phosphate uridyl transferase activity
Normal*	300-470 U/kg Hb	18.3-28.6 Beutler and Baluda units/g Hb	*Duarte variant enzyme (a normal variant) may distort these ranges. A blood transfusion within 3 mo prior to this test may invalidate the result.
Galactosemia heterozygote*	140-220	8.5-13.4	
Galactosemia homozygote	0-40	0-2.4	

Gamma-glutamyl transferase (GGT)
Kodak method at 37° C Source: liver, pancreas

<1 mo	<385 U/L
1-2 mo	<225
2-4 mo	<135
4-7 mo	<75
7 mo-15 yr	<45
>15 yr	Male <75
	Female <55

Gases
See *acid-base*

Gastrin
Fasting   <50 ng/L   pg/ml

Globulin, beta-1-C
See *C3 complement*

Globulins
By electrophoresis

	1-3 g/L 0.1-0.3 g/dl
α_1	2-7 0.2-0.7
α_2 Birth-6 mo	4-11 0.4-1.1
>6 mo	3-6 0.3-0.6
β Birth-6 mo	3-12 0.3-1.2
>6 mo	6-12 0.6-1.2
γ Birth	2-7 0.2-0.7
1-6 mo	2-9 0.2-0.9
6 mo-2 yr	4-14 0.4-1.4
>2 yr	

Continued.

Blood (Cont'd)

Reference Values

Agent or Test	SI Units	Traditional Units	Notes
Glucose (fasting)			
Infant	>2.5 mmol/L	>45 mg/dl	
Child <3 yr	2.5-5.0	45-90	
Child >3 yr	2.8-6.1	50-110	
Adolescent-adult	3.3-6.1	60-110	
Glucose-6-phosphate dehydrogenase (G-6-PD)			
Newborn	1.6-2.8 IU/ml RBC	160-280 IU/100 ml RBC	
>2 mo	1.2-1.8	120-180	Children with values between 5 and 8 may be normal, but require careful follow-up
Growth hormone After stimulation (by sleep, exercise, arginine, insulin, L-dopa, or propranolol) peak value should be: and preferably:	>5 µg/L >8	>5 ng/ml	
Haptoglobin	0.27-1.39 g/L	27-139 mg/dl	Acute-phase reactant
Hemoglobin (plasma)	<30 mg/L	<3 mg/dl	

Hemoglobin A$_{1C}$ (glycosylated hemoglobin)

Expressed as fraction of total hemoglobin

Healthy nondiabetic	0.04-0.06
Diabetic with average control	0.09-0.1

Abnormal or variant hemoglobins and hemoglobin F may give falsely elevated levels

Human chorionic gonadotropin, beta subunit (β-HCG)

Nonpregnant adult   <5 U/L

3-Hydroxybutyrate (β-hydroxybutyrate)

During documented hypoglycemia	
Expected values	1.5-2.0 mmol/L

17-Hydroxyprogesterone

Children <3 mo	<10 nmol/L
Children 3 mo to adults	<6
Borderline for non-classical CAH	6-10

	<3.3 µg/L
	<2.0
	2.0-3.3

Cord blood and samples from neonates <24 hr old are not satisfactory. Elevated values are seen in very sick newborns (up to 30 nmol/L). Values are increased in luteal phase of menstrual cycle (up to 14 nmol/L).

25-Hydroxyvitamin D

Winter	20-60 nmol/L
Summer	25-80

	8-24 ng/ml
	10-32

Values exceeding these are not necessarily diagnostic of vitamin D toxicity, nor are lower levels diagnostic of deficiency. Levels may be increased in deficient patients after exposure to ultraviolet radiation.

Continued.

Blood (Cont'd)

Immunoglobulins

Agent or Test	Reference Values SI Units	Traditional Units	Notes
IgG			
0-6 mo	2-8 g/L	200-800 mg/dl	
6 mo-1 yr	2-10	200-1000	
1-2 yr	4-12	400-1200	
2-5 yr	4-12	400-1200	
5-10 yr	6-15	600-1500	
Adult	6-15	600-1500	
IgA			After age 10 yr values for IgA and IgM increase to reach adult levels
0-6 mo	0.08-0.7 g/L	8-70 mg/dl	Lower limit of IgA increases progressively in infants from approximately 0.01 g/L at 1 mo to 0.08 g/L at 6 mo
6 mo-1 yr	0.11-0.9	11-90	
1-2 yr	0.15-1.2	15-120	
2-5 yr	0.22-1.6	22-160	
5-10 yr	0.35-2.4	35-240	
Adult	0.70-3.1	70-310	

IgM		
0-6 mo	0.2-1.0 g/L	20-100 mg/dl
6 mo-1 yr	0.3-1.5	30-150
1-2 yr	0.4-1.7	40-170
2-5 yr	0.4-2.0	40-200
5-10 yr	0.4-2.5	40-250
Adult	0.5-3.5	50-350
IgE (values are stated as < mean + 1 standard deviation)		
0-6 mo	<17.5 µg/L	<7.3 kU/L
6 mo-1 yr	<31	<13
1-2 yr	<55	<23
2-5 yr	<115	<48
5-10 yr	<204	<85
Adult	<98	<41

Upper limit of IgE increases progressively in infants from approximately 5.5 µg/L at 6 wk to 17.5 µg/L at 6 mo
After age 10 yr the value declines to reach adult levels

Insulin
Fasting <145 pmol/L <20 mU/L

Reference values may be higher in obese patients.
Hemolysis and insulin antibodies may lower values.

Intralipid
See *lipid*

Iron
Newborn	20-48 µmol/L	110-270 µg/dl
4 mo-1 yr	5-13	30-70
>1 yr	9-27	50-150
Toxicity (1 yr and older)	>53	>300

Hemolysis elevates the result

Continued.

Blood (Cont'd)

Reference Values

Agent or Test	SI Units	Traditional Units	Notes
Iron-binding capacity (IBC)			
Newborn	11-31 µmol/L	60-175 µg/dl	
>1 yr	45-72	250-400	
Lactate			
Venous	<2.5 mmol/L	<22.5 mg/dl	Delayed separation of serum from RBC and hemolysis both elevate the result. Transport sample on ice.
Lactate dehydrogenase (LDH)			
At 30° C			
Adult	45-85 U/L		Source: highest concentrations in heart, liver, skeletal muscle, erythrocytes, kidney. Elevated in hemolyzed samples. Values are poorly defined and higher in children, and method dependent.
Lead			
0-10 yr	<1.2 µmol/L blood	0-25 µg/dl blood	Concentration of lead in whole blood is 75 times greater than in serum or plasma.
>10 yr see p 480	<1.93	0-40	

Lipid
During supplementation,
values should not exceed 1.0 g/L Indication: monitoring for toxicity when exogenous intravenous lipids are administered

Lipoproteins
By electrophoresis
See *cholesterol, triglycerides*

Indication: investigation and classification of hyperlipidemia

Plasma HDL-Cholesterol
 2-17 yr 1.0-1.8 mmol/L 40-70 mg/dl
 Male
  18-29 yr 0.9-1.6 35-62
 Female
  18-29 yr 0.9-2.0 35-77
Plasma LDL-Cholesterol
 2-17 yr 1.6-2.8 62-108 mg/dl
 18-29 yr 1.7-3.0 65-115

Luteinizing hormone (LH, WHO 68/40 standard)
Male mIU/ml
 0-3 mo <23 IU/L
 4 mo-2 yr <7
 2-6 yr <4
 6-10 yr <7
 Adult <10

Values rise through puberty to adult values

Continued.

Blood (Cont'd)

Reference Values

Agent or Test	SI Units	Traditional Units	Notes
Luteinizing hormone (LH, WHO 68/40 standard)—cont'd			
Female		mIU/ml	
1-6 mo	<20 IU/L		
6 mo-2 yr	<7		
2-8 yr	<6		
8-12 yr	2-13		
Adult			
Follicular and luteal value	<45		
Ovulatory value	<100		
Magnesium			
Newborn	0.75-1.15 mmol/L	1.5-2.30 mEq/L	
Child	0.70-0.95	1.4-1.9	
Adult	0.65-1.00	1.3-2.0	
Methemoglobin			
In SI, expressed as fraction of total hemoglobin	<0.03	<3%	Alternate value, <5.0 g/L

5'-Nucleotidase	0-14 U/L	Source: liver
Osmolality	275-295 mmol/kg water	mOsm/kg water May be lower in first 5 days after birth
Parathyroid hormone	10-65 ng/L	pg/ml Immunoassay is PTH "intact" molecule type (Nichols)
Phenylalanine	<110 μmol/L	<1.8 mg/dl
Phenylalanine/tyrosine ratio		Indication: determination of heterozygosity for phenylketonuria
Normal ratio	<1.0	
Equivocal	1.0-1.2	
Hetero/homozygote	>1.2	
Phosphate	mmol/L	mg/dl
Birth-1 mo	1.62-3.10	5.0-9.6 Reported values vary widely, especially during first month of life
1-4 mo	1.55-2.62	4.8-8.1 Hemolysis causes an elevated value
4 mo-1 yr	1.30-2.20	4.0-6.8
1-4 yr	1.16-2.10	3.6-6.5
4-8 yr	1.16-1.81	3.6-5.6
9-14 yr	1.07-1.71	3.3-5.3
>14 yr	0.87-1.52	2.7-4.7

Continued.

Blood (Cont'd)

Reference Values

Agent or Test	SI Units	Traditional Units	Notes
Porphyrins			Purpose: investigation of lead poisoning, erythrohepatic protoporphyria and congenital erythropoietic porphyria—see *free erythrocyte protoporphyrin* Investigation of acute intermittent porphyria—see *uroporphyrinogen-I-synthetase*
Potassium		mEq/L	Hemolysis elevates values
Premature infants	4.5-6.5 mmol/L		
Term infants	5.0-6.5		
2 days-2 wk	4.0-6.4		
2 wk-3 mo	4.0-6.2		
3 mo-1 yr	3.7-5.6		
1-16 yr	3.5-5.2		
Prolactin		ng/ml	Level drops to adult range by 12 wk of age (term); and by 20 wk (premature)
Birth (mean)	280 µg/L		
Level drops after birth— 4 wk (mean)	75		

Children
1 yr-puberty 3-20
Adult males 2-15
Adult females 3-26

Protein
See *total protein*

Protoporphyrin, free erythrocyte
See *free erythrocyte Protoporphyrin*

Pseudocholinesterase
See *cholinesterase*

Pyruvate
Venous 80-150 µmol/L 0.7-1.32 mg/dl, as pyruvic acid Delayed separation of serum from RBCs, and hemolysis both elevate the result

Pyruvate kinase
Newborn 1.2-2.1 IU/ml RBC
Older 1.0-1.4

Continued.

Blood (Cont'd)

Reference Values

Agent or Test	SI Units	Traditional Units	Notes
Renin			Normal values vary with method, sodium intake, time of day, posture, and age
Plasma renin activity			Antihypertensive medication may alter results; if possible, *medication should be discontinued 1-3 wk prior to test*
Normal salt intake:			
<3 mo wide range; values as high as: (particularly high in premature infants)	14.00 ng/L/sec	50 ng/ml/hr	
3 mo-1 yr	<4.20	<15	
1 yr-4 yr	<2.80	<10	
4 yr-15 yr	<1.70	<6	
Adult			
Supine, after 1-12 hr rest	<0.56	<2.0	
At 1200 hr, ambulant	<1.11	<4.0	
Serum glutamic oxaloacetic transaminase (SGOT) See *aspartate aminotransferase* (AST)			
Serum glutamic pyruvate transaminase (SGPT) See *alanine aminotransferase* (ALT)			

Sodium

Premature infant	132-140 mmol/L	mEq/L
Term infant	133-142	
Child	135-143	
Adult	135-145	

Testosterone

Male

1-15 days	<6.6 nmol/L	<190 ng/dl
1-3 mo	<12.1	<350
3-5 mo	<6.9	<200
5-7 mo	<2.1	<60
7 mo-onset of puberty	<1.0	<30
Adult	12.0-38.0	350-1100

During puberty, levels correlate with pubertal stage or bone age rather than chronologic age and progressively increase to adult values

Female

Birth-onset of puberty <1.0 nmol/L <30 ng/dl
Puberty— levels increase to adult values.
Levels are higher in girls experiencing anovulatory cycles but still within normal range.

Adult	0.7-2.4	20-70

Levels during the luteal phase are higher on average than the follicular phase
Levels may rise to 3.3 nmol/L (95 ng/dl) during estrogen or progesterone therapy

Continued.

Blood (Cont'd)

Reference Values

Agent or Test	SI Units	Traditional Units	Notes
Thyroid-stimulating hormone (TSH)		μU/ml	
Cord blood	<30 mU/L		
Rises shortly after birth to peak	<50		
Child >4 days of age	<5		
Adult	<5		
Thyroxine (T₄)	115-280 nmol/L	9-22 μg/dl	Premature infants have much lower values—the more premature, the lower the value. In patients with normal thyroid function, T_4 low values may occur with absent or low levels of thyroxine-binding globulin (TBG), hypoproteinemia, drugs (e.g., phenytoin), or severe hemolysis. In patients with normal thyroid function, high T_4 values may occur with high levels of TBG, as during pregnancy or while on contraceptive or estrogen therapy.
Levels rise shortly after birth to peak at 24 hr then fall at 3 days to:			
4 days-3 wk	100-245	8-19	
3 wk-2 mo	90-205	7-16	
2 mo-1 yr	65-180	5-14	
1 yr-childhood	65-165	5-13	
Adult	50-155	4-12	

Thyroxine-binding globulin (TBG)
Adult   12-30 mg/L

Values in children are ill defined, slightly higher than adult values

Total protein
0-6 mo		4.5-7.5 g/dl
6 mo-2 yr		5.4-7.5
Children and adult		5.3-8.5

Triglycerides
2-17 yr	0.4-1.3 mmol/L	35-115 mg/dl
>18 yr	0.6-2.3	53-204

Triiodothyronine (T_3)
Do not confuse with T_3RU

Birth	<1.0 nmol/L	<70 ng/dl
Rises rapidly after birth to a value at 3 days of:	0.8-5.4	50-350
6 days-1 yr	1.4-4.6	90-300
1 yr-childhood	1.4-4.1	90-270
Adult	1.4-3.4	90-220

T_3 assay has a low sensitivity for diagnosing hypothyroidism

Continued.

Blood (Cont'd)

Reference Values

Agent or Test	SI Units	Traditional Units	Notes
Triiodothyronine resin uptake test (T₃RU) Do not confuse with T₃	0.25–0.35	25%–35%	A synthetic resin and patient's TBG (thyroxine-binding globulin) compete for radioactive T₃ T₃RU > 0.35 (>35%) indicates FEWER available binding sites in serum, as in hyperthyroidism (sites occupied by T₄) or absence or deficiency of TBG T₃RU < 0.25 (<25%) indicates MORE available binding sites, as in hypothyroidism (little T₄ available to occupy sites) or increased TBG (e.g., during estrogen therapy or pregnancy)
Urate (formerly URIC ACID) Child or adult female	120–360 μmol/L	2.0–6.0 mg/dl, as uric acid	
Adult male	180–420	3.0–7.0	

Urea (formerly BLOOD UREA NITROGEN, BUN)

Newborn	2.9-10.0 mmol/L	8-28 mg/dl as urea nitrogen
1-2 yr	1.8-5.4	5-15
2-16 yr	2.9-7.1	8-20

Uric acid
See *urate*

Uroporphyrinogen-I-synthetase

5.2-15.5 nmol/s/L RBC

Source: erythrocytes
Purpose: investigation of acute intermittent porphyria

Vitamin A

0.70-2.10 µmol/L   20-60 µg/dl

Vitamin B$_{12}$

150-670 pmol/L   200-900 pg/ml

Vitamin D
See *25-hydroxyvitamin D*
1,25-dihydroxyvitamin D

Vitamin E

12-46 µmol/L   0.5-2.0 mg/dl

Zinc

0-1 yr	11.5-22.2 µmol/L	75-145 µg/dl
2-10 yr	10.7-20.0	70-130
11-18 yr	10.0-19.0	65-124
Adult	9.2-18.4	60-120

LAB REF VALUES

Urine

Reference Values

Agent or Test	SI Units	Traditional Units	Notes
Acyl carnitines			For diagnosis of MCAD (medium chain acyl CoA dehydrogenase deficiency); measure after carnitine load
Amino acids, screen See *metabolic study*			
Bilirubin			Normally absent
Calcium	<0.1 mmol/kg body wt/day	<4 mg/kg body wt/day	
Related to creatinine	<0.56 μmol/mol creatinine	<0.2 mg/mg creatinine	
Catecholamines Norepinephrine			Drugs such as methyldopa, apresoline, quinidine, epinephrine, or norepinephrine-related drugs (e.g., L-dopa) and renal function test dyes may interfere with catecholamine excretion and affect the results
0-2 yr	95th percentile (100th percentile) 280 (375) μmol/mol creatinine	95th percentile (100th percentile) 420 (558) μg/g creatinine	

		95th percentile (100th percentile)	95th percentile (100th percentile)
	2-4 yr	80 (150)	120 (224)
	5-9 yr	60 (90)	90 (135)
	10-19 yr	55 (60)	82 (92)
	Adult	76 (90)	114 (135)
Epinephrine			
	0-2 yr	45 (150) μmol/mol creatinine	75 (246) μg/g creatinine
	2-4 yr	35 (60)	57 (97)
	5-9 yr	20 (40)	35 (66)
	10-19 yr	20 (70)	34 (110)
	Adult	14 (50)	23 (81)
Dopamine			
	0-2 yr	2220 (3480) μmol/mol creatinine	3000 (4708) μg/g creatinine
	2-4 yr	1130 (2230)	1533 (3020)
	5-9 yr	770 (990)	1048 (1342)
	10-19 yr	400 (510)	545 (692)
	Adult	400 (580)	535 (781)

Continued.

Urine (Cont'd)

Reference Values

Agent or Test	SI Units	Traditional Units	Notes
Copper			
Normal	<0.6 µmol/day	<40 µg/day	
Coproporphyrin			
See *porphyrins*			
Cortisol (urine "free" cortisol)			
4 mo-10 yr	<74 nmol/day	<27 µg/day	Most sensitive screen for increased cortisol production
11-20 yr	<152	<55	
Adult	50-220	18-80	
4 mo-10 yr	11-55 µmol/mol creatinine	35-176 µg/g creatinine	
11-20 yr	<14	<44	
Adult	4-19	13-60	

Creatinine clearance

Age-related reference ranges for creatinine clearance corrected for body surface area are shown in Figure 1. Note that SI units are printed in blue.

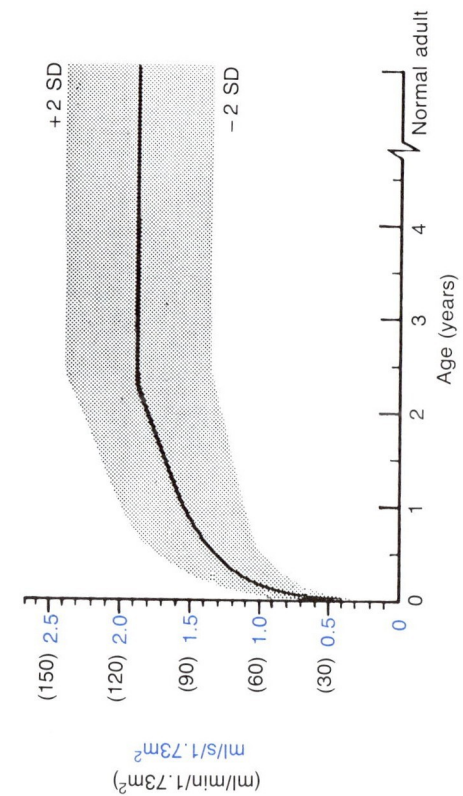

Figure 1 **Creatinine clearance.** (Adapted from McCrory WW. Developmental nephrology. Cambridge: Harvard University Press, 1972:98.)

Continued.

Urine (Cont'd)

Agent or Test	Reference Values SI Units	Traditional Units	Notes
Dinitrophenylhydrazine (DNPH) test *See metabolic study*			
Glycosaminoglycuronoglycans *See mucopolysaccharide screen*			
Hemoglobin			Normally absent; may be positive after exercise and during infectious or febrile states. Myoglobinuria may give a false-positive result.
Homovanillic acid (HVA)	95th percentile (100th percentile)	95th percentile (100th percentile)	
0-1 yr	20 (48) mmol/mol creatinine	32 (77) mg/g creatinine	
2-4 yr	14 (37)	23 (60)	

5-9 yr		9 (21)	14 (34)
10-19 yr		8 (27)	13 (43)
Adult		5 (6)	8 (10)

5 Hydroxyindoleacetic acid (5HIAA)

Adult	5-50 μmol/day	1-9.6 mg/day

Ketones

Normally absent, but may be positive in febrile or toxic states or during fasting periods

Mercury

Random specimen	<0.05 μmol/L	<0.01 mg/L
Dental fillings may elevate excretion to:	0.4	0.08

Metabolic study

The following screening tests are performed to detect metabolic disease:
1. Two-dimensional amino acid chromatography—aminoaciduria
2. Cyanide nitroprusside test—cystinuria, homocystinuria, glutathionuria, certain defects of tubule-transport
3. DNPH (dinitrophenylhydrazine) test—detects ketoacids in cases of PKU, MSUD, methionine malabsorption, tyrosinemia. Also detects ketones in normal subjects after a prolonged fast. Cyanide nitroprusside and DNPH test results are normally negative.

Continued.

Urine (Cont'd)

Reference Values

Agent or Test	SI Units	Traditional Units	Notes
Metanephrines (metanephrine and normetanephrine)			Medications like hydrocortisone and phenobarbital may cause false-positive results, whereas propranolol and theophyllines may cause false-negative results with certain laboratory techniques
<2 yr	<2.8 mmol/mol creatinine	<4.6 mg/g creatinine	
2-10 yr	<1.9	<3	
10-15 yr	<1.2	<2	
Adult	<0.6	<1	
Mucopolysaccharide screen (glycosaminoglycuronoglycans)			Normally not detectable A normal result does not rule out all mucopolysaccharidoses
Myoglobin			Normally not detectable Reacts like hemoglobin by dipstick Confirmatory tests are available
Nitroprusside test See *metabolic study*			

Organic acids

Gas chromatography—mass spectrometry results need to be interpreted by a specialist in metabolic diseases Most diagnostic if urine collected when patient is ill

Osmolality

Infant	50-600 mmol/kg water	mOsm/kg water
Child and adult: maximum (dehydration)	800-1400	
Child and adult: minimum (water diuresis)	40-80	

Values should be interpreted in conjunction with serum osmolality and clinical state of patient

Oxalate

	<8.1 μmol/kg body wt/day
	<0.73 mg/kg body wt/day, as anhydrous oxalic acid

Porphobilinogen screen
See *porphyrins*

Porphyrins

Child: ranges poorly defined

Adult

Coproporphyrin	0-380 nmol/day	0-250 μg/day
Protoporphyrin	Not detected	
Uroporphyrin	<35 nmol/day	<30 μg/day
Porphobilinogen	<15 μmol/day	<3 mg/day

Screening tests are of value only during an acute attack Urine porphobilinogen may be increased between (as well as during) attacks of acute intermittent porphyria Porphyrinuria may also occur in lead poisoning, liver disease, and conditions of increased erythropoiesis

Continued.

Urine (Cont'd)

Reference Values

Agent or Test	SI Units	Traditional Units	Notes
Potassium			Varies widely, depending on intake
Protein (quantitative)			
Over 1 yr of age	<0.10 g/m^2/day		
Protoporphyrin See *porphyrins*			
Reducing substances			Qualitative test (Clinitest tablet), detecting reducing substances such as glucose, galactose, fructose, lactose, pentoses, and homogentisic acid. Only glucose is detected by glucose-specific dipsticks (Clinistix).

Sodium

Infant	6-10 mmol/m² of body surface/day (~ 0.3-3.5 mmol/day)	mEq/m²/day	Urinary sodium should be interpreted in relation to serum sodium
Child	40-180 mmol/day	mEq/day	
Adult	80-200 mmol/day		

Specific gravity

Child >6 mo and adult	>1.020 (after fluid deprivation)	

Urate

	<60 μmol/kg body wt/day	<10 mg/kg body wt/day, as uric acid
Related to creatinine	<0.67 μmol/mol creatinine	<1 mg/mg creatinine, as uric acid

Urobilin and urobilinogen

Normally not detectable
Urobilin is the oxidation product of unstable urobilinogen
Increased in severe hemolytic jaundice and in some liver disorders

Uroporphyrin
See *porphyrins*

Continued.

Urine (Cont'd)

Reference Values

Agent or Test	SI Units	Traditional Units	Notes
Vanillylmandelic acid (VMA)			
24-hr collection	95th percentile (100th percentile)	95th percentile (100th percentile)	Nonspecific elevations occur in fever, asthma, chronic anemia, or after surgery
0-1 yr	12 (16) μmol/day	2.3 (3.1) mg/day	
2-4 yr	15 (20)	3.0 (4.0)	
5-9 yr	18 (44)	3.5 (8.7)	
10-19 yr	30 (39)	6.0 (7.7)	
Adult	34 (41)	6.8 (8.1)	
"Spot VMA"	95th percentile (100th percentile)	95th percentile (100th percentile)	Less satisfactory than 24-hr collection
0-1 yr	11 (34) mmol/mol creatinine	19 (59) mg/g creatinine	
2-4 yr	6.5 (12)	11 (21)	
5-9 yr	5 (5.5)	8 (9)	
10-19 yr	5 (8)	8 (14)	
Adult	3.5 (5)	6 (8)	

Feces

Agent or Test	Reference Values		Notes
	SI Units	Traditional Units	
Alpha-1-antitrypsin clearance	<22 ml/day		Falsely low values where lesion(s) is in the esophagus, stomach, or upper small bowel as low pH environment degrades alpha-1-antitrypsin. Collection must be free of urine. Serum alpha-1-antitrypsin required during the collection
Chymotrypsin 37° C ATEE substrate	30-750 U/g		
Coproporphyrin See *porphyrins*			

Continued.

Feces (Cont'd)

Reference Values

Agent or Test	SI Units	Traditional Units	Notes
Fat			
Fecal fat (fraction of intake)			3- or 5-day stool collection required
Premature infants	<0.20		Accurate account of dietary fat necessary during the period of stool collection
Term infants	<0.15		Regular fat study measures only the amount of LONG-chain fatty acids in the stool
>3 mo	<0.10		
Occult blood			Qualitative study
			Detected when there is 4 ml whole blood per 100 g feces (i.e., 6 mg Hgb per g feces)
Porphyrins			
Adult values (values poorly defined in children)			Fecal porphyrin may be elevated after GI bleeding

Coproporphyrin	<10 μmol/kg wet weight of stool	<655 μg/100 g wet weight of stool	Fecal porphyrin may be elevated after GI bleeding
Protoporphyrin	<25 μmol/kg wet weight of stool	<1407 μg/100 g wet weight of stool	Fecal porphyrins useful in porphyria variegata (protocoproporphyria) or hereditary coproporphyria
Protoporphyrin See *porphyrins*			Normal values in acute intermittent porphyria or cutaneous hepatic porphyria (cutanea tarda)

Cerebrospinal Fluid

Reference Values

Agent or Test	SI Units	Traditional Units	Notes
Glucose			
When blood glucose is normal	2.1-3.6 mmol/L	38-65 mg/dl	CSF glucose should be roughly 2/3 the blood glucose
Proteins			
CSF total protein			Excessively high protein concentrations (>5 g/L) can occur if spinal canal is blocked
Premature	0.15-1.3 g/L	15-130 mg/dl	
Term	0.40-1.2	40-120	
<1 mo	0.20-0.7	20-70	
>1 mo	0.15-0.4	15-40	
CSF IgG			
Normal	<0.1 of CSF total protein		

Laboratory Reference Values

Viral and Other Titers

- N.B.: Only changes in titer (≥fourfold increase or decrease over time) are diagnostic of recent infection (or reactivation)
- Adenovirus*: complement fixation <1:2 negative; ≥1:64 high
- Antihyaluronidase ≥1:300 suggestive of recent streptococcal infection
- Antistreptolysin O (ASO) ≥500 Todd units suggestive of recent streptococcal infection
- *Chlamydia trachomatis**: immunofluorescence <1:8 negative; ≥1:64 high
- Cytomegalovirus (CMV)*†: latex agglutination <1:2 negative; ≥1:32 high
- Epstein-Barr Virus (EBV)
  1. Heterophile antibody: agglutination of horse erythrocytes after absorption (monospot test) is suggestive of recent infection
  2. Immunofluorescence
     - Antibody to VCA (viral capsid antigen) ≥1:640 suggestive of recent infection; if EBNA (EBV nuclear antigen) is also positive, this suggests past infection (false-positive reactions can occur in connective tissue diseases or malignant disease)
     - Antibody to EA (early antigen)
       <1:40 negative or old infection
       ≥1:40 recent infection or reactivation
- Herpes simplex*†‡: complement fixation <1:2 negative; ≥1:64 high
- Influenza A and B*: complement fixation <1:2 negative; ≥1:64 high
- Measles*: immunofluorescence <1:8 negative; ≥1:64 high

---

*Negative: No previous exposure. High: Suggestive of recent infection or reactivation. Titers in between are suggestive of previous exposure.
†Neonates may have titers equal to, or one dilution higher, than maternal titers. Serum titers in neonates suspected of having congenital infection must be interpreted in conjunction with the maternal antibody titers.
‡In absence of CSF infection, antibody levels in serum are 200 or more times greater than in CSF.

- Mumps*: immunofluorescence <1:8 negative; ≥1:64 high
- *Mycoplasma pneumoniae:* complement fixation ≥1:32 suggestive of recent infection
- Parainfluenza*: complement fixation <1:2 negative; ≥1:64 high
- Respiratory syncytial virus*: complement fixation <1:2 negative; ≥1:64 high
- Rubella†: latex agglutination <1:2 negative; ≥1:64 possibility of recent infection; ≥1:10 considered Rubella immune
- Toxoplasmosis†: latex agglutination <1:16 negative; immunofluorescence ≥1:256 suggestive of exposure
- Varicella zoster: immunofluorescence ≥1:8 considered immune to V-Z

---

*Negative: No previous exposure. High: Suggestive of recent infection or reactivation. Titers in between are suggestive of previous exposure.

†Neonates may have titers equal to, or one dilution higher, than maternal titers. Serum titers in neonates suspected of having congenital infection must be interpreted in conjunction with the maternal antibody titers.

FIVE

FORMULARY

$$SA = W^{.5378} \times H^{.3964} \times .024265$$

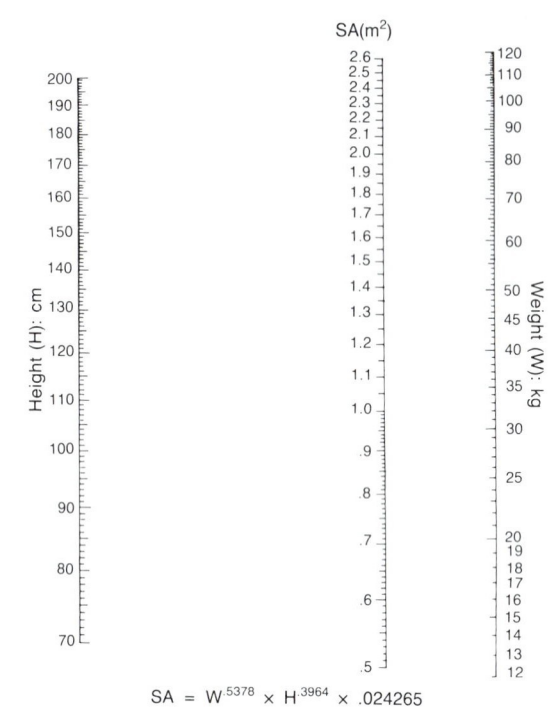

To use the nomogram, a ruler is aligned with the height and weight on the two lateral axes. The point at which the center line is intersected gives the corresponding value for surface area.

Figure 1 **Body surface area nomogram for children and adults.** (From Haycock GB, Schwartz GJ, Wisotsky DH. J Pediatr 1978; 93:62-66.)

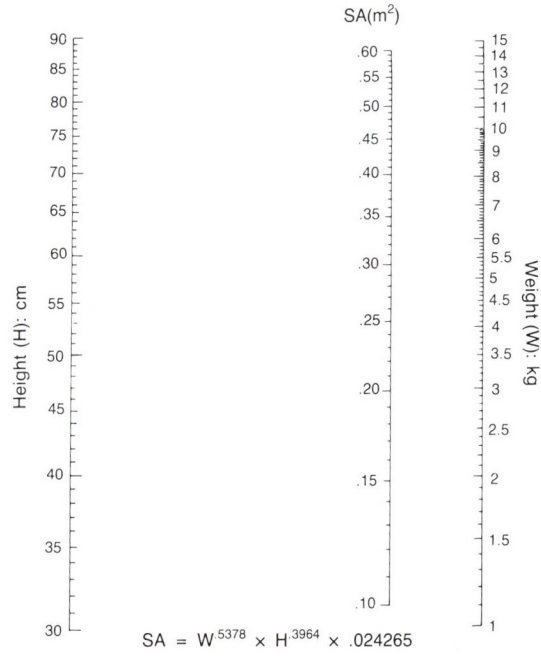

$$SA = W^{.5378} \times H^{.3964} \times .024265$$

To use the nomogram, a ruler is aligned with the height and weight on the two lateral axes. The point at which the center line is intersected gives the corresponding value for surface area.

Figure 2 **Body surface area nomogram for infants.** (From Haycock GB, Schwartz GJ, Wisotsky DH. J Pediatr, 1978; 93:62-66.)

TABLE 1 Drug Dosage Guidelines for Infants and Children

Drug	Dose	Dose Limit	Comments
Acetaminophen	40-60 mg/kg/day ÷ q4-6h PO/PR	65 mg/kg/day	Optimal single antipyretic dose = 10-15 mg/kg.
Acetylcysteine (Mucomyst)	Acetaminophen overdose: see p 472		
Acetylsalicylic acid	JA, pericarditis, rheumatic fever: 60-100 mg/kg/day PO ÷ qid Kawasaki disease: 100 mg/kg/day PO ÷ q6h until defervescence × 36 hr then 5-10 mg/kg/day PO qam	150 mg/kg/day	Monitoring of serum concentrations recommended. Not recommended for antipyresis during viral illness. Give with food. Do not give enteric-coated tablets with milk, dairy products, or antacids.
ACTH	Infantile spasms: 40-80 IU/day IM/SC once daily or ÷ bid		Close clinical monitoring for dose-related and idiosyncratic adverse effects recommended.
Activated charcoal	Initial dose: 1 g/kg PO/NG Subsequent dose: 0.5 g/kg PO/NG q4-6h PRN		Give a dose of sorbitol 70% with initial dose of activated charcoal.

Acyclovir (Zovirax)	Ointment: Apply 4-6 times daily. Herpes simplex encephalitis: 30 mg/kg/day IV ÷ q8h Other Herpes simplex: Treatment: 15-30 mg/kg/day IV ÷ q8h Adults and adolescents: 200 mg qid PO Prophylaxis: 50 mg/kg/day PO ÷ qid Varicella or Herpes zoster in immuno-compromised host: 25-50 mg/kg/day IV ÷ q8h or 1500 mg/m^2/day IV ÷ q8h Cytomegalovirus prophylaxis: 50 mg/kg/day PO ÷ qid	1 g/day PO 3 g/day PO	Maintain fluid intake. May be given PO with food. Dose interval adjustment in renal impairment as follows: moderate—q12h; severe—q24-48h.
Adenosine	Supraventricular tachycardia: 0.05 mg/kg/dose IV. May repeat PRN in the following doses Q2 min: 0.1 mg/kg, 0.15 mg/kg, 0.2 mg/kg, 0.25 mg/kg.	25 mg/dose	EMERGENCY-RELEASE DRUG.
Adrenaline	See Epinephrine		
Albumin	0.5-1 g/kg/dose IV	6 g/kg/day	
Albuterol	See Salbutamol		
Aldactazide	See Novospirozine		

Continued.

FORMULARY

TABLE 1 Drug Dosage Guidelines for Infants and Children (Cont'd)

Drug	Dose	Dose Limit	Comment
Allopurinol	400 mg/m^2/day PO ÷ tid-qid	600 mg/day	Decrease daily dose to 67% in mild and 50% in moderate renal impairment. In severe renal impairment give 3 mg/kg q2-3 days.
Alphacalcidiol	0.01-0.02 μg/kg/day PO as a single daily dose.		Adjust dose according to plasma calcium concentration
Aluminium hydroxide (aluminium and magnesium hydroxides)	Infant: 2-5 ml PO q1-2h Child: 5-15 ml PO pc and qhs Adult: 15-45 ml PO pc and qhs		
Amantadine	Influenza A prophylaxis and treatment: 5-8 mg/kg/day PO ÷ q12h	200 mg/day	Continue prophylactic therapy for at least 10 days following exposure or throughout epidemic. Active treatment should continue for 5 days after disappearance of symptoms. Avoid alcohol. Dose interval adjustment in renal impairment as follows: mild—q12-24h; moderate—q2-3 days; severe—q7 days

Drug	Dose	Notes
Amikacin	15-30 mg/kg/day IV/IM ÷ q8h	Monitoring of serum concentrations recommended. Dose interval adjustment in renal impairment as follows: mild-moderate—q12h; severe—q24-48h.
Aminocaproic acid (Amicar)	Hemophilia prior to dental extraction: 200 mg/kg/day PO ÷ q6h × 7-10 days after procedure Hemophilia, acute hemorrhage: 400 mg/kg/day PO/IV ÷ q6h	30 g/day	Decrease dose to 50 mg/kg once daily in severe renal impairment.
Aminophylline	See Theophylline		Contains 80% theophylline.
5-Aminosalicylic acid	See Mesalamine		
Amiodarone	Loading dose: 10 mg/kg/day PO as a single daily dose or ÷ bid × 7-10 days Maintenance dose: 5 mg/kg/day PO as a single daily dose	Usual adult loading dose: 800-1600 mg/day Usual adult maintenance dose: 200-400 mg/day	Reduce digoxin dose by 50% during concurrent therapy. Dose may require reduction in patients with liver impairment. Monitor thyroid, liver, lung, and eye function.
Amoxycillin	20-50 mg/kg/day PO ÷ q8h	4 g/day	May be given with food.

Continued.

TABLE 1 Drug Dosage Guidelines for Infants and Children (Cont'd)

Drug	Dose	Dose Limit	Comment
Amphotericin B	Initial: 0.25-0.5 mg/kg/day IV as a single dose. Increase by 0.25 mg/kg/day up to 0.5 mg/kg/day for *Candida* or 1 mg/kg/day for *Aspergillus* IV once daily or q2 days.	70 mg/day or 1 mg/kg/dose, whichever is less	Infuse at a concentration of ≤0.1 mg/ml in 5% Dextrose over 4-6 hr. Monitor serum potassium. Consider premedication with meperidine-diphenhydramine-hydrocortisone.
Ampicillin	Meningitis: 200-300 mg/kg/day IV ÷ q6h Other: 50-100 mg/kg/day ÷ q6h	10 g/day	Dose interval adjustment in renal failure as follows: severe—q12-16h.
Amrinone	Loading dose: 0.75-3 mg/kg/dose IV over 5 min Maintenance dose: 5-20 µg/kg/min via continuous IV infusion	Loading dose: 3 mg/kg Maintenance dose: 10 mg/kg/day	Incompatible with dextrose. Monitor liver function. Dose may require reduction in liver impairment.
Astemizole	<6 yr: 0.2 mg/kg/day PO as a single dose 6-12 yr: 5 mg PO as a single daily dose >12 yr: 10 mg PO as a single daily dose		Give on an empty stomach (1 hr ac or 2 hr pc).

Atropine	Resuscitation: see inside front cover Pre-op: 0.01-0.02 mg/kg/dose 　　　　IM/PO 　　　　30-60 min pre-op. 　　　　Minimum: 0.1 mg/dose Cholinergic crisis: 0.05 mg/kg IV 　q5min until secretions dry	0.6 mg/dose
Belladonna and opium	Ureteral spasm: $1/4$-$1/2$ suppository q4-6h PR PRN	2 mg/dose
Bisacodyl	0.3 mg/kg/dose PO 6-12 hr before desired effect <6 yr: 5 mg supp. or 2.5 ml micro-enema PR 15-60 min before desired effect >6 yr: 10 mg supp. or 5 ml micro-enema PR 15-60 min before desired effect	Do not divide or chew tablets. Do not administer PO with milk or antacid.
Budesonide	Severe acute asthma: 　Children: 0.5-1 mg bid via nebulizer 　Adults: 1-2 mg bid via nebulizer Maintenance: 　Children: 0.25-0.5 mg via nebulizer 　Adults: 0.5-1 mg bid via nebulizer	Inhalation suspension available on emergency release.

FORMULARY

Continued.

TABLE 1 Drug Dosage Guidelines for Infants and Children (Cont'd)

Drug	Dose	Dose Limit	Comment
Calcitriol (1,25-dihydroxycholecalciferol)	Hypoparathyroidism, vitamin D resistant rickets, dialysis: Initial: 0.015-0.025 µg/kg/day PO ÷ bid Maintenance: increase PRN gradually to 0.5-1 µg/day PO		
Calcium carbonate	Calcium deficiency and hyperphosphatemia prophylaxis in renal patients: Infants: 125 mg Ca/dose PO tid Children: 250 mg Ca/dose PO tid		Titrate dose according to serum PO_4. Oral suspension 200 mg/mL contains 80 mg elemental Ca/mL. Tablet 625 mg contains 250 mg elemental Ca.
Calcium	Resuscitation: see inside front cover Hypocalcemia: 0.1-0.2 mmol Ca/kg/h IV. Adjust IV rate q4h according to plasma Ca concentration		For IV administration, dilute to 0.05 mmol/ml or less. Avoid extravasation. Cardiac monitoring recommended. 100 mg calcium chloride = 28 mg elemental Ca = 0.68 mmol Ca 100 mg calcium gluconate = 9.6 mg elemental Ca = 0.23 mmol Ca

Drug	Dose	Max	Notes
Captopril	Hypertension: Initial dose: 0.45-0.9 mg/kg/day PO ÷ tid Maintenance dose: 0.3-0.6 mg/kg/day PO ÷ tid CHF: 1.5-6 mg/kg/day PO ÷ tid	6 mg/kg/day	Reduce dose to 50% in severe renal impairment.
Carbamazepine	Initial dose: 10 mg/kg/day PO once or twice daily Maintenance dose: up to 20-30 mg/kg/day PO ÷ q8h. Increase dose gradually over 2-4 wk		Chewable tablets must be thoroughly chewed and not swallowed whole. Controlled-release tablets may be split. Give with food or milk. Dose may require reduction in liver impairment. Monitoring of serum drug concentrations recommended.
Cardiac cocktail	See Catheter mixture no. 3.		
Catheter mixture no. 3	0.1 ml/kg IM 20-60 min pre-procedure	2 ml/dose No repeat or supplemental doses	Reduce dose in patients with CNS impairment. Contains meperidine 25 mg/ml, chlorpromazine 6.25 mg/ml, and promethazine 6.25 mg/ml.
Cefaclor	20-40 mg/kg/day PO ÷ q8h	1.5 g/day	May be given with food. Dose adjustment in renal impairment as follows: moderate—50-100%; severe—33%.
Cefazolin	Mild to moderate infections: 25-50 mg/kg/day IV/IM ÷ q8h Severe infections: 50-150 mg/kg/day IV/IM ÷ q8h Cardiac surgery prophylaxis: 40 mg/kg/dose q8h × 6 doses	2 g/day 6 g/day 750 mg/dose	Dose interval adjustment in renal impairment as follows: moderate—q12h; severe—q24-48h.

Continued.

TABLE 1 Drug Dosage Guidelines for Infants and Children (Cont'd)

Drug	Dose	Dose Limit	Comment
Cefixime	8 mg/kg/day PO ÷ q12-24h	400 mg/day	Inactive against staphylococci. Dose adjustment in renal impairment as follows: moderate—75%; severe—50%
Cefotaxime	Mild to moderate infections: 75-100 mg/kg/day IV/IM ÷ q6-8h Severe infections: 150-200 mg/kg/day IV/IM ÷ q6-8h Meningitis in infants 1-3 mo of age: 200 mg/kg/day IV/IM ÷ q6h	6 g/day 8 g/day 8 g/day	Dose interval adjustment in renal impairment as follows: moderate—q8-12h; severe—q12-24h.
Cefoxitin	Mild to moderate infections: 80-100 mg/kg/day IV/IM ÷ q6-8h Severe infections: 80-160 mg/kg/day IV/IM ÷ q4-6h	4 g/day 12 g/day	Dose interval adjustment in renal impairment as follows: moderate—q8-12h; severe—q24-48h
Ceftazidime	Mild to moderate infections: 75-100 mg/kg/day IV/IM ÷ q8h Severe infections: 125-150 mg/kg/day IV/IM ÷ q8h CF Patients: 200 mg/kg/day IV/IM ÷ q6h	3 g/day 6 g/day 12 g/day	Dose interval adjustment in renal impairment as follows: moderate—q48h; severe—q48-72h.

Drug	Dose	Max	Notes
Ceftriaxone	Meningitis in children > 3 mo of age: 100 mg/kg/day IV/IM ÷ q12h Uncomplicated gonorrhea: <45 kg: 125 mg/dose IM as a single dose ≥45 kg: 250 mg/dose IM as a single dose	4 g/day	Treat uncomplicated gonorrhea in children ≥45 kg with tetracycline/doxycycline as well.
Cefuroxime	75 mg/kg/day IV/IM ÷ q8h	4.5 g/day	Dose interval adjustment in renal impairment as follows: moderate—q8-48h; severe—q24-72h. Not to be used for the treatment of meningitis.
Cephalexin	25-50 mg/kg/day PO ÷ qid	4 g/day	May be given with food. Dose interval adjustment in renal impairment as follows: severe—q8-12h.
Charcoal, activated	see Activated Charcoal		
Chloral hydrate	Hypnotic: 50 mg/kg/dose PO/PR 20-45 min pre-exam Sedative: 25 mg/kg/dose PO/PR qhs PRN Sedation precardiac ultrasonography 80 mg/kg/dose PO 20-45 min pre-exam May repeat 40 mg/kg/dose in 1 hr PRN	1 g/dose 1 g/initial dose 500 mg/supplemental dose	Reduce dose in patients with CNS impairment. Dose may require reduction in liver impairment. Capsules may be given rectally.

Continued.

TABLE 1 Drug Dosage Guidelines for Infants and Children (Cont'd)

Drug	Dose	Dose Limit	Comment
Chloramphenicol	Meningitis: 75-100 mg/kg/day IV/PO ÷ q6h Other: 50-75 mg/kg/day IV/PO ÷ q6h	4 g/day	Avoid in liver impairment. Do not use chloramphenicol palmitate in infants <1 yr or in patients with cystic fibrosis. Give PO on an empty stomach (1 hr ac or 2 hr pc). Monitoring of serum drug concentrations recommended.
Chloroquine	Malaria prophylaxis: 5 mg base/kg/dose PO once weekly beginning 1 wk before and for 6 wk after last exposure Malaria: 10 mg base/kg/dose PO × 1 dose 5 mg base/kg/dose PO 6 hr later Then 5 mg base/kg/day PO as a single daily dose × 2 days or 3.5 mg base/kg/dose IM/SC Repeat × 1 in 6 hr PRN	300 mg base/dose First dose: 600 mg base Subsequent doses: 300 mg base or 7.5 mg base/day IM/SC	250 mg chloroquine phosphate = 150 mg chloroquine base. Give PO with food or milk. PO drug extremely bitter. Parenteral drug available on *emergency release.*

Drug	Dose	Max	Notes
Chlorpheniramine	0.35 mg/kg/day PO ÷ q6-12h	Usual adult dose: 4 mg PO q4-6h PRN or 8 mg PO q12h PRN (Sustained release tablets)	Give with food or milk.
Chlorpromazine	Afterload reduction: 0.1-0.25 mg/kg/dose IV Antineoplastic-induced emesis prophylaxis: 0.3-0.5 mg/kg/dose IV q4-6h PRN Nausea and vomiting: 2 mg/kg/day PO/IM/IV q4-6h 4 mg/kg/day PR ÷ q6-8h	<5 yr: 40 mg/day 5-12 yr: 75 mg/day	Monitor blood pressure after IV therapy. Administer diphenhydramine concurrently during antineoplastic-induced emesis prophylaxis to prevent extrapyramidal reactions. Give PO with food or milk.
Cholestyramine	0.24-1.1 g/kg/day PO ÷ bid/tid		May alter absorption of other drugs.
Cimetidine	20 mg/kg/day PO/IV ÷ q6h or ÷ tid with meals and qhs	2400 mg/day	Dose adjustment in renal impairment as follows: moderate—75%; severe—50%. Monitor gastric pH in patients requiring IV therapy. Coadministration of cimetidine and propranolol may decrease the effect of propranolol. Coadministration of cimetidine and either theophylline, phenytoin, or procainamide may produce toxicity due to the latter drug.
Cisapride	0.42-0.78 mg/kg/day PO ÷ tid ac or ÷ tid ac and qhs	40 mg/day	Dose may require reduction in renal or liver impairment. May alter the absorption of other drugs. *Continued.*

FORMULARY

TABLE 1 Drug Dosage Guidelines for Infants and Children (Cont'd)

Drug	Dose	Dose Limit	Comment
Clindamycin	Mild to moderate infections: 15-25 mg/kg/day IM/IV ÷ q6-8h 10-30 mg/kg/day PO ÷ q6h Severe infections: 25-40 mg/kg/day IM/IV ÷ q6-8h Chloroquine-resistant falciparum malaria: 30 mg/kg/day PO ÷ q8h × 7 days	1.8 g/day IV/IM 2 g/day PO 2.7 g/day IV/IM 1.35 g/day PO	Do not use palmitate in infants <1 yr old or in patients with CF. Give capsule PO with food or a full glass of water to avoid esophageal ulceration.
Clonazepam	≤30 kg: Initial dose: 0.05 mg/kg/day PO ÷ bid or tid increasing by 0.05 mg/kg/day every 3 days PRN up to 0.2 mg/kg/day >30 kg: Initial dose: 1.5 mg/kg/day PO ÷ tid increasing by 0.5-1 mg/day every 3 days up to 20 mg/day PO ÷ tid	20 mg/day	Dose may require reduction in liver impairment.
Cloxacillin	Mild to moderate infections: 50-100 mg/kg/day PO/IV/IM ÷ q6h Severe infections: 150-200 mg/kg/day IV/IM ÷ q6h	4 g/day PO/IV/IM 12 g/day IV/IM	Give PO on an empty stomach (1 hr ac or 2 hr pc). Oral suspension extremely bitter. Consider flucloxacillin or cephalexin if oral liquid is required.

CM-3	See Catheter mixture no. 3		
Codeine	Analgesic: 3-6 mg/kg/day PO/IM ÷ q4-6h PRN Antidiarrheal: 2 mg/kg/day PO/IM ÷ q6h Antitussive: 0.8-1.2 mg/kg/day PO ÷ q4-6h	1.5 mg/kg/dose	Max. dose should not be given for >24 hr. Avoid IM route if possible.
Cortisone acetate	Hypoadrenalism: 25 mg/m^2/day PO ÷ tid		Give with food or milk. To discontinue in patients receiving therapy for ≥10 days reduce dose by 50% q10-14 days.
Cotrimoxazole	Bacterial infection: 5-10 mg trimethoprim/kg/day PO/IV ÷ q12h (Includes 25-50 mg/kg/day sulfamethoxazole) *Pneumocystis carinii*: Treatment: 20 mg trimethoprim/kg/day IV or PO ÷ q6h (Includes 100 mg/kg/day sulfamethoxazole) Prophylaxis: HIV infected/exposed children: 150 mg trimethoprim/m^2/day PO 3 times weekly.		Maintain fluid intake. May be given PO with food. Dose interval adjustment in renal impairment as follows: moderate—q18h; severe—q24h.

Continued.

TABLE 1 Drug Dosage Guidelines for Infants and Children (Cont'd)

Drug	Dose	Dose Limit	Comment
Cotrimoxazole—cont'd	Prophylaxis: Other immunocompromised children: 2.5-5 mg trimethoprim/kg/day PO q2d or 3 times weekly as a single daily dose. Prophylaxis: Otitis media and urinary tract infection: 2-5 mg trimethoprim/kg/day PO once daily Prophylaxis: asplenia: 5 mg trimethoprim/kg/day PO once daily		
Cromoglycate sodium	1% inhalation solution (Intal): 20 mg (2 ml) dose bid-qid via nebulizer Metered-dose aerosol (Fivent): 2 mg (2 puffs) qid		

	Spincap (Intal): 60-80 mg/day via inhalation ÷ tid/qid Nasal (Rynacrom): 1-2 squeezes into each nostril, up to 6×/day	
Cyclosporine	Bone marrow transplant: 3 mg/kg/day IV ÷ q12h 12 mg/kg/day PO ÷ q12h Liver transplant: Initial dose: 3 mg/kg/day IV as a continuous infusion Renal transplant: 5 mg/kg/day PO ÷ q12h	Dose may require reduction in liver impairment. Give PO on an empty stomach (1 hr ac or 2-3 hr pc). Coadministration of cyclosporine and rifampin may decrease the effects of cyclosporine. Coadministration of cyclosporine and erythromycin or ketoconazole may produce cyclosporine toxicity. Monitoring of level recommended.
Deferoxamine mesylate (Desferal)	Acute iron intoxication: see p 476 Chronic iron overload: 50 mg/kg/dose by continuous SC infusion overnight	Titrate dose according to serum ferritin.
Desmopressin (DDAVP)	Diabetes insipidus: 5-20 µg/day intranasally once daily or ÷ bid Coagulopathy: 0.3 µg/kg/dose IV or SC Enuresis: Initial dose: 20 µg intranasally qhs × 5 doses.	
	25 µg/dose 40 µg/dose	Maintain lowest effective dose × 4 wk, then taper by decreasing dose by 10 µg q1-2 days.

Continued.

TABLE 1 Drug Dosage Guidelines for Infants and Children (Cont'd)

Drug	Dose	Dose Limit	Comment
Desmopressin (DDAVP) —cont'd	May increase dose q5 days in 10 μg increments up to 40 μg/night		
Dexamethasone	Extubation (if previous difficulties with extubation): 1-2 mg/kg/day PO, IV, or IM ÷ q6h beginning 24 hr prior to extubation and continuing 4-6 hr afterwards Increased ICP: Initial dose: 0.2-0.4 mg/kg IV Subsequent dose: 0.3 mg/kg/day IV or IM ÷ q6h. May be useful in cerebral tumors and malaria Croup: 0.6 mg/kg IV × 1	Initial dose: 10 mg	Give PO with food or milk. To discontinue in patients receiving therapy for ≥10 days, reduce dose by 50% q48h until 0.3 ± 0.1 mg/m^2/day achieved. Then reduce dose by 50% q10-14 days.
Dextromethorphan	1 mg/kg/day PO ÷ q6-8h	1 mg/kg/day Usual adult dose: 10-20 mg PO q4h PRN	

Drug	Dose	Max/Notes	Comments
Dextrose	Resuscitation: see inside front cover		
Diazepam	Status epilepticus: 0.1-0.3 mg/kg/dose IV q10min × 3 or 0.3-0.5 mg/kg/dose PR × 1 Pre x-ray >30 kg: 0.2 mg/kg/dose PO × 1 dose only Sedation: 0.1 mg/kg/dose IV 0.1-0.8 mg/kg/day PO ÷ q6h	Status epilepticus < 5 yr: 5 mg/dose ≥ 5 yr: 10 mg/dose Usual adult dose (Sedation): 2-10 mg/dose bid-qid PO 5-10 mg/dose IV	May cause hypotension and apnea when given IV. Dose may require reduction in liver impairment.
Diazoxide	Acute hypertension: 1-2 mg/kg/dose IV q5-15 min PRN	Max. total dose: 8 mg/kg or 4 doses	Give IV undiluted over 30 sec.
Digoxin	Digitalization dose: (3 doses — 1st STAT, 2nd in 6 hr, 3rd in another 6 hr) ≥37 weeks PCA—2 yr old: 0.017 mg/kg **dose** PO 0.012 mg/kg **dose** IV >2 yr: 0.013 mg/kg/dose PO 0.01 mg/kg **dose** IV	Total digitalization dose: 1.0 mg	Calculate dose according to ideal body weight. Reduce dose by 50% during concurrent administration of amiodarone, propafenone, or quinidine. Maintenance dose adjustment in renal impairment as follows: moderate—25-75%; severe—10-25%. Once daily dosing may be satisfactory, especially in patients >2 yr. Monitoring of serum drug concentrations recommended. PCA = post-conceptional age.

Continued.

TABLE 1 Drug Dosage Guidelines for Infants and Children (Cont'd)

Drug	Dose	Dose Limit	Comment
Digoxin—cont'd	Maintenance dose: ≥37 wk PCA—2 yr old: 0.01 mg/kg/day PO ÷ bid or as a single daily dose >2 yr: 0.008 mg/kg/day PO ÷ bid or as a single daily dose	Maintenance dose: 0.25 mg/day	
Dimenhydrinate	5 mg/kg/day PO, IV, IM, or PR ÷ q6h	300 mg/day	
Dimercaprol (BAL in Oil)	Lead poisoning: 50 mg/m² IM q4h		Give by deep IM injection.
Diphenhydramine	Antihistamine: 5 mg/kg/day PO, IV, or IM ÷ q6h Anaphylaxis: 1-2 mg/kg/dose IV	300 mg/day 50 mg/dose	
Dipyridamole	5 mg/kg/day PO ÷ tid	400 mg/day	Give on an empty stomach (1 hr ac or 2 hr pc).
Dobutamine	2-20 µg/kg/min IV	40 µg/kg/min	*Avoid extravasation.* Administer via central line wherever possible.

Drug	Dose	Usual/Max	Notes
Docusate sodium	5 mg/kg/day PO ÷ q6-8h or as a single daily dose	Usual adult dose: 100-200 mg/day	Dilute liquid in milk or juice. Onset of action = 24-72 hr.
Domperidone	1.2-2.4 mg/kg/day PO ÷ tid-qid. Give 15-30 min ac + qhs	80 mg/day Usual adult dose: 10 mg tid-qid	
Dopamine	5-20 μg/kg/min via continuous IV infusion	25 μg/kg/min	Avoid extravasation. Administer via central venous line wherever possible.
Doxycycline	5 mg/kg/day PO ÷ q12h	200 mg/day	May be given PO with food. Not recommended for children ≤8 yr.
Edetate calcium disodium	Lead poisoning: 1000 mg/m^2/day by continuous IV infusion		Begin therapy with second dose of dimercaprol.
Edrophonium	Supraventricular tachycardia: 0.2 mg/kg/dose IV over 3 min		Have atropine ready.
Epinephrine	Resuscitation: see inside front cover Anaphylaxis: 0.01 mg/kg/dose (0.01 ml of 1:1000 solution/kg/dose) SC q10-20 min PRN *minimum* 0.1 mg (0.1 ml)/dose		
Epinephrine (Racemic) for inhalation	0.5 ml/dose in 3 ml NS via nebulizer PRN up to max q1h	0.5 ml/dose	

Continued.

TABLE 1 Drug Dosage Guidelines for Infants and Children (Cont'd)

Drug	Dose	Dose Limit	Comment
Erythromycin	Base: 40 mg/kg/day PO ÷ q6h Stearate and estolate: 20-40 mg/kg/day PO ÷ q6-12h Ethylsuccinate: 40 mg/kg/day PO ÷ q6h Gluceptate and lactobionate: 20-50 mg/kg/day IV ÷ q6h Inflammatory acne: 500-1000 mg/day PO ÷ q6-8h May be decreased to 250 mg/day PO as a single daily dose	2 g/day PO 4 g/day IV	Use base for CF patients. Give PO on an empty stomach (1 hr ac or 2 hr pc) unless GI upset occurs.
Erythropoietin	Anemia of chronic renal failure: Initial dose: 50 U/kg/day IV or SC 3 × weekly		Titrate dose according to hemoglobin.
Ethambutol	Initial dose: 15 mg/kg/day PO as a single daily dose or 50 mg/kg/dose PO twice weekly Retreatment: 25 mg/kg/day PO as a single daily dose	Initial: 1.5 g/day Twice weekly regimen: 2.5 g/day Retreatment: 2.5 g/day	Bacteriostatic. Give with food if GI upset occurs. Dose interval adjustment in renal impairment as follows: moderate—q24-36h; severe—q48h.

Drug	Dose	Notes
Ethosuximide	Initial dose: 15 mg/kg/day PO as a single dose or ÷ bid. Increase gradually q3days PRN to maximum dose.	1.5 g/day or 40 mg/kg/day, whichever is less	Dose may require reduction in liver impairment. Monitoring of serum drug concentrations recommended.
Fansidar	Chloroquine-resistant falciparum malaria: <1 yr: ¼ tablet PO × 1 1-3 yr: ½ tablet PO × 1 4-8 yr: 1 tablet PO × 1 9-14 yr: 2 tablets PO × 1 >14 yr: 3 tablets PO × 1		Each tablet contains pyrimethamine, 25 mg, and sulfadoxine, 500 mg. Fansidar may cause Stevens-Johnson syndrome and Toxic Epidermal Necrolysis.
Ferrous sulfate	Treatment: 6 mg elemental Fe/kg/day PO tid Prophylaxis: 0.5-2 mg elemental Fe/kg/day PO as a single daily dose or ÷ bid-tid		Dilute drops prior to administration in a glass of water or juice. Administer tablets with ½ to 1 glass of water or juice. Administer 1 hr before or 2 hr after dairy products, eggs, coffee, tea, or whole grain bread or cereal.
Flecainide	2-5 mg/kg/day PO ÷ bid-tid	Sustained VT: 400 mg/day Nonsustained VT, couplets, PVCs: 600 mg/day Usual adult dose: 300-400 mg/day PO ÷ q12h	Dose adjustment in renal impairment as follows: severe—75%. Dose may require reduction in liver impairment. Digoxin dose may require reduction during concurrent flecainide therapy.

Continued.

TABLE 1 Drug Dosage Guidelines for Infants and Children (Cont'd)

Drug	Dose	Dose Limit	Comment
Flucloxacillin	25-100 mg/kg/day PO ÷ q6h	2 g/day	Give on an empty stomach (1 hr ac or 2 hr pc). Consider cephalexin if oral liquid required. Dose may require reduction in renal impairment.
Flucytosine	50-150 mg/kg/day PO ÷ q6h 100-150 mg/kg/day IV ÷ q6h		Dose interval adjustment in renal failure as follows: moderate—q12-24h; severe—q24-48h. Monitoring of serum drug concentrations recommended.
Fludrocortisone	Salt-losing hypoadrenalism: 0.05-0.2 mg/day PO ÷ q12h		Give with food or milk.
Furazolidone	Giardiasis: 5-8 mg/kg/day PO ÷ qid × 7-10 days		
Furosemide	1-2 mg/kg/day PO—may increase to 3-8 mg/kg/day PO ÷ q6-8 hr PRN 0.5-2 mg/kg/dose IV/IM	6 mg/kg/dose	Give IV over 5-10 min no faster than 20 mg/min.

Ganciclovir	CMV infection: Treatment: 10 mg/kg/day IV ÷ q12h Prophylaxis: 5 mg/kg/day IV as a single daily dose	Handle as a biohazard. Dose *and* interval adjustment in renal impairment as follows: GFR DOSE 25-50 3 mg/kg/dose q12h 10-25 3 mg/kg/dose q24h <10 1.5 mg/kg/dose q24h
Gelusil (extra strength)	See aluminium and magnesium hydroxides	
Gentamicin	7.5 mg/kg/day IV/IM ÷ q8h Cardiac surgery prophylaxis: 2 mg/kg/dose IV 1 hr preop and 8 hr postop	100 mg/dose prior to serum concentration determination. 120 mg/dose	Calculate dose according to effective body weight. Monitoring of serum drug concentrations recommended. Dose interval adjustment in renal impairment as follows: mild-moderate—q12h; severe—q24-48h.
Glucagon	Hypoglycemia in diabetes mellitus: <5 yr: 0.5 mg/dose SC >5 yr: 1 mg/dose SC May repeat in 5-20 min PRN	
GoLytely	See Peg-electrolyte liquid	
Growth hormone	0.06 mg/kg/dose IM or SC 3 × weekly	
Heparin	Initial dose: 50 U/kg IV bolus Maintenance dose: 20 U/kg/h via continuous IV infusion	Maintain PTT 1.5-2.5 times normal Antidote = protamine sulfate

Continued.

TABLE 1 Drug Dosage Guidelines for Infants and Children (Cont'd)

Drug	Dose	Dose Limit	Comment
Hydralazine	Initial dose: 0.15-0.8 mg/kg/dose IV q4-6h or 1.5 µg/kg/min IV Maintenance dose: 0.75-7 mg/kg/day PO ÷ q6h	25 mg/dose IV	Associated with development of drug-induced lupus
Hydrochloro-thiazide	2-4 mg/kg/day PO ÷ q12h	200 mg/day or 7 mg/kg/day, whichever is less	For hydrochlorothiazide in combination with spironolactone, see Novospirozine Ineffective when GFR <30 ml/min
Hydrocortisone	Acute asthma: 4-6 mg/kg/dose IV q4-6h Anaphylaxis: 5-10 mg/kg IV Hypoadrenalism Normal endogenous production = 10 ± 3 mg/m^2/day Maintenance dose: 20 mg/m^2/day PO ÷ tid or	Usual adult dose: 25-100 mg/dose PO as a single daily dose, bid or q2 days	Bioavailability of PO hydrocortisone = 50%. Triple maintenance dose during concurrent illness or stress. In CAH, administer 1/2 the daily dose at bedtime to suppress AM surge of ACTH. Give PO with food or milk.

Drug	Dose	Max	Notes
	12 mg/m^2/day IV ÷ q6h Preop 100 mg/m^2 IV × 1 preop, then 100 mg/m^2/day IV ÷ q6h Acute adrenal crisis: 100 mg/m^2 IV STAT, then 100 mg/m^2/day IV ÷ q6h		To discontinue in patients receiving therapy for ≥10 days, reduce dose by 50% q48h until 10 ± 3 mg/m^2/day achieved. Then reduce dose by 50% q10-14 days.
Hydroxy- chloroquine	Juvenile arthritis: 60 mg/kg/day PO as a single daily dose	300 mg/day	
Hydroxyzine	2 mg/kg/day PO ÷ tid or qid Chronic urticaria: 2-4 mg/kg/day PO ÷ tid or qid	400 mg/day	Give with food or milk. Avoid alcohol. Monitor visual acuity.
Imipenem- cilastatin	60-100 mg/kg/day IV or IM ÷ q6h	2 g/day or 50 mg/kg/day, whichever is less	Dose interval adjustment in renal impairment as follows: moderate—q8-12h; severe—q12h (max, 1 g/day)
Imipramine	Enuresis: ≥5 yr: 10-50 mg PO qhs ≥12 yr: 50-75 mg PO qhs	2.5 mg/kg/day	
Immune globulin (Human IV)	Hypogammaglobulinemia: 600 mg/kg/dose IV once monthly Idiopathic thrombocytopenia purpura: 1 g/kg/dose IV as a single daily dose for 1 or 2 days Kawasaki disease: 2 g/kg IV as a single dose		Supplied as Gamimune except for study patients.

Continued.

TABLE 1 Drug Dosage Guidelines for Infants and Children (Cont'd)

Drug	Dose	Dose Limit	Comment
Indomethacin	1.5-3 mg/kg/day PO ÷ tid with meals	200 mg/day	Give with food or milk. Sustained release capsules may be dosed bid.
Iodoquinol	Intestinal amoebiasis: 30-40 mg/kg/day PO ÷ tid pc × 20 days	1.95 g/day	
Ipecac	9-12 mo: 10 ml PO 1-10 yr: 15 ml PO >10 yr: 30 ml PO	≤ 1 yr: 1 single dose > 1 yr: can repeat once after 20 min	Contact Poison Center re: treatment of patients <9 mo old
Ipratropium	Metered dose aerosol: 1-2 puffs tid-qid Inhalation Solution: <4 yr: 125 µg/dose ≥4 yr: 250 µg/dose Give each dose in 3 ml NS via nebulizer tid-qid PRN. In severe acute asthma, may be given q1h PRN.	12 puffs/day Usual adult dose: 250-500 µg/dose in 3 ml NS via nebulizer q4-6h PRN	
Iron	See Ferrous sulfate		

Drug	Dose	Notes
Isoniazid	10-20 mg/kg/day PO as a single daily dose or ÷ q12 or 10-20 mg/kg/dose PO twice weekly	CNS disease: 500 mg/day Twice weekly regimen: 900 mg/day Other: 300 mg/day	Pyridoxine supplementation recommended in adolescents and adults. Give on an empty stomach (1 hr ac or 2 hr pc) unless GI upset occurs.
Isoproterenol	Resuscitation: see inside front cover		
Isotretinoin (Accutane)	Cystic scarring acne: 0.5-1 mg/kg/day PO ÷ q12h	2 mg/kg/day	*Must avoid pregnancy* for 1 mo prior to, during, and for 1 mo following therapy.
Kayexalate	See Sodium polystrene sulfonate		
Ketoconazole	5-10 mg/kg/day PO as a single daily dose or ÷ q12h	400 mg/day	Give with food.
Ketotifen	>3 yr: Initial dose: 0.5 mg PO qhs or 0.25 mg PO bid Maintenance dose: 1 mg PO bid		
Labetalol	Acute hypertension: 1-3 mg/kg IV Hypertension: 1 mg/kg/hr by continuous IV infusion	3 mg/kg/hr	Dose may require reduction in liver impairment.
Lactulose	Constipation: Initial dose: 5-10 ml/day PO once daily Double daily dose until stool is produced.	Usual adult dose: 15-30 ml/day (constipation)	For hepatic encephalopathy: decrease/discontinue if severe diarrhea develops. Treatment is effective if stool is soft with pH < 5.5. Hypernatremia or hypokalemia may occur.

Continued.

TABLE 1 Drug Dosage Guidelines for Infants and Children (Cont'd)

Drug	Dose	Dose Limit	Comment
Lactulose —cont'd	Hepatic encephalopathy: <1 yr: 2.5 ml PO bid Older children and adolescents: 10-30 ml PO tid	<1 yr: 2.5 ml PO qid	
Levothyroxine	1-6 mo: 7-12 μg/kg/day PO once daily 6-12 mo: 6-8 μg/kg/day PO once daily 1-5 yr: 4-6 μg/kg/day PO once daily 5-10 yr: 3-5 μg/kg/day PO once daily 10-20 yr: 2-3 μg/kg/day PO once daily		Adjust dose according to clinical status and thyroid function tests. Give on an empty stomach (1 hr ac or 2 hr pc).
Lidocaine	Resuscitation: see inside front cover		
Lindane (Kwellada)	Scabies: Apply cream or lotion in a thin layer to skin below the neck and leave on overnight. Bathe in 8-12 hr.		In children <2 yrs consider use of an alternative scabicide due to possible CNS toxicity.
Loperamide	0.08-0.24 mg/kg/day PO ÷ bid or tid	16 mg/day 2 mg/dose	Following the first treatment day, give 0.1 mg/kg/dose only after a loose stool.

Drug	Dose	Notes
Loratadine	<30 kg: 5 mg PO once daily <30 kg: 10 mg PO once daily	
Lorazepam	Preop: 0.05 mg/kg/dose SL Status epilepticus: 0.05 mg/kg/dose IV/PR May repeat once PRN	SL: 4 mg IV/PR 4 mg/dose 8 mg/12 hr or 0.1 mg/kg/12 hr, whichever is less	Dose may require reduction in liver impairment. For PR administration, dilute injection according to IV instructions.
Magnesium citrate	Cathartic: 4 ml/kg/dose PO	296 ml/dose	Use with caution in renal failure
Magnesium glucoheptonate	Hypomagnesemia: 20-40 mg elemental mg/kg/day PO ÷ tid		Large doses may cause diarrhea Use with caution in renal failure
Magnesium hydroxide	Cathartic: 0.5 ml/kg/dose PO	Usual adult dose: 30-60 mL	Use with caution in renal failure
Magnesium sulfate	Hypomagnesemia Initial dose: 0.21-0.42 mmol/kg/dose IV (5-10 mg/kg/dose elemental magnesium) Continuous infusion: 0.42 mmol/kg/day IV (10 mg/kg/day elemental magnesium)	40 mmol (1000 mg elemental Mg) per dose	Must be diluted before administration. Use with caution in renal failure. 500 mg magnesium sulfate = 50 mg Mg = 2 mmol Mg = 4 mEq Mg.

Continued.

TABLE 1 Drug Dosage Guidelines for Infants and Children (Cont'd)

Drug	Dose	Dose Limit	Comment
Mannitol	Test for oliguria: 0.2 g/kg/dose IV over 10 min × 1 dose Cerebral edema: 0.2-0.5 g/kg/dose IV over 10-30 min (1-2.5 ml of 20% solution/kg IV)		
Mebendazole	Pinworm: 100 mg PO × 1 dose. Repeat in 2 wk. Other nematodes: 200 mg/day PO ÷ bid × 3 days		Do not use for children <2 yr. Tablets may be chewed, swallowed whole, or crushed, and mixed with food.
Meperidine	Analgesic: 1-1.5 mg/kg/dose IV/SC/IM/PO q3-4h PRN Pre-op: 1-2 mg/kg/dose IM/SC/PO 60 min preop	IV/IM/SC: 2 mg/kg/dose or 100 mg/dose, whichever is less PO: 4 mg/kg/dose or 150 mg/dose, whichever is less	Dose reduction in renal impairment as follows: severe—50-75%. Dose may require reduction in liver impairment. May cause constipation, respiratory, or CNS depression. Dose is cumulative. Metabolite may cause seizures. For patients being converted from parenteral to oral therapy, IM:PO dose ratio = 1:4. Avoid IM route if possible.

Drug	Dose	Notes
Mesalamine (5-aminosalicylic acid, Salofalk, Asacol)	Adult dose: 4 g once daily PR 1200-2400 mg/day PO ÷ tid-qid	4 g/day PO
Methotrexate	Juvenile arthritis: 5 mg/m^2/dose PO once weekly; may double dose PRN after 6-8 wk		Give on an empty stomach (1 hr AC or 2 hr PC) Monitor liver function
Methyldopa	Initial dose: 10 mg/kg/day PO ÷ tid or qid. Increase dose gradually over several days until desired effect is achieved.	4 g/day or 65 mg/kg/day, whichever is less	Dose interval reduction in renal impairment as follows: moderate — q8-18h; severe — q12-24h.
Methylprednisolone	Pulse therapy (rheumatology, immunology): 10-30 mg/kg in 50-100 ml 5% dextrose IV over 1 hr	1 g/dose	
Metoclopramide	Small bowel intubation: 0.1 mg/kg/dose PO/IM or IV Delayed gastric emptying: <5 yr: 0.5 mg/kg/day PO ÷ tid with meals 5-14 yr: 2.5-5 mg PO tid before meals >14 yr: 5-10 mg PO tid before meals		May alter the absorption of other drugs. When used as antiemetic, concomitant diphenhydramine is recommended.

Continued.

TABLE 1 Drug Dosage Guidelines for Infants and Children (Cont'd)

Drug	Dose	Dose Limit	Comment
Metoclopramide—cont'd	Antineoplastic-induced emesis prophylaxis: 0.5-2 mg/kg/dose IV/PO q3-4h PRN	10 mg/kg/day	
Metoprolol	Wolff-Parkinson-White syndrome: 2-5 mg/kg/day PO ÷ bid-tid Hypertension: 1-4 mg/kg/day PO ÷ bid		Dose may require reduction in severe liver impairment
Metronidazole	Anaerobes, including *Clostridium difficile*: 15-30 mg/kg/day PO ÷ tid 30 mg/kg/day IV ÷ q6-8h	2 g/day PO 4 g/day IV	Give PO with food or milk. Avoid alcohol. *Trichomonas vaginalis*: partner must also be treated. Dose reduction required in severe liver impairment.
	Giardiasis: 15 mg/kg/day PO ÷ tid × 5 days or single daily dose as follows: <25 kg: 35 mg/kg/day PO × 3 days 25-40 kg: 50 mg/kg/day PO × 3 days >40 kg: 2 g/day PO × 3 days	750 mg/day 2 g/day	

Drug	Dose	Usual Max	Comments
Mexiletene	Amoebiasis: 35-50 mg/kg/day PO ÷ tid x 5-10 days *Trichomonas vaginalis* >13 yr: 2 g PO STAT	2.25 g/day	
	Loading dose: 6-8 mg/kg PO Maintenance dose: 6-16 mg/kg/day PO ÷ tid-qid	1200 mg/day Usual adult dose: 600 mg/day PO ÷ qid	Give with food, milk or antacids. Dose reduction (maintenance only) required in liver impairment.
Mineral oil (heavy)	1 ml/kg/dose qhs	Usual adult dose: 15-45 ml PO as a single dose	Avoid in children <1 yr.
Minocycline	Inflammatory acne: 50-100 mg/day PO ÷ bid	200 mg/day	May be taken with food or milk. Contraindicated in children <8 yr.
Minoxidil	0.1-1 mg/kg/day PO ÷ bid		
Morphine	Pre-procedure sedation: X-ray: 50 µg/kg/dose IV Repeat × 1 in 20 min PRN Pre-op: 50-200 µg/kg/dose IM 30-60 min preop Analgesia: Intermittent dose: 0.15-0.3 mg/kg/dose PO/PR q4h 0.05-0.1 mg/kg/dose IV/SC q2-4h.	5 mg/dose 10 mg/dose 15 mg/dose IV/IM or SC No dosing limit for palliative care	For patients being converted from parenteral to oral therapy, IM:PO dose ratio = 1:3. Avoid IM route if possible. Do not adjust maintenance dose until a constant dose has been running for at least 8 hr. If a maintenance dose of >100 µg/kg/hr or additional boluses seem to be required, contact clinical pharmacology.

Continued.

TABLE 1 Drug Dosage Guidelines for Infants and Children (Cont'd)

Drug	Dose	Dose Limit	Comment
Morphine —cont'd	May increase up to 0.2 mg/kg/dose IV/SC q2-4h PRN. Continuous IV/SC infusion preferred for management of prolonged pain requiring frequent or high-dose administration. Continuous infusion: 10-40 µg/kg/h by continuous IV/SC infusion. Breakthrough dose: 20-50 µg/kg/dose IV/SC q4h PRN. Increase infusion rate PRN in increments not greater than 25% of previous rate. Vaso-occlusive crisis in sickle cell disease: Loading dose: 150 µg/kg IV over 5 min. Maintenance dose: 40 µg/kg/hr IV. Increase dose q8h PRN in increments of 20 µg/kg/hr up to a maximum of 100 µg/kg/hr	Loading dose: 7.5 mg Maintenance dose: 100 µg/kg/hr	

Drug	Dose	Notes
Nabilone	<18 kg: 0.5 mg PO q8-12h >18 kg: 1 mg PO q8-12h	6 mg/day	Give first dose the night before antineoplastic therapy. Dose reduction may be required in liver impairment.
Nadolol	Hypertension: 1 mg/kg/day PO once daily Increase daily dose by 1 mg/kg/day q3-4 days PRN	4 mg/kg/day or 320 mg/day, whichever is less	Dose reduction in renal impairment as follows: moderate—50%; severe—25%.
Naloxone	Resuscitation: see inside front cover. Narcotic overdose: see p 479.		
Naproxen	10-20 mg/kg/day PO ÷ bid	1 g/day	Dose may require reduction in liver impairment.
Neomycin	Hepatic encephalopathy: 20-30 mg/kg/day PO ÷ q6h	2 g/day	
Neostigmine	Supraventricular tachycardia: 0.01-0.04 mg/kg/dose IV Curare antagonism: 0.02-0.08 mg/kg/dose IV	2.5 mg/dose	Have atropine at hand.
Nifedipine	Hypertension: Initial dose: 0.5 mg/kg/day PO ÷ q8h Increase gradually prn 1-1.5 mg/kg/day PO	Usual adult dose: 10-30 mg/dose	Prolonged action tablets may be dosed q12h. Do not crush or split prolonged action tablets. For more rapid action, direct patient to bite and swallow capsule.

Continued.

TABLE 1 Drug Dosage Guidelines for Infants and Children (Cont'd)

Drug	Dose	Dose Limit	Comments
Nitrazepam	Initial dose: 0.25 mg/kg/day PO once daily or ÷ tid. Increase gradually PRN to 1.2 mg/kg/day PO.		Give with food or milk.
Nitrofurantoin	5-7 mg/kg/day PO ÷ q6h	600 mg/day or 10 mg/kg/day	Give with food or milk. Do not give to infants <1 mo old. Do not give if creatinine clearance is <40 ml/min. May discolor urine rust-yellow to brown.
Nitroglycerin	0.5-10 µg/kg/min via continuous IV infusion		
Nitroprusside	0.5-8 µg/kg/min via continuous IV infusion	2.5 mg/kg/day cumulative dose	Caution regarding cyanide toxicity.
Norepinephrine	0.02-0.1 µg/kg/min via continuous IV infusion		*Avoid extravasation.* Administer via central line wherever possible.
Novospirozine	2-4 mg of each component/kg/day PO ÷ bid	Usual adult dose: 2-4 tablets/day	Give with food or milk. Contains spironolactone and hydrochlorothiazide in equal amounts. Ineffective when GFR <30 ml/min.

Drug	Dose	Notes
Nystatin	400,000-2,400,000 U/day PO ÷ q4-6h	
Orciprenaline	0.9-2 mg/kg/day PO ÷ tid-qid 0.01-0.03 ml of inhalation solution/kg/dose in 3 ml NS q4-6h via nebulizer	20 mg/dose PO Inhalation: 1 ml/dose
Oxybutinin	Neurogenic bladder: 10-15 mg/day PO ÷ bid-tid	Not recommended for children <5 yr.
Pancrelipase (Cotazym)	Infants: 1 regular capsule/120 ml formula Children and adults: regular capsules: 6/meal; 2/snack enteric-coated (EC) capsules: 3/meal; 1/snack	Do not chew or crush capsule contents. Titrate dose to stool fat content. Cotazym capsules contain lipase, 8,000 IU; amylase, 30,000 IU; and protease, 30,000 IU.
Pancuronium	Muscle paralysis for mechanical ventilation: 0.1 mg/kg/dose IV q30 min PRN Prevention of fasciculation associated with succinylcholine: 0.006-0.01 mg/kg/dose IV	If succinylcholine is used for intubation, decrease initial pancuronium dose by 33%.
Paraldehyde	200-400 mg/kg/dose (0.2-0.4 ml of undiluted paraldehyde/kg/dose) PR q4-8h. Give PR as a 30-50% solution in oil or NaCl 0.9%.	PR: 10 g/dose	Dose reduction may be required in renal or liver impairment. Undiluted paraldehyde contains 1 g/mL. Do not administer in polyvinyl chloride plastic.

Continued.

TABLE 1 Drug Dosage Guidelines for Infants and Children (Cont'd)

Drug	Dose	Dose Limit	Comment
Paraldehyde—cont'd	100-150 mg/kg/dose (2-3 ml of a 5% solution/kg/dose) IV over 15-20 min, then 20 mg/kg/hr (0.4 ml of a 5% solution/kg/hr) as a continuous IV infusion.		
Pediazole	Otitis media: 50 mg erythromycin/kg/day PO ÷ qid (includes 150 mg/kg/day sulfamethoxazole)	1600 mg erythromycin/day	Maintain fluid intake. Dose interval adjustment in renal impairment as follows: moderate—q8-12h; severe—q12-24h.
Penicillamine	Juvenile arthritis: Initial dose: 5 mg/kg/day PO as a single daily dose. Increase dose in increments of 5 mg/kg/day at 2-3-mo intervals up to 15 mg/kg/day PO ÷ bid-qid	Initial dose: 250 mg/dose Final dose: 1.5 g/day	Give on an empty stomach (1 hr ac or 2 hr pc).
Peg-electrolyte liquid (GoLytely, PegLyte)	Older children: 240 ml PO q10min until rectal effluent is clear	4 L/course	

Drug	Dosage	Notes
Penicillin G	Mild to moderate infections: 25,000-50,000 U/kg/day IM/IV ÷ q6h Severe infections: 100,000-400,000 U/kg/day IM/IV ÷ q4-6h Meningitis: 250,000 U/kg/day IM/IV ÷ q4-6h	20 MIU/day	Dose interval adjustment in renal impairment as follows: moderate—q8-12h; severe—q12-16h. 600 mg = 1 million units. Contains 1.7 mmol Na or K per 1 million units.
Penicillin G benzathine (Bicillin 1200 LA)	Rheumatic heart disease prophylaxis: 1.2 MU IM once monthly Streptococcal pharyngitis/rheumatic fever: <27 kg: 600,000 U IM × 1 >27 kg: 1.2 MU IM × 1		
Penicillin VK	Infection: Streptococcal: 25-30 mg/kg/day PO ÷ bid Other: 50-100 mg/kg/day PO q6-8h Rheumatic fever: 125-250 mg PO tid-qid × 10 days Rheumatic fever prophylaxis: >5 yr: 125-300 mg PO bid Prophylaxis in asplenics: >5 yr: 125-300 mg PO bid	3 g/day	May be given with food. Dose reduction in renal impairment as follows: moderate—75%; severe—25-50%; 250 mg ~ 400,000 units

Continued.

TABLE 1 Drug Dosage Guidelines for Infants and Children (Cont'd)

Drug	Dose	Dose Limit	Comment
Pentamidine isethionate	*Pneumocystis carinii* prophylaxis: 150 mg in 6 ml NS via inhalation q2 for wk or 300 mg in 6 ml NS via inhalation q4 wk *Pneumocystis carinii*: 4 mg/kg/day IM/IV as a single daily dose for 12-21 days	56 mg/kg cumulative dose	Use Respirgard II jet nebulizer to administer inhalation. Dose interval adjustment for IM/IV therapy in renal impairment as follows: moderate—q24-36h; severe—q48h.
Pentobarbital (Nembutal)	Pre x-ray: <15 kg: 6 mg/kg/dose IM/PR >15 kg: 5 mg/kg/dose IM/PR 20-30 min pre x-ray or 2.5 mg/kg (max 50 mg) IV over 1 min. Then 1.25 mg/kg (max 25 mg) IV over 30 sec. Wait 1 min. Then, 1.25 mg/kg (max 25 mg) IV over 30 sec. Wait 1 min. If required, an additional dose of 1 mg/kg (max 20 mg) IV may be given.	200 mg/dose 120 mg/dose	Rapid IV administration may cause respiratory depression, apnea, laryngospasm, and hypotension. Dose reduction in liver impairment may be required.

Drug	Dose	Notes
	Preop sedative: < 8 yr: 3-4 mg/kg/dose PR > 8 yr: 2-4 mg/kg/dose PO 60-120 min pre-op.	
Permethrin (Nix)	Pediculosis capitis: Shampoo, rinse, and towel dry hair as usual. Saturate hair and scalp with cream rinse and leave on hair for 10 min.	
Phenobarbital	Status epilepticus: 20 mg/kg IV × 1 Maintenance dose: <3 mo: 5-6 mg/kg/day PO once daily or ÷ bid >3 mo: 3-5 mg/kg/day PO once daily or ÷ bid adolescents: 2-4 mg/kg/day PO once daily or ÷ bid	800 mg/dose Maintenance dose: 200 mg/day	Calculate loading dose according to total body weight. Calculate maintenance dose according to ideal body weight. Dose reduction in liver impairment may be required. Monitoring of serum drug concentrations recommended. Administer IV at a rate not to exceed 60 mg/min or 1 mg/kg/min, whichever is less. Coadministration of phenobarbital and valporic acid may lead to phenobarbital toxicity.
Phenoxybenzamine	Loading dose: 1 mg/kg IV over 1 hr Maintenance dose: 0.5-2 mg/kg/day IV/PO q6-12h		Emergency-release drug
Phentolamine	Acute hypertension: 0.1-0.2 mg/kg IV		

Continued.

TABLE 1 Drug Dosage Guidelines for Infants and Children (Cont'd)

Drug	Dose	Dose Limit	Comment
Phenylephrine	Supraventricular tachycardia: Initial dose: 0.01 mg/kg/dose IV Increase in 0.01 mg/kg increments up to 0.1 mg/kg/total dose Tetralogy spell: 0.1 mg/kg IM as continuous IV infusion		For SVT and hypercyanotic spells, the final dose should be based on a successful result or a 50% increase in blood pressure over baseline

Phenytoin	Status epilepticus: 20 mg/kg IV
	Maintenance dose:
	  0.5-3 yr: 7-9 mg/kg/day PO ÷ q8-12h
	  4-6 yr: 6.5 mg/kg/day PO ÷ q8-12h
	  7-9 yr: 6 mg/kg/day PO ÷ q8-12h
	  10-16 yr: 3-5 mg/kg/day PO ÷ q8-12h
	Arrhythmia:
	Loading dose:
	  15 mg/kg/dose IV over 1 hr
	Simultaneously give 3 mg/kg/dose PO × 1; then 6 hr later give 2 mg/kg/dose PO × 1
	Start maintenance 6 hr later
	or
		Loading dose: 1 g	Calculate loading dose according to total body weight. Calculate maintenance dose according to ideal body weight. Administer IV at a rate not to exceed 1 mg/kg/min or 50 mg/min, whichever is less. Dose reduction may be required in severe liver disease. Monitoring of serum drug concentrations recommended. Coadministration of phenytoin and theophylline or valproate may decrease the effects of both drugs. Coadministration of phenytoin and cimetidine, sulfonamides, or trimethoprim may produce phenytoin toxicity. Coadministration of phenytoin and quinidine may decrease the effects of quinidine.

Piperacillin	5 mg/kg/dose PO q6h × 4 doses. Then 2.5 mg/kg/dose PO q6h × 4 doses Maintenance: 5-6 mg/kg/day PO ÷ q12h		Dose interval adjustment in renal impairment as follows: moderate—q6-8h; severe—q8h.
Piperazine	200-300 mg/kg/day IV/IM ÷ q6h CF patients: 300 mg/kg/day IV/IM ÷ q6h	24 g/day	
Pivampicillin	Roundworm: 75 mg/kg/day PO ÷ bid-tid × 2 days	3.5 g	
	Mild-moderate infections: 20-50 mg/kg/day PO ÷ bid Otitis media: 40-50 mg/kg/day PO ÷ bid Serious infections: 40-100 mg/kg/day PO ÷ q8h	1 g/dose	May be given with food. Dose interval adjustment in renal impairment as follows: severe—q12-16h.
Potassium chloride	Maintenance requirement: 30-40 mmol/m^2/day Hypokalemia: 3 mmol/kg/day + maintenance requirement IV as a continuous infusion or PO in divided doses.		Give PO with food. Dilute oral solution in water or juice and give over 5-10 min. For peripheral IV administration, dilute to at least 0.04 mmol/ml and infuse at a rate not to exceed 20 mmol/h or 0.3 mmol/kg/hr.
Potassium iodide	Radiation protection: 30 mg iodine/day PO as a single daily dose	100 mg iodine daily	Dilute in 1 glassful of water, juice, or milk. Give with food or milk. Lugol's solutions = 126 iodine/ml.

Continued.

TABLE 1 Drug Dosage Guidelines for Infants and Children (Cont'd)

Drug	Dose	Dose Limit	Comment
Prazosin	0.5-7 mcg/kg/day PO ÷ tid		Dose reduction may be required in renal impairment.
Prednisone	Asthma: 1 mg/kg/day PO as a single daily dose × 5 days Nephrotic syndrome, JA, IBD, etc: Initial dose: 1 mg/kg/day PO as a single daily dose or in divided doses.	60 mg/day	Individualize dose according to response. Give with food or milk. To discontinue in patients receiving therapy for ≥ 10 days, reduce dose by 50% q48h until 2.5 ± 0.8 mg/m^2/day achieved. Then reduce dose by 50% q10-14 days.
Primaquine	Malaria: 0.3 mg base/kg/day PO as a single daily dose × 14 days	15 mg base/day	Rule out G6PD deficiency prior to therapy. Give with food or milk. 26.3 mg primaquine phosphate = 15 mg primaquine base.
Primidone	*0-8 yr* Starting dose: 125 mg PO qhs Increase on day 7 to: 125 mg PO bid Increase on day 14 to: 125 mg PO tid Increase on day 21 to: 10-25 mg/kg/day PO ÷ tid/qid	*>8 yr* 250 mg PO qhs 250 mg PO bid 250 mg PO tid 750-1500 mg/day PO ÷ tid/qid	Monitoring of serum concentrations of primidone and phenobarbital recommended. Dose interval adjustment in renal impairment as follows: moderate—q8-12h; severe—q12-24h. Coadministration of primidone and β-adrenergic blockers or quinidine may decrease the effects of the latter drug. Coadministration of primidone and phenytoin may produce primidone toxicity.

Drug	Dose	Notes
Procainamide	Loading dose: 12-15 mg/kg/hr IV over no longer than 75 min Maintenance dose: 20-80 μg/kg/min by continuous IV infusion 15-60 mg/kg/day PO ÷ q4-6h	2 g/day IV	Dose may require reduction in severe CHF. Dose reduction in renal impairment as follows: moderate—q8-12h; severe—q8-24h. Monitoring of serum procainamide and NAPA concentrations is recommended. May be associated with SLE. IV loading dose should be switched to maintenance infusion rate prior to 75 min if arrhythmia reverts or if QRS is prolonged 50% over baseline. Give PO on an empty stomach (1 hr ac or 2 hr pc) unless GI upset occurs.
Propafenone	200-600 mg/m²/day PO ÷ tid-qid	500 mg/dose PO	
		900 mg/day Usual adult dose: 450-600 mg/day PO ÷ q8-12h	Give with food or milk. Reduce digoxin dose by 50% when initiating concurrent propafenone therapy. Dose reduction in renal impairment may be required. Reduce dose in hepatic impairment.
Propranolol	Arrhythmia: 0.01-0.15 mg/kg/dose IV q6-8h PRN Wolff-Parkinson-White syndrome: 2-10 mg/kg/day PO ÷ tid-qid Antihypertensive: 0.5-4 mg/kg/day PO ÷ tid or qid Tetralogy spell: 0.05-0.10 mg/kg/dose IV over 10 min. Maintenance dose: 1-6 mg/kg/day PO ÷ tid-qid	3 mg/dose IV	Give IV propranolol only under ECG monitoring at a rate not to exceed 1 mg/min. Reduce dose in hepatic impairment.

Continued.

TABLE 1 Drug Dosage Guidelines for Infants and Children (Cont'd)

Drug	Dose	Dose Limit	Comment
Propylthiouracil	Initial dose: 150 mg/m^2/day PO ÷ q8h or 10 mg/kg/day PO ÷ q8h Maintenance: Usually 1/3–1/2 of initial dose once patient is euthyroid	Usual adult dose: Initial dose: 300–900 mg/day Maintenance: 50–600 mg/day	Give on an empty stomach (1 hr ac or 2 hr pc).
Protamine	1 mg IV for every 100 U of heparin administered in the previous 3–4 hr at a rate not to exceed 5 mg/min	50 mg/dose	Actual protamine neutralization factor for each heparin lot is listed on manufacturer's label.
Pseudoephedrine	4 mg/kg/day PO ÷ q6h PRN	Usual adult dose: 60 mg/dose PO q4-6h PRN	Use with caution in hypertensive patients <2 yr. Dose combination products, e.g., Sudafed DM according to pseudoephedrine content.
Pyrantel pamoate	Roundworm, pinworm: 11 mg of base/kg/dose PO × 1 dose only Hookworm: 11 mg of base/kg/day PO as a single daily dose × 3 days	1 g of base/dose	For pinworm, repeat dose after 2 wk. May be given with food or on an empty stomach.

Pyrazinamide	15-30 mg/kg/day PO ÷ q6-8h or 50-70 mg/kg/dose PO twice weekly	2 g/day	Dose reduction may be required in hepatic impairment.
Pyrimethamine and sulfadoxine	See Fansidar		
Quinacrine	Giardiasis: 6 mg/kg/day PO ÷ tid pc × 5-7 days	300 mg/day	Give with a full glass of water or juice.
Quinidine	Dysrhythmia: 15-60 mg of base/kg/day PO ÷ q4-6h Chloroquine-resistant falciparum malaria: Initial: 14 mg of base/kg IV Maintenance: 21 mg of base/kg/day IV ÷ q8h	500 mg/dose Initial: 494 mg base	Dose may require reduction in severe CHF. Reduce dose to 30% in severe liver impairment. Digoxin maintenance dose requires reduction during concurrent quinidine therapy. Monitoring of serum drug concentrations recommended. Do no break or chew controlled-release tablets. Quinidine bisulfate = 66% base. Quinidine sulfate = 83% base. Infuse IV doses over 4 hours. In malaria, if patient remains severely ill after 72 hr therapy, REDUCE dose to 67% due to expected impaired hepatic clearance.
Quinine sulfate	Chloroquine-resistant falciparum malaria: 25 mg/kg/day PO ÷ tid × 3 days	1.95 g/day	Give with food or milk.

Continued.

TABLE 1 Drug Dosage Guidelines for Infants and Children (Cont'd)

Drug	Dose	Dose Limit	Comment
Ranitidine	1.25-1.9 mg/kg/day IV ÷ q6-12h 2.5-3.8 mg/kg/day PO ÷ q12h	300 mg/day except in Zollinger-Ellison syndrome. Usual adult dose: 300 mg/day as a single HS dose or ÷ q12h.	Monitor gastric pH in patients requiring IV therapy. Dose reduction in renal impairment as follows: moderate—75%; severe—50%.
Ribavirin	6 g/day; 20 mg/ml solution via inhalation over 12-18 h/day for 3-7 days		Use small particle aerosol generator (SPAG-2) for administration. Do not wear contact lenses when exposed to ribovirin aerosol.
Rifampin	Tuberculosis: 10-20 mg/kg/day PO once daily or ÷ q12h or 10-20 mg/kg/dose PO twice weekly Meningococcal prophylaxis: 20 mg/kg/day PO ÷ q12h × 2 days *H. Influenzae* prophylaxis: 20 mg/kg/day PO once daily × 4 days	600 mg/day 1200 mg/day 600 mg/day	Reduce dose in liver impairment. May discolor urine, sweat, saliva, and tears. Give on an empty stomach (1 hr ac or 2 hr pc) unless GI upset occurs. Coadministration of rifampin and either metoprolol, propranolol, cyclosporine, or quinidine may decrease the effects of the latter drug.

Drug	Dose	Max	Comments
Salbutamol	0.3 mg/kg/day PO ÷ tid/qid 0.01–0.03 ml of inhalation solution/kg/dose in 3 ml NS via nebulizer q½–4h PRN. In severe cases give initial dose of 0.03 ml/kg/dose (max, 1 ml/dose) q20 min via nebulizer. 100–200 μg TID via metered aerosol or diskhaler. Initial infusion rate: 1 μg/kg/min IV. Increase by 1 μg/kg/min q15 min PRN up to a maximum of 10 μg/kg/min.	PO: 16 mg/day Inhalation solution: 1 ml/dose Metered aerosol/Diskhaler/Rotahaler: 800 μg/day	Limit nebulized salbutamol to 4 times/day for outpatients. May cause hypokalemia. Metered aerosol: 100 μg/puff Diskhaler: 200 μg OR 400 μg/blister Rotahaler: 200 μg OR 400 μg/capsule Inhalation solution: 5 mg/mL
Sodium bicarbonate	Resuscitation: See inside front cover		
Sodium polystyrene sulfonate (Kayexalate)	1 g/kg/dose PO q6h PRN 1 g/kg/dose PR q2–6h PRN		Exchanges approximately 1 mmol/kg. Administer rectally in appropriate volume of tap water, 10% dextrose or equal parts tap water and 2% methylcellulose. Moisten resin with honey or jam for PO use.
Sorbitol	Cathartic: 1.5–2 ml/kg PO	150 ml/dose	

Continued.

TABLE 1 Drug Dosage Guidelines for Infants and Children (Cont'd)

Drug	Dose	Dose Limit	Comment
Sotalol	Arrhythmias: 2-10 mg/kg/day PO ÷ bid	480 mg/day Usual adult dose: 320 mg/day PO ÷ bid	Dose reduction in renal impairment as follows: moderate—30%; severe—15-30%. Dose may require reduction in liver impairment.
Spironolactone	1-4 mg/kg/day PO into 1, 2, 3, or 4 daily doses	Usual adult dose: 25-200 mg/day PO	For spironolactone in combination with hydrochlorothiazide, see Novospirozine. Avoid when creatinine clearance <10 ml/min.
Streptokinase	Loading dose: 10,000 IU/kg IV over 20 min Maintenance dose: 1,000 IU/kg/hr as a continuous IV infusion		
Succinylcholine	1-2 mg/kg/dose IV One dose only—no repeats		
Sucralfate (Sulcrate)	Adolescents and adults: 4 g/day PO ÷ qid (1 hour ac + qhs)		

Drug	Dose	Notes
Sulfasalazine	JA: 40-60 mg/kg/day PO ÷ bid-qid	Begin with ⅓ of recommended dose and increase q2 days to maximum required dose. Maintain fluid intake. Give with food.
Terfenadine	3-6 yr: 30 mg/day PO ÷ bid 7-12 yr: 60 mg/day PO ÷ bid >12 yr: 120 mg/day PO ÷ bid	Give with food or milk.
Tetracycline	Inflammatory acne: 1 g/day PO ÷ qid × 1 wk Then, 500 mg/day PO ÷ bid	Dose interval adjustment in renal impairment as follows: moderate—q12-24h. Avoid in severe renal impairment. Contraindicated in children <8 yr. Do not administer with milk or antacids.
Theophylline	For patients not currently receiving aminophylline or theophylline: Loading dose: 6 mg/kg IV Initial maintenance dose: 2-6 mo: 0.4 mg/kg/hr IV 6-11 mo: 0.7 mg/kg/hr IV 1-12 yr: 0.8 mg/kg/hr IV 12-16 yr: 0.7 mg/kg/hr IV >16 yr (nonsmoker): 0.6 mg/kg/hr IV Cardiac decompensation, cor pulmonale, liver dysfunction: 0.2 mg/kg/hr IV	Calculate loading dose according to effective body weight and maintenance dose according to ideal body weight. Dose reduction may be required in liver impairment. Administer IV at a rate not to exceed 20 mg/min. IV doses are conservative. Titrate dose according to serum concentration. Oral doses apply to sustained-release products, which are preferred for chronic dosing. Maximum oral doses should be attained in a stepwise fashion to prevent intolerance in patients not being converted from IV therapy. Begin at 50% of recommended doses. Give PO on an empty stomach (1 hr ac or 2 hr pc) unless GI upset occurs. Do not administer

Continued.

TABLE 1 Drug Dosage Guidelines for Infants and Children (Cont'd)

Drug	Dose	Dose Limit	Comment
Theophylline—cont'd	Maximum maintenance dose prior to TDM: 6-52 wk: [0.2 × (age in wks) + 5] mg/kg/day PO ÷ q6-8h 1-12 yr: 20 mg/kg/day PO ÷ q8-12h 12-16 yr: 18 mg/kg/day PO ÷ q12h >16 yr: 14 mg/kg/day PO ÷ q12h or 900 mg/day, whichever is less		Somophyllin-12 by NG. See pp 731-733 for further monitoring guidelines. Coadministration of theophylline and non-selective β-blockers may decrease the effects of theophylline. Coadministration of theophylline and cimetidine or erythromycin may produce theophylline toxicity. Coadministration of theophylline and phenytoin may decrease the effects of both drugs.
Ticarcillin	200-300 mg/kg/day IM/IV ÷ q4-6h CF patients: 300 mg/kg/day IM/IV ÷ q4-6h	24 g/day	Dose interval adjustment in renal impairment as follows: moderate—q6-8h; severe—q8h.
Tobramycin	7.5 mg/kg/day IV/IM ÷ q8h	100 mg/dose prior to serum concentration determination.	Calculate dose according to effective body weight. Dose interval adjustment in renal impairment as follows: mild-moderate—q12h; severe—

	CF patients: 10 mg/kg/day IV/IM ÷ q8h 80 mg TID via nebulizer	No maximum single dose.	q24-48h. Monitoring of serum drug concentrations recommended.
Tolmetin	20-40 mg/kg/day PO ÷ tid or qid	1.6 g/day	
Trimethoprim	4 mg/kg/day PO ÷ q12h	200 mg/day	Dose interval adjustment in renal impairment as follows: moderate—q18h; severe—q24h. Give on an empty stomach (1 hr ac or 2 hr pc) unless GI upset occurs.
Valproic acid	Initial dose: 15 mg/kg/day PO once daily or ÷ q8-12h. Increase dose weekly PRN by 5-10 mg/kg/day up to 30-60 mg/kg/day PO ÷ tid or qid.	60 mg/kg/day	Reduce dose in liver impairment. Monitoring of serum drug concentration recommended. Coadministration of valproic acid and either phenobarbital or primidone may result in toxicity due to the latter drug. Coadministration of valproic acid and phenytoin may decrease the effects of both drugs.
Vancomycin	Mild to moderate infections: 40 mg/kg/day IV ÷ q6h Severe infections: 40 mg/kg/day IV ÷ q6h Meningitis: 60 mg/kg/day IV ÷ q6h Pseudomembranous colitis: 50 mg/kg/day PO ÷ q6h Cardiac surgery prophylaxis: 20 mg/kg/dose IV q12h × 2 doses	2 g/day 4 g/day 4 g/day 500 mg/day 1 g/day	Calculate doses according to effective body weight. Dose interval adjustment in renal impairment as follows: mild—q8-18h; moderate—q18-72h; severe—q3-7 days. Monitoring of serum drug concentrations recommended. Injection may be used or oral dosing.

Continued.

TABLE 1 Drug Dosage Guidelines for Infants and Children (Cont'd)

Drug	Dose	Dose Limit	Comment
Varicella zoster immune globulin	125 U/10 kg/dose IM minimum: 125 U/dose	625 U	Do not administer part vials. Round dose up to the next number of whole vials. Approximately 125 U/vial.
Vasopressin	Variceal bleeding: 0.2-0.3 U/kg/dose IV over 20 minutes. Repeat in 1-2 hr if bleeding continues.		
Vitamin C	Chronic iron overload: Not to exceed 100 mg/day PO		
Verapamil (Isoptin)	0-2 yr: 0.1-0.2 mg/kg/dose IV 2-15 yr: 0.1-0.3 mg/kg/dose IV May repeat × 1 in 30 min PRN Maintenance dose: 2-10 mg/kg/day PO ÷ tid/qid	10 mg/dose IV Usual adult dose: 240-480 mg/day	Administer IV under ECG monitoring. Avoid use in early postcardiosurgical period, in severe CHF, or in presence of beta-blockers.
Vitamin K₁ (Phytonadione)	Anticoagulant overdose: Infants: 1-2 mg IV/SC/IM q4-8h PRN Children: 5-10 mg IV/SC/IM q4-8h PRN Acute fulminant liver failure: Infants: 1-2 mg IV Children: 10 mg IV		Administer IV at a rate not to exceed 1 mg/min.

Drug	Dose		Notes
Warfarin	Day 0: 0.2 mg/kg PO as a single daily dose Day 1: INR ≤1.64: 0.2 mg/kg PO as a single daily dose INR >1.64: 0.1 mg/kg PO as a single daily dose Day 2: INR ≤2.16: 0.2 mg/kg PO as a single daily dose INR >2.16 or <3.08: 0.1 mg/kg PO as a single daily dose INR ≥3.08: hold dose Day 3: INR <3.08: 0.1 mg/kg PO as a single daily dose INR ≥3.08: 0.08 mg/kg PO as a single daily dose	10 mg	Monitor INR daily. Adjust dose to maintain INR between 2.16-3.08. The therapeutic range for patients with synthetic prosthetic heart valves is not clearly established. Adjust dose only after 2 consecutive days therapy at the same dose and after 2 consecutive days of INR >3.08 but <4.77. Increase or decrease dose in 20% increments. If INR >4.77 at any time, hold dose until INR <3.08. Then restart warfarin at 20% less than previous dose.
Zidovudine	Infants: 720 mg/m²/day PO ÷ q6h Older children and adults: 200 mg Q4h PO		
Zinc	Supplementation: 0.5-1 mg/kg/day PO ÷ bid or tid Acrodermatitis enteropathica: 10-45 mg/day PO ÷ bid or tid		

TABLE 2 Neonatal Drug Dosage Guidelines*

Drug	Dose	Comments
Acetaminophen (Tempra; Tylenol)	10-15 mg/kg/dose PO or per rectum q4-6h	Max: 60 mg/kg/day
Acyclovir (Zovirax)	Herpes simplex infections: 15-30 mg/kg/day IV ÷ q8h	Reduce dose in renal impairment. Higher doses may be required in herpes zoster infections.
Albumin	0.5-1.0 g/kg/dose (10-20 ml of 5% solution/kg) IV	Dilute 25% albumin to 5% strength, e.g., 4 ml 25% albumin + 16 ml 5% dextrose, or give 5% undiluted
Alprostadil	0.05-0.1 µg/kg/min IV as a continuous infusion	May cause apnea. Formula for dilution: 500 µg in 80 ml at 1 ml/kg/hr = 0.1 µg/kg/min
Amikacin	<2 kg: 0-7 days: 15 mg/kg/day IV or IM ÷ q12h >7 days: 20 mg/kg/day IV or IM ÷ q8h	Reduce dose in renal impairment. Monitoring of serum drug concentrations is recommended. Indicated for organisms resistant to gentamicin.

	≥2 kg: 0-7 days: 20 mg/kg/day IV or IM ÷ q12h > 7 days: 30 mg/kg/day IV or IM ÷ q8h	
Amphotericin B	0.25 mg/kg/day IV as a single daily dose. Increase by 0.25 mg/kg/day up to 1 mg/kg/day IV as tolerated.	Infuse in a concentration of ≤0.1 mg/ml in 5% dextrose over 4-6 hr. May be given on alternate days. Monitor serum potassium.
Ampicillin	<2 kg: 0-7 days: Meningitis: 100 mg/kg/day IV ÷ q12h Other: 50 mg/kg/day IV ÷ q12h >7 days: Meningitis: 150 mg/kg/day IV ÷ q8h Other: 75 mg/kg/day IV ÷ q8h ≥2kg: 0-7 days: Meningitis: 150 mg/kg/day IV ÷ q8h Other: 75 mg/kg/day IV ÷ q8H > 7 days: Meningitis: 200 mg/kg/day IV ÷ q6h Other: 100 mg/kg/day IV ÷ q6h	Reduce dose in severe renal impairment.

Continued.

*These dosage guidelines apply to all neonates until a postconceptional age of >38 weeks *and* a postnatal age of >4 weeks have been achieved.

FORMULARY

TABLE 2 Neonatal Drug Dosage Guidelines* (Cont'd)

Drug	Dose	Comments
Atropine	Resuscitation: 0.01-0.02 mg/kg/dose IV, IM, SC, or ETT q20 min PRN	ETT route to be used only if IV access not possible.
Caffeine	Loading: 10 mg/kg PO or IV Maintenance: 2.5 mg/kg/dose PO or IV once daily	Monitoring of serum drug concentrations recommended.
Calcium gluconate	Resuscitation: 1.5 ml/kg/dose of a 2% solution = 30 mg/kg/dose q10-20 min PRN Maintenance: 200-400 mg/kg/day (2-4 ml of 10% solution/kg/day) IV	Avoid extravasation. Preferable to use a central line when giving a 10% solution. Administer at a rate not to exceed 10 mg/min. 10% solution: 1 ml = 100 mg of calcium gluconate = 9.3 mg elemental calcium = 0.23 mmol of calcium.
Calcium lactate	For infants <2 kg receiving >50% of daily requirements as breast milk, starting at 2 wks of age, supplement as follows:	Give after feeds. Discontinue when infant reaches 1800 g or 35 weeks post conceptional age.

	Dose:	
Cefazolin	Patient's weight: <1000 g: 40 mg q2h PO 1000-1250 g: 60 mg q2h PO 1251-1500 g: 70 mg q2h PO 1501-1800 g: 120 mg q3h PO <2 kg regardless of age and ≥2 kg aged 0-7 days: 40 mg/kg/day IV/IM ÷ q12h ≥2 kg aged > 7 days: 60 mg/kg/day IV/IM ÷ q8h	Reduce dose in renal impairment.
Cefotaxime	0-7 days: 100 mg/kg/day IV ÷ q12h >7 days: 150 mg/kg/day IV ÷ q8h	Reduce dose in renal impairment.
Ceftazidime	<2 kg: 0-7 days: 100 mg/kg/day IV/IM ÷ q12h >7 days: 150 mg/kg/day IV/IM ÷ q8h ≥2 kg: 0-7 days: 100 mg/kg/day IV/IM ÷ q8h >7 days: 150 mg/kg/day IV/IM ÷ q8h	Reduce dose in renal impairment.

Continued.

*These dosage guidelines apply to all neonates until a postconceptional age of >38 weeks *and* a postnatal age of >4 weeks have been achieved.

FORMULARY

TABLE 2 Neonatal Drug Dosage Guidelines* (Cont'd)

Drug	Dose	Comments
Chloral hydrate	25-50 mg/kg/day PO/PR ÷ q6h	Reduce dose in patients with CNS impairment. Dose may require reduction in liver impairment.
Chloramphenicol	<2 kg: 25 mg/kg/day IV as single daily dose ≥2 kg: 0-7 days: 25 mg/kg/day IV as single daily dose >7 days: 50 mg/kg/day IV ÷ q12h	Monitoring of serum drug concentrations is recommended. Avoid in liver impairment.
Cimetidine	≤7 days: 10-15 mg/kg/day PO/IV ÷ q4-6h Infants >7 days: 20 mg/kg/day PO/IV ÷ q4-6h	Reduce dose in renal impairment.
Clindamycin	<2 kg: 0-7 days: 10 mg/kg/day IV ÷ q12h >7days: 15 mg/kg/day IV/PO ÷ q8h	Do not administer PO to infants <7 days old. Do not administer clindamycin palmitate PO.

	≥2 kg:	0-7 days: 15 mg/kg/day IV ÷ q8h >7 days: 20 mg/kg/day IV/PO ÷ q6h
Cloxacillin	<2 kg:	0-7 days: Meningitis: 100 mg/kg/day IV ÷ q12h Other: 50 mg/kg/day PO/IV ÷ q12h >7 days: Meningitis: 150 mg/kg/day IV ÷ q8h Other: 75 mg/kg/day PO/IV ÷ q8h
	≥2 kg:	0-7 days: Meningitis: 150 mg/kg/day IV ÷ q8h Other: 75 mg/kg/day PO/IV ÷ q8h >7 days: Meningitis: 200 mg/kg/day IV ÷ q6h

Continued.

*These dosage guidelines apply to all neonates until a postconceptional age of >38 weeks *and* a postnatal age of >4 weeks have been achieved.

TABLE 2 Neonatal Drug Dosage Guidelines* (Cont'd)

Drug	Dose	Comments
Cloxacillin—cont'd	Other: 100 mg/kg/day PO/IV ÷ q6h	
Dexamethasone (Decadron)	Subglottic stenosis or inflammation: 0.5-0.1 mg/kg/dose IV/PO up to 3 doses/day	Do not use for longer than 1 day.
Dextrose	Transient hypoglycemia: 5-7 mg/kg/min IV Acute hypoglycemia: Loading dose: 0.1-1.2 g/kg IV Maintenance dose: 5-7 mg/kg/min IV	
Diazepam (Valium)	Seizure: 0.1-0.2 mg/kg/dose IV	Administer at a rate not to exceed 0.05 mg/kg/min.
Digoxin	Digitalization dose: (3 doses – 1st STAT, 2nd in 6 hours, 3rd in another 6 hours). <37 wks PCA†: 0.007 mg/kg/dose PO 0.005 mg/kg/dose IV	Do not administer IM. Reduce dose by 50% during concurrent indomethacin therapy. When digitalizing to terminate tachycardia, the total digitalization dose is divided 1/2, 1/4, 1/4. Decrease maintenance dose in renal

	≥37 wks PCA: 0.017 mg/kg/dose PO 0.012 mg/kg/dose IV	impairment. Monitoring of serum drug concentrations is recommended.
	Maintenance dose:	
	<37 wks PCA: 0.004 mg/kg/day PO ÷ q12h 0.003 mg/kg/day IV ÷ q12h	
	≥37 wks PCA: 0.01 mg/kg/day PO ÷ q12h 0.007 mg/kg/day IV ÷ q12h	
Dobutamine	5-25 μg/kg/min IV	
Dopamine	Renal: 2-5 μg/kg/min IV Inotropic: 5-20 μg/kg/min IV Vasoconstrictive: >20 μg/kg/min IV	Neonates may be less sensitive to dopamine. See pp 550-551 for infusion details.
Doxapram	0.5 mg/kg/hr IV. May increase gradually up to 2.5 mg/kg/hr IV.	Caffeine or theophylline should be given concurrently. Monitor abdominal girth, blood pressure, and blood glucose.
Epinephrine	Resuscitation: 0.1 ml/kg/dose of 1:10,000 IV, ETT, or SC	1:10,000 = 0.1 mg/ml

Continued.

*These dosage guidelines apply to all neonates until a postconceptional age of >38 weeks and a postnatal age of >4 weeks have been achieved.
†PCA-postconceptional age.

FORMULARY

TABLE 2 Neonatal Drug Dosage Guidelines* (Cont'd)

Drug	Dose	Comments
Erythromycin estolate	<2 kg: 0-7 days: 20 mg/kg/day PO ÷ q12h >7 days: 30 mg/kg/day PO ÷ q8h ≥2 kg: 0-7 days: 20 mg/kg/day PO ÷ q12h >7 days: 30-40 mg/kg/day PO ÷ q8h	
Erythromycin gluceptate or lactobionate	20-40 mg/kg/day IV ÷ q6h	
Flucytosine	50-150 mg/kg/day IV or PO ÷ q6h	Reduce dose in renal impairment. Monitoring of serum drug concentrations is recommended. Injection is available as an emergency-release drug.
Furosemide	1-2 mg/kg/dose IV or PO	

Gentamicin	≤1 kg: 3.5 mg/kg/day IV or IM once daily <37 weeks PCA and > 1 kg: 5 mg/kg/day IV or IM ÷ q12h ≥37 weeks GA† and ≤ 7 days old: 5 mg/kg/day IV or IM ÷ q12h ≥37 weeks GA and > 7 days old: 7.5 mg/kg/day IV or IM ÷ q8h	Reduce dose in renal impairment. Monitoring of serum drug concentrations is recommended.
Glucagon	1.0-1.5 mg/day IV as a continuous infusion	Dilute in 5% or 10% dextrose.
Heparin	Maintenance of indwelling lines: 1 U/ml run at 1-2 ml/hr Thrombosis: Loading dose: 50-100 U/kg IV Maintenance dose: 20-30 U/kg/hr IV via continuous infusion	Monitor PTT and titrate infusion rate accordingly.
Hydralazine	1.7-3.5 mg/kg/day IV ÷ q4-6h	

Continued.

*These dosage guidelines apply to all neonates until a postconceptional age of >38 weeks *and* a postnatal age of >4 weeks have been achieved.
†GA = gestational age.

TABLE 2 Neonatal Drug Dosage Guidelines* (Cont'd)

Drug	Dose	Comments
Indomethacin	Patent ductus arteriosus: Age at 1st dose: <48 hr: 0.2 mg/kg/dose IV followed 12 hrs later by 0.1 mg/kg/dose q12h IV × 2 doses >48 hr: 0.2 mg/kg/dose IV q12h × 3 doses	Reduce doses of aminoglycosides and digoxin to half until good urine output returns. Infuse over 20 min.
Insulin	0.01-0.02 U/kg/hr IV as a continuous infusion	Titrate infusion rate according to blood glucose. Use regular insulin only.
Isoproterenol	0.05-1.0 µg/kg/min IV as continuous infusion	Stop or slow infusion if heart rate >200/min.
Lorazepam	Seizures: 0.05 mg/kg/dose IV or PR May repeat once PRN	For PR administration, dilute injection according to IV instructions.
Mannitol	1 g/kg/dose IV (5 ml of 20% solution/kg/dose)	

Drug	Dose	Notes
Metoclopramide	Initial dose: 0.1 mg/kg/day PO or IV ÷ q8h Maximum: 0.5 mg/kg/day	Extrapyramidal side effects may be reversed with diphenhydramine, 1 mg/kg/dose IV.
Morphine	Pain: Loading dose: 0.1-0.2 mg/kg IV Maintenance dose: 0.01-0.02 mg/kg/hr IV as a continuous infusion	
Naloxone	0.1 mg/kg/dose IV/ETT. Repeat PRN.	Contact Poison Control in cases of narcotic overdose.
Novospirozine	2-4 mg of each component/kg/day PO ÷ q12h	Contains equal amounts of hydrochlorothiazide and spironolactone.
Pancuronium (Pavulon)	0.05-0.1 mg/kg/dose IV PRN	
Paraldehyde	150 mg/kg/hr (3 ml of 5% solution/kg/hr) IV over 2 hr once daily 300 mg/kg (0.3 ml of undiluted paraldehyde/kg) × 1 PO 300 mg/kg (0.3 ml of undiluted paraldehyde/kg) × 1 per rectum diluted in oil or normal saline to make a 30-50% solution	Make a 5% solution by adding 1.75 ml of paraldehyde to 5% dextrose to make a total volume of 35 ml in a syringe. Undiluted paraldehyde contains 1 g/ml.

Continued.

FORMULARY

*These dosage guidelines apply to all neonates until a postconceptional age of >38 weeks *and* a postnatal age of >4 weeks have been achieved.

TABLE 2 Neonatal Drug Dosage Guidelines* (Cont'd)

Drug	Dose	Comments
Penicillin G (Benzylpenicillin)	<2 kg: 0-7 days: Meningitis: 100,000 U/kg/day IV ÷ q12h Other: 50,000 U/kg/day IV ÷ q12h >7 days Meningitis: 150,000 U/kg/day IV ÷ q8h Other: 75,000 U/kg/day IV ÷ q8h ≥2 kg: 0-7 days: Meningitis: 150,000 U/kg/day IV ÷ q8h Other: 50,000 U/kg/day IV ÷ 8qh >7 days: Meningitis: 200,000 U/kg/day IV ÷ q6h Other: 100,000 U/kg/day IV ÷ q6h	Reduce dose in severe renal impairment.
Phenobarbital	Loading dose: <37 wk PCA: 10-20 mg/kg IV; may repeat dose of 5-10 mg/kg/ IV up to max total dose of 25 mg/kg	Reduce dose in liver impairment. Administer undiluted at a rate not to exceed 1 mg/kg/min. Monitoring of serum drug concentrations is recommended.

	≥ 37 weeks PCA: 10-20 mg/kg IV; may repeat dose of 10 mg/kg IV up to max total dose of 30 mg/kg Maintenance dose: 4-6 mg/kg/day IV or PO once daily	
Phenytoin	Loading dose: 20 mg/kg IV Maintenance dose: 4-8 mg/kg/day PO or IV once daily or ÷ bid	Reduce dose in liver impairment. Monitor for hypotension during infusion. Administer undiluted at a rate not to exceed 1 mg/kg/min. Poorly absorbed orally in the infant. Monitoring of serum drug concentrations is recommended.
Piperacillin	<2 kg: 0-7 days: 150 mg/kg/day IV ÷ q12h >7 days: 225 mg/kg/day IV ÷ q8h ≥2 kg: 0-7 days: 225 mg/kg/day IV ÷ q8h >7 days: 300 mg/kg/day IV ÷ q6h	Reduce dose in severe renal impairment.
Propranolol	Resuscitation: 0.01-0.10 mg/kg/dose IV Other: 0.5-1.0 mg/kg/day PO ÷ q6h	

Continued.

---

*These dosage guidelines apply to all neonates until a postconceptional age of >38 weeks and a postnatal age of >4 weeks have been achieved.

TABLE 2 Neonatal Drug Dosage Guidelines* (Cont'd)

Drug	Dose	Comments
Prostaglandin E$_1$	see Alprostadil	
Pyridoxine (vitamin B$_6$)	50-100 mg/dose IV	Monitor EEG concurrently.
Ranitidine	1.25-1.9 mg/kg/day IV ÷ q6-12h 2.5-3.8 mg/kg/day PO ÷ q12h	Reduce dose in renal impairment.
Sodium bicarbonate	IV dose (mmol) = wt. (kg) × 0.3 × base deficit 1-3 mmol/kg IV over 5 min in mild asphyxia 3-5 mmol/kg IV over 5 min in severe asphyxia	4.2% = 0.5 mmol/ml 8.4% = 1 mmol/ml Dilute 8.4% 1:1 with sterile water or 5% dextrose or use 4.2% undiluted.
Sodium polystyrene sulfonate (Kayexalate)	1 g/kg/dose PO or per rectum	Mix in water or 5% dextrose. Exchanges ~ 1 mmol K$^+$/g.
Spironolactone	2-4 mg/kg/day PO ÷ q12h	For spironolactone in combination with hydrochlorothiazide, see Novospirozine.

Theophylline	For patients not currently receiving aminophylline or theophylline: Loading dose: 5 mg/kg IV or PO Maintenance dose: 2 mg/kg/day IV or PO ÷ q12h	Monitoring of serum theophylline and caffeine concentrations is recommended. Administer at a rate not to exceed 0.4 mg/kg/min.

Ticarcillin	<2 kg: 0-7 days: 150 mg/kg/day IV ÷ q12h
	        > 7 days: 225 mg/kg/day IV ÷ q8h
	≥2 kg: 0-7 days: 225 mg/kg/day IV ÷ q8h
	        >7 days: 300 mg/kg/day IV ÷ q6h
		Reduce dose in severe renal impairment.

Tobramycin	≤1 kg: 3.5 mg/kg/day IV or IM once daily <37 weeks PCA and >1 kg: 5 mg/kg/day IV or IM ÷ q12h ≥37 weeks GA and ≤7 days old: 5 mg/kg/day IV/IM ÷ q12h ≥37 weeks GA and >7 days old: 7.5 mg/kg/day IV or IM ÷ q8h	Reduce dose in renal impairment. Monitoring of serum drug concentrations is recommended.

Continued.

*These dosage guidelines apply to all neonates until a postconceptional age of >38 weeks *and* a postnatal age of >4 weeks have been achieved.

TABLE 2 Neonatal Drug Dosage Guidelines* (Cont'd)

Drug	Dose	Comments
Tolazoline (Priscoline)	Loading dose: 1-2 mg/kg IV Maintenance dose: 0.5-2 mg/kg/hr IV via continuous infusion	Monitor blood pressure. Emergency-release or investigational agent. Should be used in critical care areas only.
Trimethoprim	UTI prophylaxis: 2 mg/kg/day PO ÷ bid or as a single daily dose	
Vancomycin	*Post-* *Weight (g) conceptional Dosage* *Age (wks)* <800 or <27 27 mg/kg/dose IV q36h 800-1200 or 27-30 24 mg/kg/dose IV q24h 1201-2000 or 31-36 18 mg/kg/dose IV q12h	Reduce dose in renal impairment. Monitoring of serum drug concentrations is recommended.

| | | or | 27 mg/kg/dose IV q18h | |
| | >2000 | or | >37 | 22.5 mg/kg/dose IV q12h | |

Vitamin K₁ (phytonadione)	Hemorrhagic disease of the newborn: Prophylaxis: 0.5-1.0 mg IM or SC at birth Treatment: 1 mg/dose IM or IV	Administer IV at a rate not to exceed 1 mg/min.

*These dosage guidelines apply to all neonates until a postconceptional age (PCA) of >38 weeks *and* a postnatal age of >4 weeks have been achieved.

†GA = gestational age.

TABLE 3 Recommendations for Endocarditis Prophylaxis

1. Dental procedures, oropharyngeal surgery, instrumentation of the respiratory tract, including children with prosthetic tissue or heart valves:

Children able to receive penicillin

Ampicillin 50 mg/kg (max 2 g) IV/IM 30 min before procedure, then 25 mg/kg (max 1 g) IV/IM 6 hr later. The second dose may be replaced by pivampicillin 25 mg/kg (max 1.5 g) PO 6 hr later, except in neonates

or

Pivampicillin 50 mg/kg (max 3 g) PO 1 hr before procedure, then 25 mg/kg (max 1.5 g) 6 hr later. Neonates should not receive oral prophylaxis. Use IV/IM regimen above.

Children allergic to penicillin or on continuous penicillin prophylaxis for rheumatic fever or who have been treated with antibiotics more than once in the past month:

Clindamycin 10 mg/kg IV (max 300 mg) 30 min before procedure, then 5 mg/kg IV/PO (max 150 mg) 6 hr later

or

Clindamycin 10 mg/kg PO (max 600 mg) 1 hr before procedure. No repeat dose. Neonates should not receive oral prophylaxis. Use IV/IM regimen above.

2. Gastrointestinal and genitourinary procedures or instrumentation, including children with prosthetic tissue or heart valves

If the urine is infected, an antibiotic should be chosen which is active against the infecting pathogen as well as against enterococci.

Children able to receive penicillin

Major procedures:
Ampicillin 50 mg/kg (max 2g) IV/IM 30 min before procedure then 8 hr later.

plus

Gentamicin* 2 mg/kg (max 100 mg) IV/IM 30 min before procedure, then 8 hr later
The second doses may be replaced by pivampicillin 25 mg/kg (max 1.5 g) 6 hr after initial doses, except in neonates

Minor procedures:
Pivampicillin 50 mg/kg (max 3 g) PO 1 hr before procedure, then 25 mg/kg (max 1.5 g) 6 hr later. Neonates should not receive oral prophylaxis. Use IV/IM regimen above.

Children allergic to penicillin or on continuous penicillin prophylaxis for rheumatic fever or who have been treated with antibiotics more than once in the past month

Major procedures:
Vancomycin* 20 mg/kg (max 1 g) IV over 1 hr starting 1 hr before procedure and 8 hr later

plus

Gentamicin* 2 mg/kg (max 100 mg) IV/IM 30 min before procedure, then 8 hr later

Minor procedures:
Clindamycin 10 mg/kg (max 600 mg) PO 1 hr before procedure. No repeat dose. Neonates should not receive oral prophylaxis. Use IV/IM regimen above.

Continued.

TABLE 3 Recommendations for Endocarditis Prophylaxis (Cont'd)

3. Surgical procedures on infected and contaminated tissues including incision and drainage of abscesses where *Staphylococcus aureus* is suspected, including children with prosthetic tissue or heart valves

Children able to receive penicillin:

Major procedures:
  Cloxacillin 50 mg/kg (max 2 g) IV/IM 30–60 min before procedure and 6 hr later

  plus

  Gentamincin* 2 mg/kg (max 100 mg) IV/IM 30 min before procedure and 6 hr later

Minor procedures:
  Flucloxacillin 25 mg/kg (max 1 g) PO 1 hr before procedure and 6 hr later

Children allergic to penicillin or on continuous penicillin prophylaxis for rheumatic fever, or who have been treated with antibiotics more than once in the past month:

Major procedures:
  Clindamycin 10 mg/kg IV (max 300 mg) 30 min before procedure. No repeat dose.

  plus

  Gentamicin* 2 mg/kg (max 100 mg) IV/IM 30 min before procedure and 8 hr later

Minor procedures:
  Clindamycin 10 mg/kg (max 600 mg) 1 hr before procedure. No repeat dose.

*Reduce or omit second dose appropriately in patients with renal impairment.
Adapted from The Recommendations of the British Society of Antimicrobial Therapy (Lancet 1990; 335:88) and the American Heart Association (JAMA 1990; 264:2929).

Therapeutic Drug Monitoring

TDM CONCEPTS FOR PEDIATRICIANS IN PRACTICE

- The elimination half-life of a drug is defined as the time taken for the serum concentration to decrease to half its original value. This parameter is a useful index of dose requirements, dosage interval, and time to steady state, but the "normal" listed values are subject to interindividual variability
- Routine drug levels should not be measured prior to attainment of steady-state conditions (normally equivalent to a duration of constant therapy involving five elimination half-lives), unless failure of the therapeutic response or onset of toxicity is suspected
- If individualization of therapy is a critical factor in the acute phase of patient care, two blood samples drawn approximately one half-life apart (in the first dosage interval or during constant rate infusion) can provide useful information about maintenance dose requirements
- The adequacy of oral therapy can be most reliably assessed by steady-state trough level analysis
- The time of sampling is less critical for patients receiving long-term therapy if the drug has a long elimination half-life and is given by regular intermittent dosing, or if constant rate infusions are used
- If lack of efficacy or suspicion of toxicity is transient and occurs at a regular point in the dosage interval, TDM samples should be collected at these times
- To facilitate TDM interpretation, all TDM serum samples should have accurately recorded on the requisition and on the patient's permanent record:
  — The time that the sample was drawn
  — The actual time that the previous dose was drawn

TABLE 4 TDM Concepts for Pediatricians in Practice

Drug	Time to Steady State (Elimination Half-Life) Neonates	Time to Steady State (Elimination Half-Life) Infants >1 mo	Time to Steady State (Elimination Half-Life) Children >1 yr	Physician's Routine Inpatient Orders (Earliest Time for Initial TDM and Suggested Frequency with Maintenance Therapy)	Optimal Serum Concentration Range	Comments
Amikacin	24 hr* (6 hr)	24 hr (1.5 hr)	24 hr (1.5 hr)	Initial: TROUGH and PEAK with third regular dose Maintenance: TROUGH—twice weekly PEAK—baseline, then as required	TROUGH: 2.5-1.0 mg/L PEAK: 20-35 mg/L	Half-life may be prolonged in patients with renal dysfunction. Both clearance and volume of distribution may be increased in cystic fibrosis
Caffeine	14 days (3 days)	24 hr (2.5 hr)	24 hr (1.5 hr)	Initial: TROUGH—after 1 week of therapy Maintenance: TROUGH—twice weekly	30-100 µmol/L (5-20 mg/L)	Half-life of up to 100 hr in premature neonates decreases gradually throughout infancy to reach normal adult values by approximately 9 months of age
Carbamazepine	30 days (12 hr)	30 days (10 hr)	30 days (8 hr)	Initial: TROUGH—1 week after initial dose then twice weekly until stable TROUGH—Day 3 after dose change Maintenance: TROUGH—once weekly	17-50 µmol/L (4-12 mg/L) Monitoring of the active metabolite, carbamazepine 10,11 epoxide is not routine but may be of assistance TROUGH: 5-12 µmol/L	Owing to enzyme autoinduction, half-life during chronic dosing may be considerably shorter than after first dose. Consequently, within the first 2-4 wk of therapy, dose may be need to be increased to maintain therapeutic levels.
Chloramphenicol	72 hr (15 hr)	48 hr (10 hr)	24 hr (5 hr)	Initial: TROUGH and PEAK on Day 2 of therapy Maintenance: TROUGH—twice weekly PEAK—twice weekly	TROUGH: 2-10 mg/L PEAK: 15-25 mg/L	Pharmacokinetics in pediatric patients vary greatly and are unpredictable
Cyclosporine	—	—	36 hr (6 hr)	Initial: TROUGH—Day 2 of therapy Maintenance: TROUGH—every 24 hr during the acute phase	At present, this requires definition on a local basis to take account of sample matrix, analytic method, clinical indication, and time since transplantation	Monitoring is considered mandatory to avoid extremely low or high levels, which may precipitate therapeutic failure or nephrotoxicity, respectively

Drug					
Digoxin	10 days† (2.5 days)	7 days (1.5 days)	7 days (1.5 days)	Initial: TROUGH—Neonate: baseline; per first dose No risk factors: Day 5 Risk factors present: 48 hr post load Risk factors include clinical suspicion of toxicity, renal or hepatic impairment, poor response, drug interactions or noncompliance Maintenance: TROUGH—once weekly	1-2.5 nmol/L (0.8-2.0 μg/L) In neonates, serum level results may show interference with an endogenous digoxin-like substance (EDLS)	Half-life may be prolonged in renal impairment. In infants and children, the concentration-effect relationship is somewhat imprecise, particularly in renal and hepatic impairment, owing to cross-reactivity of standard assays with digoxin metabolites
Ethosuximide	—	—	7 days (1.5 days)	Initial: TROUGH—after 1 week of therapy Maintenance: TROUGH—once monthly	280-710 μmol/L (40-100 mg/L)	
Gentamicin	24 hr‡ (7 hr)‖	24 hr (4 hr)	24 hr (2 hr)§	Initial: TROUGH and PEAK with third regular dose Maintenance: TROUGH—twice weekly PEAK—baseline, then as required	TROUGH: 0.6-2.0 mg/L PEAK: 5-10 mg/L	Selected patients may tolerate and benefit from serum levels that are significantly higher than the "recommended maximum limit" Target Peak (mg/L) Indication 3-5 UTI 4-6 Prophylaxis post surgery 5-7 Pyelonephritis, cellulitis, neutropenia with fever 6-8 Pneumonia, wound infection 7-9 Positive culture with neutropenia
Methotrexate	Not applicable Monitoring of high single doses only			Dependent on specific chemotherapy protocol	Calcium leucovorin therapy normally continues until methotrexate levels are less than 0.1 μmol/L	Refer to individual protocol for target levels at specific points after initiation of high-dose infusion. Concentrations are elevated by impairment of renal filtration or secretion

*Prolonged in premature neonates to 36 hr.
†Prolonged in premature neonates from 12 to 14 days.
‡Prolonged in premature neonates from 36 to 48 hrs.
§Prolonged in patients with renal impairment; reduced in patients with cystic fibrosis.
‖May be prolonged by birth asphyxia.

Continued

TABLE 4. TDM Concepts for Pediatricians in Practice (Cont'd)

Drug	Time to Steady State (Elimination Half-Life) Neonates	Infants >1 mo	Children >1 yr	Physician's Routine Inpatient Orders (Earliest Time for Initial TDM and Suggested Frequency with Maintenance Therapy)	Optimal Serum Concentration Range	Comments
Phenobarbital	14 days (5 days)‖	7 days (2.5 days)	10 days (3 days)	Initial: TROUGH—Day 3 of therapy then twice weekly during stabilization Maintenance: TROUGH—once weekly	65–130 μmol/L (15–30 mg/L)	Specific patients tolerate and may benefit from serum levels that are significantly higher than the "recommended maximum limit"
Phenytoin	7 days Half-life is dose and concentration dependent, which makes time to steady state highly variable and unpredictable	5 days	7 days	Initial: TROUGH—Day 3 of therapy then twice weekly until stable Maintenance: TROUGH—once weekly	40–80 μmol/L** (10–20 mg/L)	Simultaneous monitoring of free phenytoin levels is not routine but may be of assistance: TROUGH—4–8 μmol/L (1–2 mg/L)
Primidone	No data available			Initial: TROUGH—Day 3 of therapy then twice weekly Maintenance: TROUGH—once weekly	23–55 μmol/L (5–12 mg/L)	Phenobarbital is the major metabolite of primidone in vivo and therefore should be monitored concurrently. The expected parent drug to metabolite ratio varies from 1:4 to 1:2
Quinidine	—	24 hr (4 hr)	24 hr (4 hr)	Initial: TROUGH—just before fifth regular dose Maintenance: TROUGH—twice weekly	7–18 μmol/L†† (2–6 mg/L)*††	Monitoring is particularly important in the presence of cardiac, hepatic, or renal impairment. Reduce the digoxin dose and monitor digoxin levels when quinidine is added to digoxin therapy

Drug	Half-life		Sampling Time	Therapeutic Range	Comments
Salicylate (ASA)	7 days	7 days	Initial: TROUGH—Day 3 Maintenance: TROUGH—once weekly Overdose: see p 469	JRA: 1.1-2.2 mmol/L (150-300 mg/L) Kawasaki disease, pericarditis: <2.2 mmol/L (<300 mg/L)	A nonlinear relationship may exist between dose and concentration owing to "capacity-limited" protein binding and hepatic metabolism
	Approximate values only. (Half-life is dose and concentration dependent)				
Theophylline	5 days (1 day)		Infusion therapy: 1. Predose if currently receiving theophylline 2. 4-8 hr after start 3. Daily as required Intermittent PO or IV: TROUGH—Day 2 then q48h during acute phase PEAK (NOT ROUTINE)—Day 2 for initial assessment of new dose 1. 1-2 hr after IV or oral liquid 2. 4-5 hr after sustained-release oral products	Neonatal apnea: 30-70 µmol/L (5-12 mg/L) Infants and children with bronchospasm: 55-110 µmol/L (10-20 mg/L)	Because theophylline is partially methylated to caffeine in the neonatal period, the levels of both methylxanthines should be monitored. Half-life may be prolonged by deficiencies in cardiac output or hepatic function
	36 hr (6 hr)	24 hr (4 hr)			
Tobramycin	Refer to gentamicin guidelines				
Valproic acid	10 days (2 days)	72 hr (15 hr)	36 hr (8 hr)	Initial: TROUGH—Day 3 Maintenance: TROUGH—twice weekly	350-700 µmol/L (50-100 mg/L)	Half-life may be prolonged in patients with hepatic disease and may be shortened in patients receiving other anticonvulsant drugs
Vancomycin	36 hr (7.5 hr)	24 hr (4.0 hr)	24 hr (2.5 hr)	Initial: TROUGH and PEAK with fourth regular dose Maintenance: TROUGH—twice weekly PEAK—baseline, then as required	TROUGH: 5-10 mg/L PEAK: 25-40 mg/L	Half-life may be prolonged in premature low-birthweight neonates and in patients with renal impairment

**Neonates may respond to lower levels.
††Therapeutic range may be lower with more specific assays.

FORMULARY

OPTIMAL SAMPLING GUIDELINES FOR TDM

- *Earliest time for first TDM:* refers to the first routine opportunity for sampling after a new order or order change; normally represents the attainment of steady state
- *Regular dose:* refers to the prescribed frequency and does not include doses administered during the adjustment to standard medication times
- *Ideal sampling time* is that which permits direct comparison with the normal therapeutic range
- Results of tests conducted on samples collected at other than the IDEAL times must be *interpreted cautiously*
- Sample collection (stat or routine) is not advised within the respective time frames described as "IMPROPER." Results cannot be interpreted reliably and may be misleading.
- Samples for antibiotic monitoring may be collected at times that do not coincide with the ideal times when
  1. Patients have unstable or poor renal function, *or*
  2. Therapy has been discontinued as a result of a previous high level, *and*
  3. The samples are labeled to indicate special circumstances.
- Except where indicated, a minimum of 0.5 mL blood (either heparinized or clotted) is required for each drug assayed. Local laboratory guidelines should be consulted to ensure that appropriate collection tubes are used and adequate blood volumes are drawn

TABLE 5 Optimal Sampling Guidelines for TDM

Drug	Earliest Time for First TDM	Ideal Sampling Time	Improper Sampling Time	Comments
Acetaminophen	No restrictions		Less than 4 hr from acute ingestion	See p 472
Amikacin TROUGH	Just before third regular dose	0-30 min before dose	More than 60 min before or any time during drug infusion	
PEAK	Third dose	IV: 30-60 min after finish of drug flush IM: 60 min post flush	Less than 30 or more than 90 min after finish of drug flush	
Caffeine	1 wk	TROUGH: 0-4 hr before dose	More than 6 hr before next dose	
Carbamazepine Initial dose Dose change	1 wk Day 3	TROUGH: 0-1 hr before dose	Less than 4 hr from last dose	

Continued.

TABLE 5 Optimal Sampling Guidelines for TDM (Cont'd)

Drug	Earliest Time for First TDM	Ideal Sampling Time	Improper Sampling Time	Comments
Chloramphenicol TROUGH	Day 2	0-30 min before dose	More than 60 min before dose or any time during drug infusion	If a bacteriologic assay is used, identify concurrent antibiotics
PEAK	Day 2	60-90 min after finish of PO dose or drug flush	Less than 45 or more than 120 min after finish of drug flush	
Cyclosporine Constant infusion	Day 2	No restrictions	No restrictions	Sampling protocol is dependent on sample matrix, analytic method, clinical indication, and time since transplantation
Intermittent	Day 2	TROUGH: 0-60 min before dose	All other times are unacceptable for inpatients	

Digoxin			
After loading	48 hr	TROUGH: 0-60 min before dose	Less than 8 hr from last dose (including cases of suspected toxicity)
Maintenance	Day 5		1 mL sample volume
Ethosuximide	Day 7	TROUGH: 0-1 hr before dose	Less than 4 hr from last dose
Gentamicin			
TROUGH	Just before third regular dose	0-30 min before dose	More than 60 min before or any time during drug infusion
PEAK	Third dose	IV: 30-60 min after finish of drug flush IM: 60 min post flush	Less than 30 or more than 90 min after finish of drug flush
Methotrexate	Sampling procedures dependent on treatment protocol		
Phenobarbital			
IV loading	No restrictions in acute phase		Less than 1 hr from last dose
Maintenance	Day 3 (day 7 for steady state)	TROUGH: 0-2 hr before dose	Less than 4 hr from last dose

Continued.

TABLE 5 Optimal Sampling Guidelines for TDM (Cont'd)

Drug	Earliest Time for First TDM	Ideal Sampling Time	Improper Sampling Time	Comments
Phenytoin				
IV loading	No restrictions in acute phase		Less than 1 hr from last dose	
Maintenance	Day 3 (day 7 for steady state)	TROUGH: 0-1 hr before dose	Less than 4 hr from last dose	
Primidone	Day 3	TROUGH: 0-1 hr before dose	More than 90 min before dose	Take concurrent phenobarbital level
Quinidine	Just before fifth regular dose	TROUGH: 0-1 hr before dose	Less than 4 hr from last dose	
Salicylate				
Toxicology	No restrictions		Less than 6 hr from acute ingestion	See p 469
Therapeutic	Day 3	TROUGH: 0-1 hr before dose	Less than 4 hr from last dose	Time to peak varies and is prolonged with the enteric-coated product

Theophylline (see pp 731-733)			
Infusion	4-8 hr of constant rate infusion	After 12-24 hr of constant rate infusion	Less than 1 hr from loading dose
Intermittent (PO or IV)			
TROUGH	Day 2	0-30 min before dose	More than 60 min before dose
PEAK	Day 2	1. 1-2 hr after IV or oral liquid 2. 4-5 hr after sustained-release oral products	Required only for initial assessment of new dose
Tobramycin			NOT ROUTINE
TROUGH	Just before third regular dose	0-30 min before dose	More than 60 min before dose or any time during drug infusion

Continued.

TABLE 5 Optimal Sampling Guidelines for TDM (Cont'd)

Drug	Earliest Time for First TDM	Ideal Sampling Time	Improper Sampling Time	Comments
Tobramycin—cont'd PEAK	Third dose	30-60 min after finish of drug flush	Less than 30 or more than 90 min after finish of drug flush	
Valproic acid	Day 3	TROUGH: 0-1 hr before dose	Less than 4 hr from last dose	
Vancomycin TROUGH	Just before fourth regular dose	0-30 min before dose	More than 60 min before or any time during drug infusion	
PEAK	Fourth dose	IV: 60-90 min after finish of drug flush	Less than 45 or more than 120 min after finish of drug flush	

DECISION STEPS FOR MANAGEMENT OF THEOPHYLLINE THERAPY
DAY 1

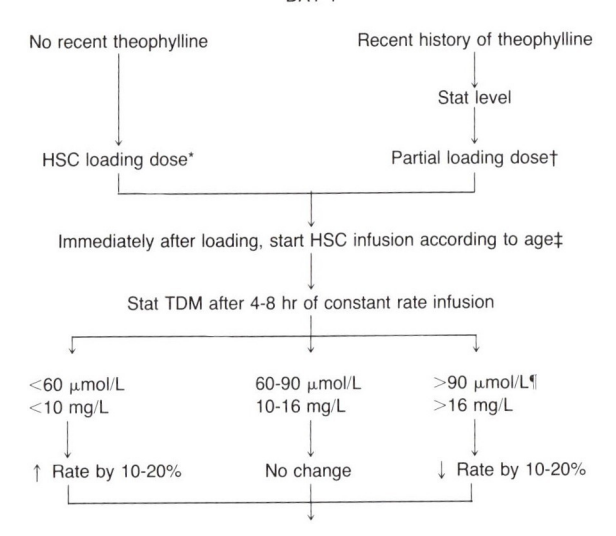

```
No recent theophylline                    Recent history of theophylline
         |                                              |
         |                                          Stat level
         |                                              |
   HSC loading dose*                           Partial loading dose†
         |_____|
                            |
   Immediately after loading, start HSC infusion according to age‡
                            |
            Stat TDM after 4-8 hr of constant rate infusion
         _____|_____
         |                 |                 |
   <60 μmol/L        60-90 μmol/L       >90 μmol/L¶
   <10 mg/L          10-16 mg/L         >16 mg/L
         |                 |                 |
   ↑ Rate by 10-20%    No change      ↓ Rate by 10-20%
         |_____|_____|
                            |
       Routine TDM after 12-24 hr of constant rate infusion
```

---

*6 mg/kg of theophylline
Administer at a rate not to exceed 20 mg/min or 0.4 mg/kg/min.
Use effective body weight for this calculation if patient is obese.
†Partial loading dose requirement can be determined as follows: each 1 mg/kg of theophylline will increase the serum level by 10 μmol/L (2 mg/L).
‡Initial maintenance dose:
1-12 yr: 0.8 mg/kg/hr IV
12-16 yr: 0.7 mg/kg/hr IV
>16 yr: (nonsmoker): 0.6 mg/kg/hr IV
In the presence of cardiac decompensation, cor pulmonale, liver dysfunction, or any drug interaction likely to inhibit hepatic metabolism, a more cautious approach to initial maintenance dosing is required—e.g., 0.2-0.4 mg/kg/hr.
¶These results are not "steady state" (i.e., the duration of constant dosing has been insufficient to assess its full impact), but they represent an "early warning" of the requirement to change the rate. An individual approach may be necessary for levels <50 or >110 μmol/L (<9 or >20 mg/L).

DECISION STEPS FOR MANAGEMENT OF THEOPHYLLINE THERAPY
IV MAINTENANCE INFUSION TO PO CHANGEOVER

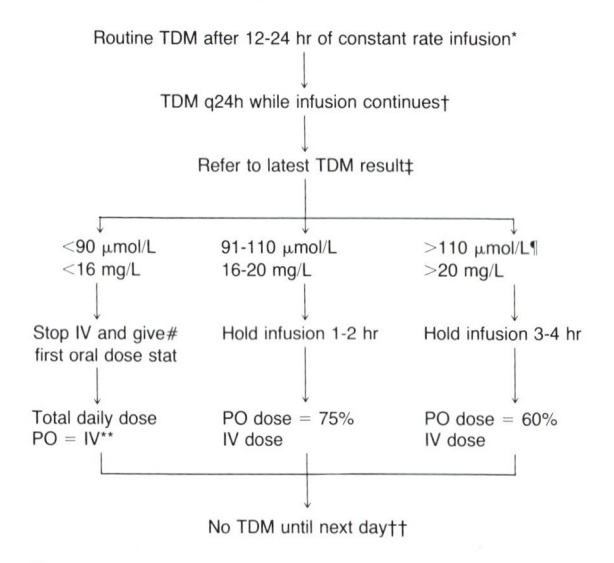

Routine TDM after 12-24 hr of constant rate infusion*

↓

TDM q24h while infusion continues†

↓

Refer to latest TDM result‡

<90 μmol/L <16 mg/L	91-110 μmol/L 16-20 mg/L	>110 μmol/L¶ >20 mg/L
Stop IV and give# first oral dose stat	Hold infusion 1-2 hr	Hold infusion 3-4 hr
Total daily dose PO = IV**	PO dose = 75% IV dose	PO dose = 60% IV dose

↓

No TDM until next day††

---

*Collect, if possible, within normal hours of TDM laboratory service. After a minimum of 12-hr infusion with a constant dose, the full impact of the therapy on serum levels (and clinical response) can be assessed. If this result is considered unsatisfactory, the infusion rate can be increased or decreased in proportion to the desired concentration change.

†For patients stabilized on IV infusion, a TDM level every 24-36 hr is considered sufficient.

‡The guidelines assume a 12-hr minimum of constant rate dosing.

¶A more individual approach may be required for levels in excess of 120 μmol/L (>22 mg/L).

#This approach is based on Somophyllin-12 absorption characteristics. Extrapolation to other formulations has not been validated.

**For example, if a steady infusion level of 80 μmol/L (14 mg/L) has been observed in association with an infusion rate of 20 mg/hr, then the equivalent oral dose will be 480 mg/day (250 mg q12h).

Normally, Somophyllin-12 doses are divided q12h; in a patient who shows evidence of high-infusion dose requirements (for age and weight), q8h dosing could be considered as an alternative, i.e., 150 mg q8h in this example.

If it is not possible to switch patients from IV to PO at one of the standard medication times, it is recommended that an interim dose of Somophyllin-12 be given stat to cover the infusion shortfall until regular dosing can begin, e.g., 250 mg PO q12 has been prescribed at 0800 hr and 2000 hr. If infusion is stopped at 1400 hr, give 125 mg stat, then 250 mg at 2000 hr, and so forth.

††No TDM assessment is necessary during first dose interval.

DECISION STEPS FOR MANAGEMENT OF THEOPHYLLINE THERAPY
MONITORING PO LONG ACTING THEOPHYLLINE

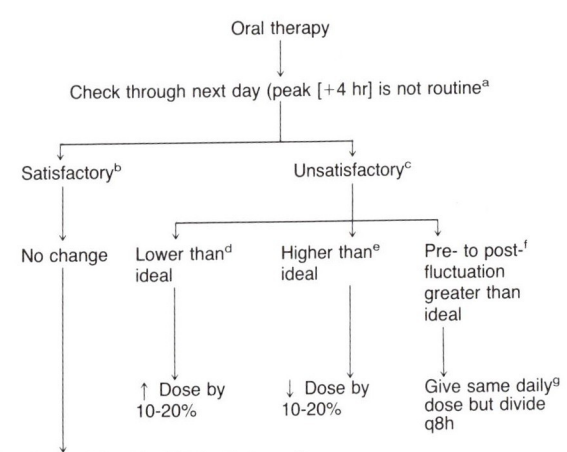

Oral therapy
↓
Check through next day (peak [+4 hr] is not routine[a]

- Satisfactory[b] → No change → Check trough (only) q48h to discharge[h]
- Unsatisfactory[c]:
  - Lower than[d] ideal → ↑ Dose by 10-20%
  - Higher than[e] ideal → ↓ Dose by 10-20%
  - Pre- to post-[f] fluctuation greater than ideal → Give same daily[g] dose but divide q8h

---

[a] The time of the peak level is unpredictable.
[b] Dependent on clinical response, this result would probably be in the range 50-90 μmol/L (9-16 mg/L).
[c] From a serum level and clinical viewpoint.
[d] Low trough level with incomplete therapeutic response.
[e] High trough level with evidence of adverse effect.
[f] Peak level exceeds trough level by 100% or more.
[g] For example, if original dose was 150 mg q12h, revised dose should be 100 mg q8h.
[h] Dependent on stability of clinical status.

Index

An *f* following a page number indicates a figure; *t* indicates a table.

A

Abdominal distension
  acute, 117, 118*f*
  chronic, 119-120, 121*f*
Abdominal pain, recurrent, 122*t*
Abrasion
  of cornea, 418
  and plastic surgery, 457
Abscess
  incision and drainage, 567
  periodontal, 56
  pulpal necrosis with, 56
Abuse, child, 553-554, 555*t*
Access
  intraosseous, 563
  venous, 562
Acetaminophen (Tempra; Tylenol), 642*t*, 698*t*, 725*t*
  for febrile seizures, 380
  for headache, 389
  and liver injury, 224*t*
Acetaminophen (Paracetamol) poisoning, 472, 473*f*
Acetylcysteine (Mucomyst), 642*t*
Acetylsalicylic acid, 642*t*
Acid-base disorders, 98
Acid-base status
  apnea, 326, 327-329*t*
  cyanosis of the newborn, 330, 331*f*
  drug withdrawal, 345-346
  duct-dependent cardiac lesions, 333
  dysrhythmia, 332
  hyperglycemia, 320
  hypocalcemia, 322
  hypoglycemia, 321
  infection, 344-345
  jaundice
    exchange transfusion, 341, 342*t*
    phototherapy, 338, 339*f*
  metabolic acidosis, 320
  metabolic alkalosis, 320
  nutrition, 343, 344*t*
  patent ductus arteriosus (PDA), 332
  respiratory acidosis, 319
  respiratory alkalosis, 319
Acidosis
  metabolic, 98, 100*f*, 320
  respiratory, 319
Acne, 60-61
ACTH, 642*t*
Activated charcoal, 642*t*
Acyclovir (Zovirax), 643*t*, 698*t*
Adenosine, 643*t*
Adenotonsillectomy, 446-447
Adolescent medicine
  eating disorders, 4-5*t*
  history and examinations, 2-3
  substance abuse, 6-13*t*
Adrenaline, 643*t*
Adrenal insufficiency, 83
Adults, body surface area for, 640*f*
AIDS, 258
  CDC classification system for HIV infection, 260-261*t*
  confirmation of HIV infection, 259
  features suggestive of HIV infection, 259
  management of, 259
  pediatric risk groups for, 259
  therapeutic considerations, 262
Alanine aminotransferase (ALT), 209
Albumin, 643*t*, 698*t*
Albuterol, 643*t*
Alcohol, 6-7*t*
Aldactazide, 643*t*
Alkaline corrosives, poisoning by, 478
Alkaline phosphatase (ALP), 209
Alkalosis
  metabolic, 320
  respiratory, 319
Allergen avoidance, 16
Allergic conjunctivitis, 17*t*
Allergic rhinitis, 17*t*, 18
Allergy and immunology
  adverse drug reactions, 19
  allergen avoidance, 16
  allergic rhinitis, 17*t*, 18
  challenge testing, 15

Index

Allergy and immunology—cont'd
  food allergy, 18
  immunotherapy, 16
  management, 16
  other measures, 16
  pharmacologic management, 17t
  skin testing, 14
  suspicion of allergic disorder, 15
  in vitro testing–radioallergosorbent test (RAST), 15
Allopurinol, 644t
Alopecia, 61-62
Alopecia areata, 62
Alphacalcidiol, 644t
Alprostadl, 698t
Aluminum, 644t
Aluminum hydroxide, 644t
Alveolar-arterial (A-a) gradient, 484, 485f
Amantadine, 644t
Ambiguous genitalia, 81, 82f
Amikacin, 645t, 699t, 720t
  PEAK, 725t
  TROUGH, 725t
Aminocaproic acid (Amicar), 645t
Aminophylline, 645t
5-Aminosalicylic acid, 645t
Aminotransferase, 209
Amiodarone, 645t
Amoxycillin, 645t
Amphetamines, 6-8t
Amphotericin B, 646t, 699t
Ampicillin, 646t, 699t
Amrinone, 646t
Anal warts, causes of, 136t
Anaphylaxis, 17t, 533
Anemia, 180
  aplastic, 190
  approach to, 182f
  hematologic parameters in types of, 181t
  hemolytic, 185
  hypochromic microcytic, 480
  iron-deficiency, 183
  sickle cell, 186, 187f
  thalassemia syndromes, 183-184
Aneuploidy, 123
Animal bites, 251-252
Anisocoria, 419
Anorexia nervosa, clinical features of, 4-5t
Antibiotics
  for acne, 60-61
  for bacterial meningitis, 262, 266
  for bites, 252
  for cellulitis, 253
  for cervical adenitis, 254
  for osteomyelitis, 250
  for pertussis, 270
  for rheumatic fever, 51
  for septic arthritis, 248, 249t
  for septic shock, 272
  for sinusitis, 273
  for streptococcal pharyngitis, 271
Anticholinergic drugs, in asthma, 499, 502
Anticonvulsants, overdose of, 475
Antidiuretic hormones, 83-84
APGAR score, 308t
Aplastic anemia, 190
Apnea, 326, 327-329t
Appendicitis, 526
Arterial blood sampling, 577
Arthritis
  approach to the child with, 509-510
  juvenile, 512-513
    differential diagnosis of, 516-517f
    subgroups of, 514-515t
  septic, 247-248
    etiologic organisms and antibiotic selection for, 249t
Aspartate aminotransferase (AST), 209
Aspirin, and liver injury, 224t
Astemizole, 646t
Asthma
  acute, 498-500
  chronic, 500-502
Ataxia, acute, 382
Atopic dermatitis, 17t, 62
Atresia
  biliary, 527
  duodenal, 521
  esophageal, 521
  small intestinal, 522
Atrial ectopic tachycardia, 42t
Atrial fibrillation, 43ft
Atrial flutter, 42t
Atrial premature beat, 41f
Atrial tachycardia, 42f
Atropine, 647t, 700t
AV block
  first degree, 43f
  second degree, 44f
  third-degree, 45f

B

Baby bottle syndrome, 57
Back pain, 442
Bacterial meningitis, 262, 266
  antibiotics for, 265t
  CSF findings in, 264t
Bacterial overgrowth, 108t

Bacterial sepsis, 190
Barbiturates, overdose of, 475
Barlow (dislocation) test, 437f
B-Cell defects, 24-25t, 26t
Belladonna, 647t
Benzathine (Bicillin 1200 LA), 681t
Benzoyl peroxide, 60
Biliary atresia, 527
Birth control pills, 144, 148t
Bisacodyl, 647t
Bites, 251-252
  animal, 251-252
  human, 252
  snake, 482-483
  spider, 483
Black dot alopecia, 69
Black widow spider bite, 483
Bladder
  catheterization, 574
  neurogenic, 151
  suprapubic aspiration, 575
Blood, reference values, 487-621t
Blood gas abnormality, 99t
Blood products, clinical use of, 198t
Blow-out fracture, 421
Body surface area
  nomogram for children and adults, 640f
  nomogram for infants, 641f
Bone infarction, differentiation between osteomyelitis and, 189t
Bottle feeding, 392
  fluoride supplement in, 392t
Breast feeding, 391
  fluoride supplement in, 392t
Bronchiolitis, 493-494
Brown recluse spider bite, 483
Budesonide, 647t
Bulimia, clinical features of, 4-5t
Bundle branch block, 46
Burns, 459-463
  corrosive, of upper GI tract, 451-452
  criteria for hospitalization of, 460
  of eye, 417
  severity of, 460
  water temperature and duration of exposure producing third degree, 463t

C

Cafazolin, 649t
Caffeine, 700t, 720t, 725t
Caftriaxone, 651t
Calcitriol (1,25-dihydroxychole-calciferol), 648t
Calcium, 648t

Calcium carbonate, 648t
Calcium gluconate, 700t
Calcium lactate, 700-701t
Candida, 64
Candidiasis, intraocular, 420
Capillary (strawberry) hemangioma, 65, 66
Captopril, 649t
Carbamazepine, 649t, 720t, 725t
  and liver injury, 224t
Carbohydrate malabsorption, reducing substances in stool to defect, 579
Carbohydrates, in total parental nutrition, 391
Carbuncle, 63
Cardiac cocktail, 649t
Cardiac dysrhythmia, identification of, 41-46f
Cardiac failure, 334
  jaundice, 336-337t
  persistent pulmonary hypertension of the newborn (PPHN), 335
Cardiac lesions, duct-dependent, 333
Cardiac procedures, corrective, 52
Cardiology
  abbreviations in, 29-30
  acute pericarditis, 53-54
  chamber enlargement, 36t
  congestive heart failure, 30-31
  corrective cardiac procedures, 52
  cyanotic spells in tetralogy of Fallot catheterization data, 54, 55t
  dysrhythmia, 41-46f
  ECG standards, 37-38f
  electrocardiography, 32-33
    disturbances related to, 35t
    lead placement for, 34t
  endocarditis, 50
  hexaxial and horizontal reference system, 39f
  hyperkalemia, 39f
  hypokalemia, 39f
  myocarditis, 53
  quadrant location, 40f
  rheumatic fever, 51-52, 51t
  treatment of supraventricular tachycardia, 47, 48-49t
Cardiomyopathy, 31
Cardiopulmonary resuscitation, 530
  advanced life support, 531
  basic life support, 530
  continuing support, 532
  drug therapy, 532t
Catheterization
  bladder, 574
  normal cardiac, 55t

Index

Catheterization—cont'd
  umbilical artery, 571
  umbilical vein, 568, 569f, 570f
Catheter mixture no. 3, 649t
Cavernous hemangioma, 65, 66
Cefaclor, 649t
Cefazolin, 701t
Cefixime, 650t
Cefotaxime, 650t, 701t
Cefoxitin, 650t
Ceftazidime, 650t, 701t
Cefuroxime, 651t
Celiac disease, 108t, 109
Cellulitis, 253
  periorbital and orbital, 253
Cephalexin, 651t
Cephalosporins, 20
  characteristics of, 274t
Cerebrospinal fluid (CSF)
  in bacterial meningitis, 264t
  cell count, 576-577
  reference values, 636t
  shunt, blocked, 384-386
Cervical adenitis, 254
Challenge testing, 15
Chamber enlargement, criteria for, 36t
Charcoal, activated, 651t
Chemosis, 417
Chemotherapy agents, side effects of
  common, 202-204t
Chest tube insertion, 566
Chicken pox. See Varicella
Child abuse, 553-554
  indicators, 555t
Childhood exanthems, 282-287
Children. See also Infants
  body surface area for, 640f
  choking in, 533-534
  drug dosage guidelines for, 642-697t
  metabolic disease in, 288-289, 294-297t
  ophthalmology for, 412
Chlamydia, 415
Chlamydia trachomatis, 135, 137t
  treatment of, 137t
Chloral hydrate, 651t, 702t
Chloramphenicol, 652t, 702t, 720t, 726t
Chloroquine, 652t
Chlorpheniramine, 653t
Chlorpromazine, 653t
  for headache, 389
Choking, 533
  in child, 533-534
  in infant, 534
Cholestasis, 209
Cholestyramine, 653t
Christmas disease, 196

Chromosome analysis, 124
Chronic renal failure, 353
Chronic treatment, 47
Cimetidine, 653t, 702t
Cisapride, 653t
Cleft lip and palate, 458
Clindamycin, 654t, 702-703t
Clonazepam, 654t
Clostridium difficile, 254-255
Cloxacillin, 654t, 703t
CM-3, 655t
Coagulation disorders, 193f
  investigation of acquired, 195t
  investigation of inherited, 194t
Coagulation values, 486t
Cocaine, 8-10t
  and liver injury, 224t
Codeine, 655t
Cold diuresis, 542
Colitis, ulceratis, 116
Coloboma, 419
Coma
  and altered level of unconsciousness, 535-536, 538-539
  causes of, 535t
  distinguishing diffuse versus focal causes of, 538
  modified glasgow scale, 537t
Complement deficiencies, 24-25t, 27t
Condyloma acuminata, 70
Congenital infections, 255, 256-257t
Congestive heart failure
  clinical features and investigations, 30
  management of, 31
Conjunctivae, 415, 416t, 417
Contraception
  availability of, in Canada, 146-147t
  birth control pills, 144
  methods of, 145t
Cornea, 417-418
Corticosteroids, in asthma, 499, 502
Cortisone acetate, 655t
Cotrimoxazole, 655-656t
Cover-uncover test, for tropia, 422f
Cow's milk protein intolerance, 109
Creative clearance, 625f
Crohn's disease, 116-117
Cromoglycate sodium, 656-657t
Croup (acute laryngotracheobronchitis), 492-493
Cryptorchidism, 527
Cyanotic spells in tetralogy of fallot, 54
  investigations, 54
  treatment, 54
Cyanosis of the newborn, 330, 331f
Cyclosporine, 657t, 720t, 726t

Cyproheptadine, for headache, 390
Cystic fibrosis, 502-504
   nutritional management for, 505t

D

Deep venous thrombosis, 199-200
Deferoxamine mesylate (Desferal), 657t
Dehydration, 88, 90t, 92
   clinical features of, 91t
   hypertonic, 96
   hypotonic, 94
Dentistry, 57
   acute herpetic gingivostomatitis, 59
   chronology of human dentition, 178-179t
   dental pain, 57
   dental postoperative hemorrhage, 58
   dental trauma, 58
Dermatitis
   atopic, 62
   diaper, 64
   irritant, 64
   poison ivy contact, 64
   seborrheic, 64, 68
Dermatology
   acne, 60-61
   alopecia, 61-62
   alopecia areata, 62
   atopic dermatitis, 62
   diaper dermatitis, 64
   emollients, 71
   erythema multiforme, 65
   furunculosis, 63
   hemangiomas, 65-66
   impetigo, 63
   lice, 66-67
   molluscum contagiosum, 67
   pityriasis rosea, 67
   poison ivy contact dermatitis, 64
   scabies, 68
   seborrheic dermatitis, 68
   staphylococcal scalded skin syndrome (SSSS), 68
   tinea capitis, 69
   topical steroids, 70, 71t
   urticaria, 69
   verrucae, 69
Dermatomes, 385, 386f
Desmopressin (DDAVP), 657t-658t
Dexamethasone, 658t, 704t
Dextromethorphan, 658t
Dextrose, 659t, 704t
Diabetes insipidus, 83-85
Diabetes mellitus, 72-73
   hypoglycemia in, 76-77
Diabetic ketoacidosis, 73-74

Diaper dermatitis, 64
Diaphragmatic hernia (Bochdalek), 524
Diarrhea
   acute, 102-103, 104f
   chronic, 106-107, 108t
Diazepam (Valium), 659t, 704t
   in febrile seizures, 381
   in seizures, 378
Diazoxide, 659t
Digoxin, 31, 659t-660t, 704t-705t, 721t, 726t
Dimelaprol, 660t
Dimenhydrinate, 660t
   for headache, 389
Dimercaprol, 661t
Diphenhydramine, 660t
Diphtheria, immunization for, 232-233
Dipyridamole, 660t
Disseminated intravascular coagulation (DIC), 199
Diuretics, 31
Dobutamine, 660t, 705t
Docusate sodium, 660t
Domperidone, 661t
Dopamine, 661t, 705t
Doxapram, 705t
Doxycycline, 661t
Drowning, near, 543-545
Drug(s)
   abuse of, 6-13t
   adverse reactions to, 18
   allergies, 20, 21f
   therapeutic monitoring, 719, 720-723t, 724, 725-730t
   withdrawal in neonatals, 345-346
Drug dosage guidelines
   for infants and children, 642-697t
   neonatal, 698-715t
Drug hepatotoxicity, 224-225t
Drug overdose
   anticonvulsants, 475
   barbiturates, 475
   narcotics, 479
Duct-dependent cardiac lesions, 333
Duodenal ulcer, 112
Dysrhythmia, 332

E

Ear
   foreign body in, 447
   mastoiditis, 456
   otitis externa, 449-450
   otitis media
      acute, 453, 454 6t
      recurrent, 455
      serous, 455-456

Ear—cont'd
  traumatic perforation of tympanic membrane, 456
ECG standards, 37-38f
Edema, pulmonary, 31
Edetate calcium disodium, 661t
Edrophonium, 661t
Elbow, pulled, 443
Electrocardiography, 32-33
  disturbances related to, 35t
  lead placement for, 34t
Electrolytes. *See also* Fluids and electrolytes
  practical approach to correction of deficits, 93t
  in total parental nutrition, 402
Emollients, 71
Encephalitis, herpes simplex, 258
Encephalopathy
  lead, 480
  stages of, in Reye's Syndrome, 212t
Endocarditis prophylaxis, recommendations for, 716-718t
Endocarditis, subacute bacterial, 50
  investigation of, 50
  management of, 50
Endocrinology
  adrenal insufficiency, 83
  ambiguous genitalia, 81, 82f
  antidiuretic hormone, 83-84
  diabetes mellitus, 72-73
  diabetic ketoacidosis, 73-74
  hypercalcemia, 81
  hypocalcemia, 79, 81
    plasma chemistry findings in, 80t
  hypoglycemia, 76-77
  management of intercurrent illness, 74, 75t
    plasma chemistry findings in, 80t
  short stature, 84-85, 85t
  thyroid disease, 86f
Endotracheal intubation, 572-573
Enteral nutrition, 404-405, 406-409t
Enterobiasis, examination for, 580t
Enterokinase deficiency, 108t
Enteropathy, protein-losing, 109
Enuresis, 370-371
Environmental illnesses
  near drowning, 543-545
  frostbite, 543
  hyperthermia and heat illnesses, 540-541
  hypothermia, 541-543
  smoke inhalation, 545-546
Environmentally induced abnormalities, 124

Epididymitis, 140
  causes of, 136t
Epiglottitis, 492
Epilepticus, status, 378-379
Epinephrine, 661t, 705t
  for inhalation, 661t
Epiphysis, slipped femoral capital, 440
Epistaxis, 450
Erythema multiforme, 65
Erythromycin, 662t
  and liver injury, 225t
Erythromycin estolate, 706t
Erythromycin gluceptate, 706t
Erythromycin lactobionate, 706t
Erythropoietin, 662t
Esophagus, foreign body in, 449
Ethambutol, 662t
Ethanol, poisoning by, 476
Ethosuximide, 663t, 721t, 726t
Exanthems, childhood, 282-287
Exchange transfusion, 341, 342t
Exocrine pancreatic insufficiency, 108t
Eye. *See* Ophthalmology
Eye alignment, abnormal, 421, 422-423f
Eyelids
  chalazion, 414
  hordeolum (stye), 414
  trauma, 414

F

Facial nerve paralysis, 452
Factor IX deficiency (Christmas disease), 196
Factor VIII deficiency (Hemophilia A), 196
Failure to thrive, 395-396
Fansidar, 663t
Feces, reference values, 633-635t
Ferrous sulfate, 663t
Fever, management of, 282
Flecainide, 663t
Flucloxacillin, 664t
Flucytosine, 664t, 706t
Fludrocortisone, 664t
Fluids. *See also* Fluids and electrolytes
  practical approach to correction, 93t
Fluids and electrolytes, 315
  conversions, 87
  dehydration, 88, 90t, 92
  electrolyte composition of gastrointestinal fluids, 90t
  guidelines for therapy, 315t, 316t
  in hyperkalemia, 318-319
  in hypernatremia, 317-318
  in hypokalemia, 318

in hyponatremia, 317
  maintenance requirements, 87, 88t
  parenteral solution composition, 89t
Fluoride supplement, for breast- and formula-fed infants, 392t
Food allergy, 18
Foot shape concerns, 430, 431t
Foreign body
  in cornea, 417
  in ear, 447
  in esophagus, 449
  ingested, 526
  in larynx, 448
  in nose, 448
  in tracheobronchial tube, 448
Fractures, 444
  facial, and plastic surgery, 458
  of nose, 451
Frostbite, 543
Furazolidone, 664t
Furosemide, 664t, 706t
Furuncle, 63
Furunculosis, 63

G

Galeazi's sign, 437f
Gammaglobulin infusion, for Guillain-Barré syndrome, 390
Gammaglutamyl transpeptidase (GGT), 210
Ganciclovir, 665t
Gastroenteritis, 88, 109
Gastroenterology
  abdominal distension, 117, 118f, 119-120, 121f
  acute diarrhea, 102-103, 104f
  chronic diarrhea, 106-107, 108t
  inflammatory bowel disease, 116-117
  oral rehydration fluids, 105t
  protein-losing enteropathy, 109
  vomiting, 109, 110f, 111
Gastroesophageal reflux, 111
Gastrointestinal bleeding, 112-113, 114-115f
Gastrointestinal fluids, electrolyte composition, 90t
Gelusil (Extra strength), 665t
Genetics
  biochemical tests, 125
  chromosome analysis, 124
  diagnostic categories, 123-124
  inborn error of metabolism (IEM), 125-126
  photographs, 125
Genital warts, causes of, 136t

Genitalia, ambiguous, 81, 82f
Genital ulcer disease, causes of, 136t
Genitourinary disease
  acute scrotum, 150
  labial fusion, 134
  neurogenic bladder, 151
  perimenarchal, 128
  postmenarchal, 129-130
  premenarchal, 127-128
  sexual assault, 149-150
  sexually transmitted diseases, 134
    causes of, 136t
    chlamydia trachonatis, 135, 137t
    epididymitis, 140
    neisseria gonorrhoea, 135, 137, 138-139t
    pelvic inflammatory disease, 135, 140t
    syphilis, 141, 142-143t
  vaginal bleeding, 127
  vulvovaginitis, 131-133
Gentamicin, 665t, 707t, 721t, 727t
Giardiasis, 109
Gingivostomatitis, acute herpetic, 59
GI tract, corrosive burns of upper, 451-452
Glomerulonephritis, 354-355
  causes of, 354t
Glucagon, 665t, 707t
Go-lytely, 665t
Gram stain, 578
Granuloma, umbilical, 527
Growth and development
  emerging patterns of behavior, 153-157t
  female height and weight charts, 162-163f, 166-167f, 169f, 171f, 173f, 175f, 176f
  human dentition, 178-179t
  male height and weight charts, 160-161f, 164-165f, 168f, 170f, 172f, 174f
  male penile length, 177
  physician's speech and language checklist, 158-159t
Growth hormone, 665t
Guillain-Barré Syndrome, 390

H

Haemophilus influenzae type B, prophylaxis for, 236
Halothane, and liver injury, 225t
Headache, 388-390
Heat exhaustion, 541
Heat illnesses, 540-541

Index

Heat stroke, 541
Hemangiomas, 65-66
Hematology and oncology
  anemia, 180, 181t, 182f, 183
  clinical uses of blood products, 198t
  coagulation disorders, 193f, 194t, 195t
  deep venous thrombosis, 199-200
  differentiation between osteomyelitis and bone infarction, 189t
  differentiation between pneumonia and pulmonary infarction, 188t
  disseminated intravascular coagulation, 199
  factor IX deficiency, 196
  hemophilia
    factor replacement in, 197t
  hemophilia A, 196
  hepatic failure, 199
  references values
    blood, 487-621t
    coagulation values, 486t
    hemoglobin, hemocrit, RBC count, reticulocytes, 582-583t
    hemoglobin electrophoresis, 484t
    platelet count, 584t
    white blood cell count and differential, 485t
  sickle cell disease, 186, 187t, 190-191
  side effects of chemotherapy agents, 202-204t, 205-207
  thalassemia syndromes, 183-184
  thrombocytopenia, 191-192
  transfusion reactions, 200-201
  tumor lysis syndrome, 201
  vitamin K deficiency, 199
  von Willebrand disease, 196
Hematuria, 370
Hemocrit, references values, 582-583t
Hemoglobin, reference values, 582-583t
Hemoglobin electrophoresis, 484t
Hemolytic anemia, 185f
Hemolytic uremic syndrome, 354
Hemophilia, initial doses of factor replacement, 197t
Hemophilia A, 196
Hemophilia B, 196
Hemorrhage
  dental postoperative, 58
  retinal, 420
  subconjunctival, 417
Henoch Schönlein purpura, 518
Heparin, 665t, 707t
Hepatic failure, 199
Hepatitis, viral, 278-279

Hepatitis B, prophylaxis for, 238, 239-240t
Hepatobiliary disease, serum markers of, 209-210
Hepatocellular necrosis, 209
Hepatology
  acute fulminant liver failure, 214-215f
  drug hepatotoxicity, 224-225t
  hepatosplenomegaly, 222-223f
  liver disease
    clinical guide to, 216-221t
    normal values for, 209f
    nutrition in, 227
    symptoms and signs of, 208f
    total parenteral nutrition, 226
  Reye's syndrome, 211, 212t, 213
  serum markers of hepatobiliary disease, 209-210
Hepatosplenomegaly, 222-223f
Hernia
  diaphragmatic, 524
  inguinal, 526
Heroin, 10-11t
Herpes simplex encephalitis, 258
Hip problems, 434-435t
Hirschberg test, 423f
Hirschsprung's disease, 524
HIV infection. See AIDS
Human bites, 252
Hydralazine, 666t, 707t
Hydrochlorothiazide, 666t
Hydrocortisone, 666-667t
Hydroxychloroquine, 667t
Hydroxyzine, 667t
Hypercalcemia, 35t, 81
Hyperglycemia, 320
Hyperkalemia, 35t, 201, 318-319
  ECG findings of, 39f
Hypernatremia, 317-319
Hyperphosphatemia, 201
Hypertension, 359
  drug therapy for acute, 368
  investigations, 366
  management, 367
  measurements in, 360-363f
  persistent pulmonary, of newborn, 335
  treatment, 366
Hyperthermia, 540-541
Hypertonic dehydration, 96
Hypertrophic pyloric stenosis, 524-525
Hyperuricemia, 201
Hyphema, 418
Hypocalcemia, 35t, 79, 81, 201, 322
  plasma chemistry findings in, 80t
Hypochromic microcytic anemia, 480

Hypoglycemia, 77, 321
  in diabetes mellitus, 76-77
  diagnoses of, 78t
Hypokalemia, 35t, 97-98, 318
  ECG findings of, 39f
Hypomagnesemia, 35t
Hyponatremia, 95f, 317
Hypopyon, 419
Hypothermia, 541-543, 543
Hypotonic dehydration, 94
  acid-base disorders, 98
  blood gas abnormality, 99t
  hyperkalemia, 98
  hypertonic dehydration, 96
  hypokalemia, 97-98
  hyponatremia, 95f
  metabolic acidosis, 98, 100f
  pseudohyponatremia, 97
  salt poisoning, 97
  urinary alkalinization, 101
Hypoventilation, 542

I

Idiopathic thrombocytopenic purpura (ITP), 192
Idiosyncratic reaction, 20
Imipenemcilastatin, 667t
Imipramine, 667t
Immune globulin (Human IV), 667t
Immunizations, 228, 229t, 230-231t. *See also* Infectious diseases
  for diphtheria, 232-233
  for *Haemophilus* influenzae type B, 236
  for hepatitis A, 237
  for hepatitis B, 238, 239-240t
  for influenza, 241-242
  for measles, 234-235
  for mumps, 234
  for *Neisseria meningitides*, 237
  for pertussis, 232-233
  for poliomyelitis, 232-233
  for rabies, 243, 244-245t, 246t
  for rubella, 234-235
  for *streptococcus pneumoniae*, 243-244
  for tetanus, 232-233
  for varicella, 247
Immunocompromised host, infections in, 279
Immunodeficiency disorders
  classification of, 26-27t
  clinical, 21
  clinical differentiation, 24-25t
  diagnosis of, 232
  management of, 23

Immunodeficiency syndrome, 24-25t
Immunotherapy, 16
Impetigo, 63
Inborn error of metabolism (IEM), 125-126
Indomethacin, 668t, 708t
Ineperidine, for headache, 389
Infants. *See also* Children
  body surface area for, 641f
  bottle feeding, 392t
  breast feeding, 391
  choking in, 534
  drug dosage guidelines for, 642-697t
  failure to thrive, 395-396
  introduction of solids, 394, 395t
  metabolic disease in, 288-289, 292-293t, 294-297t
  ophthalmology for, 411
Infection
  congenital, 255, 256-257t
  in neonatal, 344-345
  parasitic, 268-269t
  upper airway, 491t
Infectious disease, 228. *See also* Immunizations
  bacterial meningitis, 262, 266
  bites, 251-252
  cellulitis, 253
  cervical adenitis, 254
  childhood exanthems, 282-287
  clostridium difficile, 254-255
  congenital infections, 255, 256-257t
  contraindications, 228
  extrapulmonary tuberculosis, 276
  herpes simplex encephalitis, 258
  HIV infection and AIDS, 258-259, 260-261t, 262
  immunocompromised host, 279
  infectious mononucleosis, 262
  meningitis
    empiric antibiotic selection for, 265
    interpretation of CSF findings in, 264
  mumps, 267
  osteomyelitis, 250-251
  parasitic infections, 268-269t
  pertussis, 270-271
  post-measles exposure prophylaxis, 235
  post-rubella exposure prophylaxis in pregnant women, 235
  septic arthritis, 247-248, 249t
  septic shock, 271, 272t
  sinusitis, 273
  streptococcal pharyngitis, 270
  tuberculosis, 275, 276t
  varicella (chicken pox), 278

Infectious disease—cont'd
  viral hepatitis, 278-279
Infectious disease syndromes
  common risk groups and, 280t
Infectious mononucleosis, 262
Inflammatory bowel disease, 108t, 109, 116-117
Influenza, prophylaxis for, 241-242
Ingested foreign body, 526
Inguinal hernias, 526
Insecticides, poisoning by, 479
Insulin, 708t
Insulin adjustment, during intercurrent illness, 75t
Intoeing, 424-425, 426-429f
Intraocular candidiasis, 420
Intraosseous access, 563
Intravenous cutdown, 563
Intravenous fluid therapy, guidelines for, 316t
Intussusception, 525
In vitro testing—radioallergosorbent test (RAST), 15
Iodoquinol, 668t
Ipecac, 668t
IPPV, management of nonresponse to, 325t
Ipratropium, 668t
Iritis, 418-419
Iron, 668t
  poisoning by, 476
Irritant dermatitis, 64
Isoniazid, 669t
  and liver injury, 225t
Isoproterenol, 669t, 708t
Isotretinoin (Accutane), 61, 669t

J

Jaundice, 336-337t
Juvenile arthritis (JA), 512-513
  differential diagnosis, 516-517t
  subgroups of, 514-515t

K

Kasabach-Merritt syndrome, 65, 66
Kawasaki disease, 518-519
Kayexalate, 669t
Kerion, 69
Ketoconazole, 669t
Ketotifen, 669t
  for asthma, 502
Kidney. *See* Nephrology
Klippel Trenaunay syndrome, 66
Knee pain, 433
KOH preparation, 578
Kyphosis, 442

L

Labetalol, 669t
Labial fusion, 134
Laboratory investigations, initial, 289-290
Laboratory reference values
  cerebrospinal fluid, 636t
  creatinine clearance, 625f
  feces, 633-635t
  hematology
    blood, 487-621t
    coagulation values, 486t
    hemoglobin, hemocrit, RBC count, reticulocytes, 582-583t
    hemoglobin electrophoresis, 484t
    platelet count, 584t
    white blood cell count and differential, 485t
  urine, 622-624t, 626-632t
  viral and other titers, 637-638
Lacerations
  of cornea, 418
  and plastic surgery, 457-458
Lactase deficiency, 108t
Lactulose, 669-670t
Laryngotracheobronchitis, acute, 492-493
Larynx, foreign body in, 448
Lead encephalopathy, 480
Lead poisoning, 480-481
Legg-Perthes disease, 439
Leukocoria, 419
Levothyroxine, 670t
Lice, 66-67
Lidocaine, 670t
Lindane (Kwellada), 670t
Lipids, in total parental nutrition, 402
Liver disease
  nutrition in, 227
  symptoms and signs of, 208f
Liver failure, acute fulminant, 214-215f
Liver function, tests of, 210
Liver spans, normal values for, 209f
Loperamide, 670t
Loratadine, 671t
Lorazepam, 671t, 708t
  in febrile seizures, 381
  in seizures, 378
LSD, 10-11t
Lumbar puncture, 575-576
  in encephalitis, 258
  in meningitis, 262

M

Magnesium citrate, 671t
Magnesium glucoheptonate, 671t

Magnesium hydroxide, 644t, 671t
Magnesium sulfate, 671t
Malformation syndromes, 123
Mannitol, 672t, 708t
Marcus-Gunn, 419
Marijuana, 12-13t
Mastoiditis, 456
Measles immunization, 234
  post-exposure prophylaxis, 235
Mebendazole, 672t
Meningitis
  empiric antibiotic selection for, 265
  interpretation of CSF findings in, 264
Meperidine, 672t
  for headache, 389
Mesalamine (5-aminosalicylic acid, Salofalk, Asacol), 673t
Metabolic acidosis, 98, 100f, 201, 320
Metabolic alkalosis, 320
Metabolic disease
  in infancy and childhood, 288–289, 294-297t
  initial laboratory investigations, 289-290
  in the newborn, 288, 292-293t
  recognition and management of inherited, 288
Methotrexate, 673t, 721t, 727t
  and liver injury, 225t
Methyldopa, 673t
Methylprednisolone, 673t
Metoclopramide, 673-674t, 709t
Metoprolol, 674t
Metronidazole, 674-675t
Mexilitene, 675t
Migraine, management for, 389-390
Milk-soy protein intolerance, 109
Mineral oil (heavy), 675t
Minerals, in total parental nutrition, 402
Minocycline, 675t
Minoxidil, 675t
Molluscum contagiosum, 67
Mononucleosis, infectious, 262
Morphine, 675-676t, 709t
Mumps, 267
Myelomeningocele, 387
Myocarditis, 31, 53
  management, 53

N

Nabilone, 677t
Nadoiol, 677t
Naloxone, 677t, 709t
Naproxen, 677t
Narcotics, overdose of, 479
Naso lacrimal duct obstruction, 414

Near drowning, 543-545
Needle aspiration of pneumothorax, 565
Neisseria gonorrhoea, 135, 137
  therapy for, 138-139t
Neisseria meningitides, prophylaxis for, 237
Neomycin, 677t
Neonatal hemangiomatosis, 66
Neonatal respiratory distress, 322, 323t, 324f
Neonatal seizures, 313, 314t
Neonatal thrombocytopenia, 192
Neonatology
  abbreviations in, 301
  acid-base status, 319-322
  APGAR score, 308t
  conjunctivitis in, 415
  delivery of the high-risk neonate, 309
  drug dosage guidelines, 698-715t
  fluids and electrolytes, 315t, 316t
    hypernatremia, 317-318
    hypokalemia, 318
    hyponatremia, 317
  growth parameters in, 302-303f
  hyperkalemia, 318-319
  modified Dubowitz assessment, 304-305f
  ophthalmology for premature, 411
  Parkin assessment of gestational age, 306-307t
  respiratory distress, 322, 323t, 324f
Neostigmine, 677t
Nephrology
  acute renal failure, 348, 349f, 350
  chronic renal failure, 353
  enuresis, 370-371
  glomerulonephritis, 354-355
    causes of, 354t
  hematuria, 370
  hemolytic uremic syndrome, 354
  hypertension, 359
    drug therapy for acute, 368
    investigations, 366
    management of, 367
    measurements in, 360-363f
    treatment, 366
  nephrotic syndrome, 357-358
  peritonitis in chronic ambulatory peritoneal dialysis (CAPD), 371-372
  proteinuria, 356
  renal function tests, 372-373
  urinalysis, 373
  urinary tract infection (UTI), 350
Nephrotic syndrome, 357-358
Neurogenic bladder, 151

Index

Neurology
  acute ataxia, 382
  acute spinal cord lesion, 388-389f
  blocked CSF shunt, 384-385
  febrile seizures, 380-381
  Guillain-Barré syndrome, 390
  headache, 388-390
  myelomeningocele, 387
  seizures, 374t, 375-376t, 377t
  status epilepticus, 378-379
  stroke, 383-384
Neutropenia, management of, 282
Neutrophil disorders, 24-25t
Nevus flammeus, 65
Newborns. *See* Infants
Nifedipine, 677t
Nitrazepam, 678t
Nitrofurantoin, 678t
Nitroglycerin, 678t
Nitroprusside, 678t
Non-Mendelian malformation syndromes, 124
Nonpetroleum-distillate hydrocarbons, 474
Nonresponse, management of, 325t
Nonscarring alopecia, 69
Norepinephrine, 678t
Nose
  foreign body in, 448
  fracture of, 451
Novospirozine, 678t, 709t
5' Nucleotidase (5NT), 210
Nursing bottle syndrome, 393
Nursing caries, 57
Nutrition
  bottle feeding, 392t
  breast feeding, 391
  enteral, 404-405, 406-409t
  failure to thrive, 395-396
  introduction of solids, 394, 395t
  in liver disease, 227
  in management of cystic fibrosis, 505t
  in neonatitis, 343, 344t
  obesity, 410
  recommended nutrient intakes for Canadians, 398-401t
  total parenteral nutrition, 397, 398-401t, 402, 403t
  vegetarian diet, 395
Nystatin, 679t

O

Obesity, 410
Oncology. *See* Hematology and oncology
Ophthalmology
  anterior chamber, 418-419
  basic principles, 412-413
  conjunctivae, 415, 416t, 417
  cornea, 417-418
  eyelids, 414
    chalazion, 414
    hordeolum (stye), 414
    trauma, 414
  iris, 419
  naso lacrimal duct obstruction, 414
  optic nerve, 420-421
  poison in contact with eye, 468
  pupils, 419
  retina, 420
  routine procedures and screening
    1-5 yr, 412
    infant, 411
    perinatal, 411
    premature neonates, 411
  strabismus, 421, 422-423f
Opium, 647t
Optic atrophy, 421
Optic nerve, 420-421
Oral rehydration fluids, 105t
Orbital cellulitis, 253
Orciprenaline, 679t
Orthopaedics
  back pain, 442
  infection, 445
  injuries, 444-445f
  lower limb
    congenital dislocation of hip, 436-437f, 438
    diagnostic approach to the limping child, 432f
    foot shape concerns, 430, 431t
    hip problems, 434-435f
    intoeing, 424-425, 426-429f
    knee pain, 433
    Legg-Perthes disease, 439
    Osgood Schlatter's disorder, 433
    osteochondritis dissecans, 433
    out-toeing, 430
    peripatellar pain syndrome, 433
    recurrent dislocation of the patella, 433
    slipped femoral capital epiphysis, 440
    transient synovitis, 439
  neck
    congenital muscular torticollis, 443, 444f
  spine
    kyphosis, 442
    scoliosis, 440-441f

upper limb
  pulled elbow, 443
Ortolani (reduction) test, 436f
Osgood Schlatter's disorder, 433
Osteochondritis dissecans, 433
Osteomyelitis, 250-251
  differentiation between bone infarction and, 189t
Otitis externa, 449-450
Otitis media
  acute, 453, 454t
  recurrent, 455
  serous, 455-456
Otolaryngology
  adenotonsillectomy, 446-447
  corrosive burns of upper GI tract, 451-452
  epistaxis, 451
  facial nerve paralysis, 452
  foreign body in ear, 447
  fractured nose, 451
  mastoiditis, 456
  otitis externa, 449-450
  otitis media
    acute, 453, 454t
    recurrent, 455
    serous, 455-456
  traumatic perforation of tympanic membrane, 456
Out-toeing, 430
Oxybutinin, 679t

P

Pancrelipase (Cotazym), 679t
Pancuronium (Pavulon), 679t, 709t
Papilledema, 420
Papillitis, 420
Paraldehyde, 679-680t, 709t
  in febrile seizures, 381
  in seizures, 379
Paralysis, of facial nerve, 452
Parasitic infections, 268-269t
Parenteral solutions, composition of some common, 89t
Parkin assessment of gestational age, 306-307t
Patella, recurrent dislocation of, 433
Patent ductus arteriosus (PDA), 332
Pediazole, 680t
Pediculosis capitis, 66-67
Pediculosis pubus, 66-67
Peg-electrolyte liquid (Golytely PegLyte), 680t
Pelvic inflammatory disease (PID), 135
  causes of, 136t
  treatment of, 140
Penicillamine, 680t
Penicillin, 20
  sensitivity to, 21f
Penicillin G (Benzylpenicillin), 681t, 710t
Penicillin VK, 681t
Pentamidine isethionate, 682t
Pentobarbital (Nembutal), 682t
Pericarditis, acute
  investigations, 53
  treatment, 54
Perimenarchal, 128
Perinatal ophthalmology in, 411
Periodontal abscess, 57
Periorbital cellulitis, 253
Peripatellar pain syndrome, 433
Peritonitis in chronic ambulatory peritoneal dialysis (CAPD), 371-372
Permethrin (Nix), 683t
Persistent pulmonary hypertension of the newborn (PPHN), 335
Pertussis, 270-271
  immunization for, 233
Petroleum-distillate hydrocarbons (PDHs), 474
Phagocytic disorders, 26-27t
Pharyngitis, streptococcal, 270
Phenobarbital, 683t, 710-711t, 722t, 727t
  in febrile seizures, 381
  in seizures, 379
Phenoxybenzamine, 683t
Phentolamine, 683t
Phenylephrine, 684t
Phenytoin, 684t, 711t, 722t, 728t
  and liver injury, 225t
Phototherapy, 338, 339f
  in neonatal hyperbilirubinemia, 339f, 340f
Pinworm, examination for, 580t
Piperacillin, 685t, 711t
Piperazine, 685t
Pityriasis rosea, 67
Pivampicillin, 685t
Pizotyline, for headache, 390
Plantar wart, 70
Plasmapheresis, for Guillain-Barré syndrome, 390
Plastic surgery
  abrasions, 457
  burns, 459-463
    criteria for hospitalization of, 460
    severity of, 460

Plastic surgery—cont'd
  burns—cont'd
    water temperature and duration of exposure producing third-degree, 463t
  cleft lip and palate, 458
  facial fractures, 458
  lacerations, 457
    facial, 457-458
    hand, 457
Pleural effusion, 506, 507t
Pneumonia, 494-495
  antibiotic therapy for, 497t
  causes of, 494-495, 496t
  differentiation between pulmonary infarction and, 188t
Pneumothorax, 508
  needle aspiration of, 565
Poisoning
  contact with skin or eye, 468
  ingested, 464-465
  inhaled, 468
  injected, 468
  by rectal route, 468
  salt, 97
  signs and causes of, 466-467t
  specific
    acetaminophen (paracetamol), 472, 473f
    alkaline corrosives, 478
    anticonvulsants, 475
    barbiturates, 475
    ethanol, 476
    insecticides, 479
    iron, 476
    lead poisoning, 480-481
    narcotics, 479
    nonpetroleum-distillate hydrocarbons, 474
    petroleum-distillate hydrocarbons (PDHs), 474
    salicylate intoxication, 467-468, 469f
    snake bites, 482-483
    spiders, 483
    theophylline, 478
    tricyclic antidepressants, 475-476
  toxicology tests, 468-469
  unknown, 465
Poison ivy contact dermatitis, 64
Poliomyelitis, immunization for, 233
Postmenarchal, 129-130
Postpubertal vaginitis
  causes of, 136t
Potassium chloride, 685t
Potassium iodide, 685t
Prazosin, 688t

Prednisone, 688t
Premenarchal, 127-128
Prepubertal vaginitis, causes of, 136t
Primaquine, 688t
Primidone, 688t, 722t, 728t
Procainamide, 689t
Proctitis, causes of, 136t
Propafenone, 689t
Prophylaxis. *See* Immunization
Propranolol, 689t, 711t
  for headache, 390
Propylthiouracil, 688t
Protamine, 688t
Protein-losing enteropathy, 108t, 109
Proteinuria, 356
Pseudoephedrine, 688t
Pseudohermaphrodite, 82t
Pseudohyponatremia, 97
Pulmonary edema, 31
Pulmonary function testing, 486f
  patterns of observed, 487t, 488
Pulmonary infarction, differentiation between pneumonia and, 188t
Pulpal necrosis with abscess, 57
Pulpitis, 57
Pyrantel pamoate, 688t
Pyrazinamide, 689t
Pyridoxine (vitamin B_6), 712t
Pyrimethamine, 689t, 692t

Q

Quinacrine, 689t
Quinidine, 689t, 722t, 728t
Quinne sulfate, 689t

R

Rabies, prophylaxis for, 243, 244-245t
Radioallergosorbent test (RAST), 15
Ranitidine, 690t, 712t
Red blood cells, reference values for, 582-583t
Relative afferent pupil defect (RAPD), 419
Renal failure
  acute, 348, 349f, 350
  chronic, 353
Renal function tests, 372-373
Respiratory acidosis, 319
Respiratory alkalosis, 319
Respiratory disease
  acute asthma, 498-500
  alveolar-arterial (A-a) gradient, 484, 485f
  bronchiolitis, 493-494
  chronic asthma, 500-502

croup (acute laryngotracheobronchitis), 492-493
cystic fibrosis, 502-504
  nutritional management for, 505t
epiglottitis, 492
pleural effusion, 506, 507t
pneumonia, 494-495
  antibiotic therapy for, 497t
  causes of, 494-495, 496t
pneumothorax, 508
pulmonary function testing, 486f
  patterns of, observed, 388
respiratory distress, 488-489
upper airway infection, 491t
upper airway obstruction, 490
Respiratory distress, 488-489
  neonatal, 322, 323t, 324f
Respiratory procedures, 564
Reticulocytes, reference values for, 582-583t
Retina, 420
Retinal hemorrhages, 420
Reye's syndrome, 211, 212t, 213
  risk of, 241
Rheumatic fever, 51
  management of, 51-52
Rheumatology
  arthritis
    approach to the child with, 509-510
    juvenile, 512-513, 514-517t
  Henoch Schönlein purpura, 518
  Kawasaki disease, 518-519
  synovial fluid analysis, 511t
Rhinitis, allergic, 18
Ribavirin, 690t
Rifampin, 690-691t
  and liver injury, 225t
  post-exposure prophylaxis with, 236
Rubella immunization, 234
  post-exposure prophylaxis in pregnant women, 235

S

Salbutamol, 691t
Salicylate, 722t, 728t
Salicylate intoxication, 467-468, 469f
Salt depletion, 541
Salt poisoning, 97
Scabies, 68
Scoliosis, 440-441f
Scrotum, acute, 150
Seborrheic dermatitis, 64, 68

Seizure(s)
  classification of, 374t
  febrile, 380-381
  long-term management of, 377t
  neonatal, 313, 314t
  in status epilepticus, 378-379
  syncope, breath holding, differentiation, 375-376t
Septic arthritis, 247-248, 249t
Septic shock, 271, 272t
Sexual assault, 149-150
Sexually transmitted diseases, 134
  causes of, 136t
  Chlamydia trachonatis, 135, 137t
  epididymitis, 140
  Neisseria gonorrhoea, 135, 137, 138-139t
  pelvic inflammatory disease, 135, 140t
  syphilis, 141, 142-143t
Shock
  clinical features of, 548
  investigations, 552
  management of, 548-549, 550-551f, 552
  monitoring, 552
  types of, 547t
Short gut, microvillus atrophy, 108t
Short stature, 84-85, 85t
SIADH, 84
Sick child, transport of, 556-558
Sickle cell disease, 186, 187t
Sinus bradycardia, 542
Sinusitis, 273
Sinus rhythm, regular, 41f
Skin, poison in contact with, 468
Skin testing, 14
Smoke inhalation, 545-546
Snake bites, 482-483
Sodium bicarbonate, 691t, 712t
Sodium cromoglycate, for asthma, 501
Sodium polystyrene sulfonate (Kayexalate), 691t, 712t
Solid foods, introduction of, 393, 394t
Sotaiol, 692t
Speech and language checklist, 158-159t
Spiders, 483
Spinal cord compression, 207
Spinal cord lesion, acute, 385-386f
Spironolactone, 692t, 712t
Sprains, 444
Staphylococcal scalded skin syndrome (SSSS), 68
Status epilepticus, 378-379
Stenosis, 521
  hypertrophic pyloric, 524-525

Index

Steroids
 topical, 70, 71t
 for tuberculosis, 276
Stool, reducing substances in to detect carbohydrate malabsorption, 579
Stool smear, 579
Strabismus, 421, 422-423f
Streptococcal pharyngitis, 270
Streptococcus pneumoniae, prophylaxis for, 243-244
Streptokinase, 692t
Stroke, 382-383
Sturge-Weber syndrome, 66
Stye, 413
Subconjunctival hemorrhage, 417
Succinylcholine, 692t
Sucralfate (Sulcrate), 692t
Sulfadoxine, 682t, 692t
Sulfasalazine, 693t
Sulfonamide, 20
 and liver injury, 225t
Suprapubic bladder aspiration, 575
Supraventricular tachycardia, 42t
 acute treatment of, 47
Surgery
 emergencies in older children
  appendicitis, 526
  biliary atresia, 527
  cryptorchidism, 527
  ingested foreign body, 526
  inguinal hernias, 526
  intussusception, 525
  umbilical granuloma, 527
 neonatal abdominal emergencies, 520
  diaphragmatic hernia (Bochdalek), 524
  duodenal atresia or stenosis, 521
  esophageal atresia, 521
  general management principles, 520
  Hirschsprung's disease, 524
  hypertrophic pyloric stenosis, 524-525
  malrotation with midgut volvulus, 522
  meconium ileus, 522-523
  necrotizing enterocolitis, 523
  small intestinal atresia, 522
Sympathomimetic drugs, in asthma, 499, 501
Synovial fluid analysis, 511t
Syphilis, antibiotic therapy for, 142-143t

T

Tachycardia, differentiation of, 48-49t
T-cell defects, 24-25t, 26t
Teeth. See Dentistry
Terfenadine, 693t
Tetanus, immunization for, 233
Tetracycline, 693t
Tetralogy of Fallot
 cyanotic spells in, 54
Thalassemia syndromes
 α-Thalassemia minor, 183
 β-Thalassemia major, 184
 β-Thalassemia minor, 183
Theophylline, 693-694t, 713t, 723t, 728-729t
 for asthma, 500, 502
 poisoning by, 478
Theophylline therapy, management of, 731-733f
Thoracocentesis, 565
Thrombocytopenia, 190
 neonatal, 192
Thrombosis, deep venous, 199-200
Thyroid disease, 86f
Ticarcillin, 692t, 713t
Tinea capitis, 69
Tobramycin, 692-693t, 713t, 723t, 729t
Tolazoline (Priscoline), 714t
Tolmetin, 693t
Toluene, 12-13t
Topical steroids, 70, 71t
Torticollis, congenital muscular, 443, 444f
Total parenteral nutrition, 397, 398, 399-401t, 403t
 carbohydrates, 397
 complications, 402
 electrolytes, vitamins and minerals, 402
 indications for centra venous line, 402
 lipids, 402
 monitoring, 402
Total parenteral nutrition (TPN) associated liver disease, 226
Toxicology tests, 468-469
Tracheotomy, 567
Tracheobronchial tree, foreign body in, 448
Transfusion reactions, 200-201
Transient synovitis, 439
Trauma, eyelid, 414
Trauma patient, triage of the multiple, 558-560
Treponema pollidum (syphilis), 141

Triage, of multiple trauma patient, 558-560
Tricyclic antidepressants, overdose of, 475-456
Trimethoprim, 693t, 714t
Tropia, cover-uncover test, 422f
Tuberculosis, 275, 276t
  extrapulmonary, 276
Tumor lysis syndrome, 201, 205-206
Tympanic membrane, traumatic perforation of, 456

U

Ulcer, duodenal, 112
Ulcerative colitis, 116
Umbilical artery catheterization, 571
Umbilical granuloma, 527
Umbilical vein catheterization, 568, 569f, 570f
Unconsciousness. *See under* Coma
Uremic syndrome, hemolytic, 354
Urethritis, causes of, 136t
Urinalysis, 373
Urinary alkalinization, 101
Urinary tract infection, 350-352
Urine, reference values, 622-624t, 626-632t
Urticaria, 17t, 20, 69

V

Vaginal bleeding, 127
Valproic acid, 693t, 723t, 730t
  and liver injury, 225t
Vancomycin, 693t, 714-715t, 723t, 730t
Varicella (chicken pox), 278
Varicella zoster immune globulin, 696t
Vasopressin, 696t

Vegetarian diet, 395
Venous access, 562
  intraosseous access, 563
  intravenous cutdown, 563
  long-term central venous lines, 564
Ventricular premature beat, 45f
Ventricular tachycardia, 46f
Verapamil (Isoptin), 696t
Verrucae, 69
Viral and other titers, 637-638
Viral hepatitis, 278-279
Vitamin A acid, 60
Vitamin C, 696t
Vitamin K_1 (Phytonadione), 696t, 715t
Vitamin K deficiency, 199
Vitamins, in total parental nutrition, 402
Vomiting, 109, 110f, 111
Von Willebrand disease (VWD), 196
Vulvovaginitis, 131-133

W

Warfarin, 697t
Wart, 69
  anal, 136t
  genital, 136t
  plantar, 70
Wenckebach phenomenon, 44f
White blood cell count and differentials, reference values for, 585t
Wolff-Parkinson-White syndrome, 46, 47
Wound management, tetanus prophylaxis in, 246t

Z

Zidovudine, 697t
Zinc, 697t